ROUTLEDGE LIBRAR'
HEALTH, DISEASE &

Volume 3

HEALTH AND VITAL STATISTICS

HEALTH AND VITAL STATISTICS

B. BENJAMIN

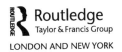

Routledge
Taylor & Francis Group

LONDON AND NEW YORK

First published in 1968 by George Allen & Unwin Ltd.

This edition first published in 2022
by Routledge
4 Park Square, Milton Park, Abingdon, Oxon OX14 4RN

and by Routledge
605 Third Avenue, New York, NY 10158

Routledge is an imprint of the Taylor & Francis Group, an informa business

© 1968 George Allen & Unwin Ltd.

British Library Cataloguing in Publication Data
A catalogue record for this book is available from the British Library

ISBN: 978-0-367-52469-2 (Set)
ISBN: 978-1-032-25170-7 (Volume 3) (hbk)
ISBN: 978-1-032-25176-9 (Volume 3) (pbk)
ISBN: 978-1-003-28190-0 (Volume 3) (ebk)

DOI: 10.4324/9781003281900

Publisher's Note
The publisher has gone to great lengths to ensure the quality of this reprint but points out that some imperfections in the original copies may be apparent.

Disclaimer
The publisher has made every effort to trace copyright holders and would welcome correspondence from those they have been unable to trace.

HEALTH AND VITAL STATISTICS

B. BENJAMIN
B.SC., PH.D., F.I.A., F.S.S.

Director of Research and Intelligence,
Greater London Council,
Formerly Director of Statistics, Ministry of Health.

Ruskin House

GEORGE ALLEN & UNWIN LTD

MUSEUM STREET LONDON

FIRST PUBLISHED IN GREAT BRITAIN IN 1968

© *George Allen and Unwin Ltd., 1968*

PRINTED IN GREAT BRITAIN
in 10/11 point Times Roman Type
BY UNWIN BROTHERS LIMITED
WOKING AND LONDON

PREFACE

My earlier textbook, entitled simply *Elements of Vital Statistics* in deference to the great work by Sir Arthur Newsholme which it attempted to replace, was published in 1959. When it ran out of print it was decided to revise the book radically and to give it a title more consonant with its modern theme and purpose—an account of methods of measurement of health and of health service activity. The best of the earlier volume remains but there has been a pruning of inessential non-statistical text and of certain tabulations which were difficult to update and were only of marginal illustrative value. New material has been introduced to cover recent developments in the various sub-fields of the subject especially in the use of hospital records and in the approach to community health records, and an attempt has been made to recast material from the earlier volume where this seemed necessary to improve lucidity. I have corrected, I hope, all those errors in the first volume which readers were kind and patient enough to point out to me.

The same basic approach is retained; of trying to look at the measurement problems that arise in health and welfare services in their day-to-day operation, the sources that may be available to supply the requisite data for their solution and the methods of analysis most appropriate to the particular situation encountered. Little or no mathematical knowledge beyond simple arithmetic is assumed on the part of the reader though on occasion the non-mathematical reader has been deliberately tempted to extend, from other sources, his knowledge of statistical theory. Availability of electronic computers has been assumed in a number of instances, but though a heavy computer user myself I have nevertheless refused to treat computer applications as a subject in itself. I firmly believe that a computer is an invaluable means to an end and not an end in itself. I have tried in this book to concentrate on ends.

For most of my professional life I have been concerned with medical and population problems. This book is based on that experience. This means that it is also based on help and guidance over a long period from colleagues too numerous to mention by name. I am deeply grateful to them.

CONTENTS

A*

CHAPTER 1

INTRODUCTORY

Statistics

1.1 Statistics originally denoted inquiry into the condition of a State but because this inevitably involved the description of social facts in quantitative terms the meaning of 'statistics' was gradually broadened to cover all types of numerical description of social, economic and biological phenomena. The statistical method is the method of comparison, of differentiation and of classification; it is the method by which aggregates of units as distinguished from units themselves can be measured. The method is essential to the study of a society consisting as it does of distinct units, all different from each other yet all related to each other. By embracing aspects of similarity and in expressing differences as variation from an average, variation to which mathematical limits can be prescribed, the statistical method enables us to form an intelligible mental picture of what would otherwise be incomprehensible, a picture of large conglomerations of units.

Vital statistics

1.2 Vital statistics are, conventionally, numerical records of marriage, births, sickness and deaths by which the health and growth of a community may be studied. Just as the biological study of a single man would be the record of a series of episodes of birth, infancy, adolescence, maturity, reproduction and ultimate decay, of illness, accidents, anxieties, triumphs, in one human life; so the biological study of groups of human beings involves the statistical summary, the numerical aggregation of a large number of episodes arising continuously in a large number of lives. This study inevitably leads to the observation of other aspects of society which react upon health or reproductivity, since in regarding society as a living complex organism, account must be taken of all factors which may be influencing its vitality. It is common therefore today to speak of *demography* as the science of which vital statistics already form a large part.

Demography

1.3 Demography is concerned with the growth, development and movement of human populations as aggregates. Its raw material ranges from the statistics of heights and weights or of blood pressure in men, to the distribution of the rents they pay for their housing accommodation or to the classes of education they give their children. As a science it impinges on the imagination of all who are at any time concerned with the survival of nations; it forms the basis for economic planning so far as it is essential to the measurement of manpower and affects the distribution of employment of the collection of taxes and the assessment of rates; it is the means by which the size and scope of health and welfare and all other community services are determined. The 'counting of heads' is an essential preliminary of democratic government itself. Whether we speak of demography or of vital statistics we are dealing with an intensely utilitarian science, because the very organization of society depends upon it.

Historical Development in Great Britain

1.4 The analysis of population statistics has not always been as actively pursued as at the present time. It was not until society reached an economic stage of development at which problems of organization, of welfare (especially, for example, the spread of infectious disease) pressed sufficiently to demonstrate the need for adequate data to sustain the study of, and produce the solution to, these problems that the Government took steps to get the information and make it available. The evolution of the science was not, however, as sharp as this might imply, but a gradual process in which, as in many other developments, pioneers played an important part.

1.5 The first London Bills of Mortality were compiled in the reign of Henry VIII, about 1538. The main continuous weekly series began with those for the year 1603 and their resumption in that year after a break from 1594 was caused by the desire for information as to Plague which was then prevalent. Thus Plague gave an impetus to vital statistics, just as the first invasion of cholera in 1831 hastened the establishment of national registration of deaths (p. 48). It was John Graunt who in his book *Natural and Political Observations . . . upon the Bills of Mortality* showed how these basic records might be analysed to indicate the prevalence of epidemic and chronic disease in the population. He and his contemporary, William Petty, may be regarded as developing the early crude population measures.

1.6 The earliest recorded attempt to estimate the population of Great Britain was made by Gregory King (1648–1712) working from tax returns of houses and using multipliers to translate houses into people, varying the multipliers to suit different housing characteristics in different areas; he also distributed the estimated population by age. Modern statisticians have examined his results and consider them to be remarkably good.

1.7 The more recondite technique of life tables was developed by Edmund Halley whose table bears his name; Dr Richard Price who constructed the Northampton Table; and Joshua Milne who was responsible for the Carlisle Table. (See p. 105).

1.8 As statistician ('compiler of Abstracts') in the General Register Office, from 1839, it was William Farr who pioneered the proper analysis of the more adequate registration data and census material which had then become available. His commentaries on current vital statistics which may be found in the Annual Reports of the Registrar General were masterly and classical. Farr made an immense contribution to the improvement of the precision of death certification and laid the foundations of scientific classification of causes of death. (See p. 77.)

International

1.9 At the London International Exhibition of 1851, the first International Statistical Congress was suggested. It met in Brussels in 1853, the opening address being made by Quetelet who welcomed a new era of unity and combination in research. At the St Petersburg meeting in 1872 a Permanent Commission of the International Statistical Congress was established; and in 1885 the International Statistical Institute was formed (a permanent office followed in 1913).

1.10 In 1907 the Office International d'Hygiene Publique (OIHP) was set up at Paris as the first permanent international health organization though primarily concerned with quarantine. (In 1902 a similar body, the Pan-American Sanitary Bureau had been established in Washington but this dealt only with the Western Hemisphere.) The OIHP was controlled by a Permanent Committee consisting of technical representatives of the participating States. The first objects of the office were to provide a means of sharing advances in medical science and public health questions, and to ensure that international sanitary conventions were kept up to date. A monthly bulletin was published.

1.11 In the history of vital statistics in particular there are two outstanding developments on the international plane. One of the early acts of the League of Nations, formed after the World War of 1914–18, was the establishment in 1923 of a Health Organization consisting of a Health Committee; an Advisory Council appointed by OIHP; and the Health Section, the executive organ which was an integral part of the League Secretariat. An Epidemiological Intelligence Service had been organized as early as 1921 and this began to publish periodical reports of infectious diseases in European countries. The first *Monthly Epidemiological Report* of the Health Section appeared in 1923. To promote the standardization of statistical methods, the Health Committee convened in 1923, 1924 and 1925 meetings of the directors of the demographic services in the principal European countries. At the 1925 meeting they agreed to draw up common rules relating to the registration of the causes of death. In conjunction with the International Statistical Institute this committee played an important part in preparing for the fourth decennial revision of the International List of Causes of Death (1929) (see p. 77). The committee also devoted its attention to the notification of communicable diseases.

1.12 The second development occurred after the World War of 1939–45 in the formation of the World Health Organization. This organization was set up as the result of an International Health Conference at New York in 1946, to which sixty-one governments sent representatives.

1.13 The work of the Organization is carried out by three organs: The World Health Assembly, the supreme authority, to which all Member States send delegates; the Executive Board, the executive organ of the Health Assembly, consisting of eighteen persons designated by as many Member States; and a Secretariat under the Director-General.

1.14 The World Health Organization (WHO) is a specialized agency of the United Nations and represents the culmination of efforts to establish a single inter-governmental body concerned with health. As such, it inherits the functions of antecedent organizations such as the Office International d'Hygiene Publique, the Health Organization of the League of Nations, and the Health Division of UNRRA (the wartime relief organization of the United Nations).

13

1.15 The scope of WHO's interests and activities exceeds that of any previous international health organization and includes, in addition to major projects relating to malaria, tuberculosis, venereal diseases, maternal and child health, nutrition, and environmental sanitation, special programmes on public health administration, epidemic diseases, mental health, professional and technical training, and other public health subjects. It is also continuing work begun by earlier organizations on biological standardization, unification of pharmacopoeias, addiction-producing drugs, health statistics, international sanitary regulations, and the collection and dissemination of technical information, including epidemiological statistics.

1.16 Among the important technical publications of WHO there is a monthly *Epidemiological and Vital Statistics Report* containing statistics on infectious diseases and birth and death rates and articles on epidemiological and demographic subjects. Subscription to this also gives access to a *Weekly Epidemiological Record* containing notifications concerning diseases designated as 'pestilential' in the International Sanitary Conventions as well as other information about the application of these conventions.

1.17 Of equal importance is the establishment of the Statistical Office of the United Nations which collects population statistics from all over the world and publishes annually a *Demographic Yearbook*. This volume provides, for an increasing number of contributing countries, detailed statistics of population, births and deaths with careful notes of conditions affecting validity or comparability. From time to time the Statistical Office publishes manuals setting out the basic principles of census taking and vital statistics systems not only for the guidance of less developed countries but to assist in the improvement of existing systems.

1.18 Recognition of the international character of problems arising from population pressure in those less developed parts of the world where available resources in their current economic state are too meagre to match the existing population let alone its high rate of natural increase, led the United Nations in 1946 to establish a Population Commission to advise on these problems and other population matters including methodology of measurement. As a counterpart to this commission the permanent office maintains a population branch staffed by experts, which carries out studies and advises member governments, at their request, upon the bearing of population factors upon plans of economic development; this branch has made notable contributions to the development and application of population statistics, both by the conduct of seminars and conferences and the publication of methodological studies.

CHAPTER 2

POPULATION

2.1 Statistical measurement of the health of the community is not only concerned with the number of persons in the community, but involves consideration of heterogeneity and it is necessary to classify the population with respect to many characteristics, e.g. age, sex, marital status, birthplace, occupation, housing conditions. We cannot compare two communities in relation to their mortality from cancer, which is age selective, unless we know what are the proportions of old people in the populations. We cannot assess the mortality from tuberculosis in printers by merely counting their deaths from this disease; we need to know the number of printers who have been 'at risk' of death from tuberculosis. It will be seen later (p. 72), that precision in determining the denominator of a death rate is no less important than the fixing of the numerator.

2.2 The actual population is known only by census enumerations, though it is common practice to make estimates for intercensal years.

Censuses in Great Britain

2.3 In England and Wales and Scotland the first census was in 1801 and was repeated thereafter at decennial intervals. World war rendered it inexpedient to have a census in 1941 and so there was a gap between 1931 and 1951 of twenty years. The census of 1801 counted the number of males and females of each house and family and the number of persons engaged in agriculture, trade, manufacture or handicraft and other occupations not specially classified. In 1821 information was first sought as to ages, but it was left optional whether this should be furnished or not. Before the 1841 census the civil registration of births, deaths and marriages had been instituted in England and Wales and the newly appointed local registrars replaced the parish overseers as the officers responsible for conducting the census. In addition, the duty of completing the enumeration form for each family was delegated to the head of household instead of to an official, thus enabling simultaneous entry to be made of every person. In Scotland civil registration was not established until 1855 and the census of 1841 was entrusted to the official schoolmaster or other fit person. The census of 1851 was carried out under Farr's supervision and was more detailed than earlier enumerations. Information was obtained of occupation, birthplace, relationship (husband, wife, etc.), marital condition (married, widowed, bachelor, etc.), education and the number of persons deaf and dumb or blind. At this census under the powers given by the Census Act, the precise age at last birthday of each person in the country was first demanded. The Scottish Census of 1861 was the first to be conducted by the Registrar-General for Scotland.

2.4 In the census report of 1881, the age and sex distribution of the population of each urban and rural sanitary authority as constituted that year was given for the first time.

2.5 At the census of 1891 the schedule contained new questions as to number of rooms and of their occupants in all tenements with less than five rooms, and the important economic distinction between employers, employees and those working on their own account.

2.6 In 1901 no further additions were made to the subjects of inquiry, but provision was made in a single enactment for taking the census throughout Great Britain. In 1911 a number of important changes were made. The difficulty of defining a 'house' was avoided by the enumeration for each urban and rural district of the number of various classes of buildings used as dwellings—ordinary dwelling houses, blocks of flats and the separate flats or dwelling composing them, shops, institutions, etc., with the corresponding populations. The limited accommodation enquiry of the 1891 Census was extended to tenements of all sizes. The industry as well as the occupation of each worker was recorded. The tabulations gave ages in single years of life instead of groupings. The most important development was a detailed enquiry into fertility. The following questions were asked in respect of every married woman.

(1) Duration of marriage in completed years.
(2) The number of children born alive to the present marriage who:
    (*a*) were still alive at the census;
    (*b*) had died before the census.

2.7 This information when related to other census data as to age, marital status, occupation, etc., enabled a study of area and social class differences in marriage and child bearing experience to be attempted. (See p. 66).

2.8 Up to 1911 each census had been covered by a separate Act of Parliament, but the Census Act of 1920 gave power to hold periodical enumerations at intervals of not less than five years and covered not only the 1921 Census but future censuses. The Act states that the questions to be asked at any census are to be prescribed by Order in Council, but must fall within the following general scope.

(*a*) Names, sex, age.
(*b*) Occupation, profession, trade or employment.
(*c*) Nationality, birthplace, race, language.
(*d*) Place of abode, character of dwelling.
(*e*) Condition as to marriage, relation to head of family, issue born in marriage.
(*f*) Any other matters with respect to which it is desirable to obtain statistical information with a view to ascertaining the social or civil condition of the population.

2.9 In designing the schedule for the census of 1921 it was thought that a point had been reached in progressive enlargement of census enquiries at which any further addition to the total quantity of information might lead to indifference or resistance and consequent inaccuracy. Most of the changes were therefore in the nature of substitutions. The fertility enquiry of 1911 was not repeated on the grounds that in 1921 such an enquiry would have reflected not normal experience but the disturbance of the 1914–18 war. Instead the schedule was designed to seek dependency information, i.e. details of all living children and step-children under the age of 16 for each married man, widower or widow on the schedule (whether these children were enumerated on the same schedule or not). Such information of the numbers and ages of existing children according to age and marital status of parent was essential to the institution of national widows' and orphans' pensions then contemplated. The questions as to infirmities (blind, deaf, dumb and lunatics) of earlier censuses were dropped since it was generally recognized that there was a natural reluctance to disclose that members of the family were afflicted in these ways and that data could not be expected to be reliable; but a new question was added as to place of work.

2.10 New industrial and occupational classifications were employed.

The 1931 Census

2.11 Although as at previous censuses the 1931 enumeration was on a *de facto* basis, i.e. each person was enumerated where found at the time the census was taken instead of at the usual place of residence (referred to as the *de jure* basis), for the first time a question was inserted in the schedule asking for a statement of the address of usual residence of each person enumerated in the household.

2.12 The 1931 schedule omitted any enquiry into education, workplace and either dependency or fertility, and was thus simpler than in 1921. This reduction in scope was made partly for economy and also because it was anticipated that in future more frequent enumerations would be made and that emphasis would be placed at different times on different additions to the minima in order to spread the complete survey over several censuses. [It was intended to hold a census in 1936 but it was later decided not to fulfil this intention.] As a reflection of the economic depression of the time the 1931 schedule was extended to include particular mention of those 'out of work'.

National Registration 1939

2.13 As part of general security measures during the war of 1939–45 every civilian person in Great Britain on September 29, 1939 had to be recorded on a National Register. The head of each household was required to complete a schedule similar to that of a normal census, showing the name, age, sex, date of birth, marital condition, occupation and national service commitment of every member of the household. For individual identification each person received a card bearing a registered number, name and address and date of birth. In 1944 the *National Register Volume* was published showing the civilian population of each area, in sex and age groups; no information was given as to occupation.

The 1951 Census of Great Britain

2.14 The enumeration was carried out as at midnight April 8/9, 1951 in England, Wales and Scotland. Arrangements were made for the General Register Office for England and Wales and the General Registry Office for Scotland to publish jointly one per cent sample tablulations for Great Britain as a whole in addition to their separate publications for England and Wales, and Scotland. In addition to the customary questions as to age, sex, marital condition, occupation, etc., certain special questions were included. These were:

Fertility: Married women under the age of fifty were asked to state
    (i) the date of present marriage (and if married more than once the date of the first marriage)
    (ii) the total children born alive to her (all marriages)
    (iii) whether she had given birth to a live-born child during the last twelve months.

Education: All persons were asked whether they were attending an educational establishment for the purpose of instruction at the date of the census and if so whether full-time or part-time. Persons not then receiving full-time instruction were asked to state the age at which such full-time education ceased.

Household arrangements: Heads of households were asked to indicate the availability to the household of the following facilities
    (i) a piped water supply within the dwelling (as distinct from a tap in the yard or public standpipe)
    (ii) cooking stove with an oven
    (iii) kitchen sink with drainpipe leading outside (not a wash basin)
    (iv) water closet (not an earth or chemical closet)
    (v) a fixed bath with waste pipe leading outside.

2.15 The question on place of work, last asked at the 1921 Census, was re-introduced.

2.16 As in earlier census enumerations the schedule was completed by the head of household and was collected by a paid enumerator who gave such assistance as was necessary on matters of interpretation regarding the completion of the form.

2.17 An important innovation was the preparation of advance tabulations of the census results almost within a year of the census date by selecting and processing a one per cent sample of the schedules. Two volumes of tables were produced during 1952. The first (*Census, 1951, Great Britain, One per cent Tables, Part I*) gave a detailed description of the method adopted to ensure that the sample was representative, of the design of the tabulations and of the factors to be borne in mind in their interpretation; it included tabulations of ages, marital condition, occupations, industries, housing and household arrangements. The second volume (Part II) covered household composition, birthplace, education and fertility. Naturally, the amount of detail given and the degree of area breakdown were limited by the fact that the data were restricted in number to one per cent of the total and the tabulations were preliminary and did not replace the full tabulations which were to come.

The 1961 Census in Great Britain

2.18 The enumeration of 1961 was notable for the following innovations:

18

(1) Three important additions to the range of questions asked at previous censuses. These were:

(i) Tenure of dwelling (whether (a) owner-occupied, or (b) rented and if so, whether from a private landlord, or local authority, or with a farm, shop, or business premises, or (c) by virtue of employment). This was to provide a measure of the sizes of these groups so that the Government would know the strengths of the various interests it had to protect.

(ii) Change of usual address in the previous year. This was to fill a long felt gap in knowledge about internal migration in the country; the main streams of movement and the characteristics of the movers (types of household, ages, occupations).

(iii) Scientific and technological qualifications. This was to provide more comprehensive statistics on scientific manpower than was previously available.

(2) The use of sampling in the enumeration for the first time. In 1951 a 1 per cent sample had been used to produce advance tabulations but every household had been required to complete the full schedule. In 1961 it was decided to reduce the burden on the public by imposing a full schedule on only 10 per cent of households, selected systematically and to require the remainder to answer only a limited range of personal questions (sex, age, marital condition, birthplace, citizenship, and, for married women, number of live-born children).

(3) Provision in the 10 per cent sample schedule for statement of members of the household absent on census day, so that for the first time the *de jure* household could be compared with the *de facto* household to which previous censuses had been restricted.

(4) The conduct of a post-enumeration survey to detect errors of response. This was on a sample basis and in two parts (a) a careful re-trawl of the selected areas as a check that every household was enumerated, (b) interviews with a small subsample of households to check any errors of response to individual questions.

For details of these innovations, reference should be made to the published volumes of the 1961 Census.

The 1966 Census of Great Britain

2.19 The census held in 1966 was entirely on a 10 per cent household sample basis and included new questions on the ownership and garaging of motor cars, means of travel to work, and employment supplementary to main occupation.

American census enumerations

2.20 The first general census of the United States was made in 1790 and the enumeration has been repeated at regular decennial intervals since that year. A permanent Census Bureau was created in 1902.

2.21 In 1950 new questions addressed to all households asked about piped water supply, type and usage (exclusive or shared or no toilet) of toilet, and access to fixed bath or shower; questions added on a sampling basis of one household in five referred to heating, lighting, refrigeration, radio and television, cooking fuel, use of kitchen sink and age of structure of dwelling. In 1960 questions were added to cover length of residence and migration within the previous five years (for school pupils) the nature of schooling (public or private) and the extent of education in years, mother tongue, access to unit cooking equipment, water heating fuel, clothes washing machine and drier, air conditioning, home food freeze, number of bathrooms, source of water, sewage disposal, telephone and automobiles. Answers were also sought to questions on numbers of bedrooms, availability of elevator, and the mobility of trailers. Except for relationship to head, sex, race, date of birth and marital condition, all questions were asked on a 25 per cent sample basis, the housing unit being the sampling unit.

2.22 The most recent census was taken as at April 1, 1960. The population of the United States, its territories, possessions, etc., was about 179,320,000 at that date.

Practical difficulties

2.23 The census is taken on a particular day, at intervals of several years, of a population which is not only continually changing in total size, but is also changing in constitution (age, sex, occupation, etc.) and in its geographical disposition within the national boundary. In times of industrial crisis or of mobilization of military forces violent changes may be taking place; on a minor level sharp changes in regional distribution occur in the usual holiday seasons. It would be advisable therefore to fix a time at which such changes are minimal so that on the one hand the actual enumeration may be facilitated by stable conditions, and on the other the results may be more likely to reflect the average condition of the population about the time of the census, i.e., the census will be representative of that era and intercensal changes will typify broad trends rather than sharp and often transient fluctuations. Unfortunately, choice of census year is determined by the overriding considerations of continuity and regularity, i.e. the desirability of maintaining in Britain equal (decennial) intervals from the first census in 1801, and in America from 1790. Unequal intervals would create difficulties in the comparison of consecutive intercensal changes.

2.24 In any particular year the day chosen should be such as to find most people at their usual occupation and in their usual residence (so as to narrow the gap between *de facto* and *de jure* enumerations), but it is difficult to suggest what frequency of absence from usual residence could be regarded as 'average'. While it is desirable to choose a week-end out of the holiday season so as to minimize absences from home for holiday, social, or business reasons, it is also desirable to carry out the enumeration at a time of the year when the weather is not inclement and the evenings are light so as to facilitate the task of the enumerators. There are statistical advantages in choosing a date near the middle of the year so that little adjustment is needed to produce a mid-year estimate. In Britain the choice of a Sunday in April is a compromise which attempts to take account of all these considerations. In 1961 the census was held on April 23rd (midnight). In the U.S.A. the 1960 census date was April 1st, but the actual enumeration was spread over a period of weeks by paid enumerators.

2.25 If enumeration is spread over a period of weeks rather than made on a single day, certain problems are created. Some persons who move during the enumeration period may be missed altogether, since the area in which they originally lived may not be canvassed before they move and enumeration may be completed in the area of their new home by the time they arrive; there is also equally the possibility of double enumeration. The USA Census Bureau consider that the net result is under-enumeration of movers. Furthermore, enumerators tend to ignore the nominal date of enumeration and to record information as at the date of the visit; in spite of instructions it is found that some infants are included in the census though born after the census date, and some persons who died after the census date are excluded.

De facto *and* de jure *populations*

2.26 As has already been indicated a person may for purposes of local enumeration be recorded according to usual residence (*de jure*) as in America, or according to where he is at the time of the census (*de facto*) as in Great Britain. It is more in accordance with the consideration outlined above that a *de jure* enumeration should be made, especially if the populations are to be used for the calculation of birth and death rates in countries where birth and death registration is on a *de jure* basis as in Great Britain. On the other hand, where the schedule is to be completed by the head of the household, it is clearly simpler to request the enumeration of all persons in the household at the time of the census; it avoids awkward distinctions between permanent and temporary residence, and the special treatment of instances where, for example, a family live in one house in the summer and another in the winter. The *de facto* enumeration is least satisfactory in health resorts and other districts where transient waves of migration periodically occur. In most areas in Great Britain, since the census takes place everywhere in a single night (so that no person can be enumerated in two places) the two populations do not differ greatly. In the United States and Canada the enumerator is responsible for filling up each schedule over a period of time and the population is counted on a *de jure* principle.

De facto *and* de jure *comparison in England and Wales*

2.27 The inclusion of the 'usual residence' question at the 1931 and 1951 Censuses of England and Wales (see p. 17) did provide considerable information about the probable difference between *de jure* and *de facto* populations. Of the total population enumerated in England and Wales in 1951, 1,013,567 persons (2·3 per cent of the whole population) stated that their 'usual residence' was elsewhere than in the borough, urban or rural district in which they were enumerated. Of this figure 107,600 were foreign or other visitors to England and Wales with their homes outside, while the balance of 905,967 represented the amount of the displacements within the national boundary on census night.

2.28 Areas where the enumerated (*de facto*) population exceeds the resident (*de jure*) population are those which include holiday resorts favoured in the spring time as well as hospitals with patients resident elsewhere and coastal ports with visiting seamen. Areas with differences in the opposite direction are those which include residential schools and colleges from which the students are absent on vacation at census day, or areas with Defence Establishments from which personnel are absent at sea or on leave at census day.

2.29 In 1961 a more direct attempt was made to establish the size and characteristics of the *de jure* population. The schedule completed by a 10 per cent sample of households asked for a list and answers to the full range of census questions in respect of persons who were normally part of the household but were absent on census night and were enumerated elsewhere. A particular point of interest, especially for housing statistics purposes, was the possible difference in the size distributions of *de facto* and *de jure* households.

Limitation of schedules

2.30 Merely to ask an additional question in the census schedule does not ensure a correct answer. Any progressive elaboration of the schedule is likely to reach a stage at which indifference, if not resentment, will introduce inaccuracy and this may cause doubt to be cast on the validity of the whole enumeration. If the number of aspects on which population statistics are sought (additional to the routine minima) are too numerous to be covered for the entire population at one census without any excessive complexity in the schedule it is better to cover them some at a time either by a set of supplemental questions at successive censuses, especially if these, by virtue of simplicity can be held more frequently than every ten years; or by a system of sampling using a different battery of questions for different samples of the population, though an important limitation is imposed by the fact that questions the answers to which are to be cross-classified must appear in the same battery. This is a very important consideration where the householder is required to complete the schedule, but even where paid canvassers are employed, steps are taken to reduce the burden of questions to be directed to any one household.

Errors in census data

2.31 In spite of publicity about the nature of the questions to be answered on the schedule, and in spite of care taken in the framing of the questions, there may be persons who do not understand the questions, who do not trouble to ascertain the precise answer, or find the official concepts unacceptable. Inaccuracy cannot be entirely eliminated.

2.32 Error in the total number of persons enumerated is probably small. At the 1931 Census the estimate carried through the intercensal period to 1931 was less than the enumerated population by barely $\frac{1}{2}$ per 10,000 though this agreement was admitted to be fortuitously close. After the 1951 Census it was stated (General Register Office, 1954) that an estimate at census date exceeded the final count of nearly 44 million, by 134,000, a difference of less than 3 per 1,000. These comparisons are not a true test of census coverage. The estimates involved are built up from the base population with recorded births and deaths and estimated migrants, the latter being much less accurately assessed than the other elements. The comparisons are thus primarily a test of migration estimates but, since errors in the latter could account for the whole of the differences revealed, they do at least suggest that any error in census coverage is quite trivial, and certainly too slight to be measured by the available

22

standards. In 1961 a more exhaustive identification of the population in a sample of areas, carried out immediately after the census, gave no evidence of any significant under- or over-enumeration. It has to be borne in mind that Great Britain is highly urbanized and concentrated and there is little opportunity for people to escape enumeration.

2.33 A particular feature of any shortfall and one which commonly occurs and is easy to recognize is a deficiency of very young infants as compared with those expected from recent birth registrations after allowing for mortality. In 1921, 795,000 infants aged 0 and 826,000 infants aged 1 were enumerated compared with 819,000 and 848,000 expected from registration records, a total error for the two ages of 46,000. It was thought that the error arose from difficulty in entering on the census schedule newly born children who were unchristened or unnamed. In 1931 therefore a note was inserted to the effect that such infants should be described as 'baby'. As a result the error was reduced to 11,000 at age 0 and 2,000 at age 1. In 1961 the corresponding deficiencies were 11,000 and 12,000.

2.34 When the age distribution of an enumerated population is examined a distinctive type of irregularity becomes obvious; there are inordinately large numbers returned at ages with certain digital endings, especially 0 and 8, but sometimes at 5. It may be that where there is uncertainty as to age there is a tendency to approximate to the nearest ten or to an even number close to a multiple of ten. In addition there is an error arising from the fact that those within a short period of a birthday tend to return the higher age instead of the attained age. These errors have decreased at successive censuses. At earlier censuses there was some evidence (based on a comparison of the enumerated population with that derived from past births, allowing for mortality and migration) that females tended to understate their ages when approaching middle age. There has been much less evidence of this in recent censuses.

2.35 The recording of occupations is subject to errors or defects of three kinds, (1) there is a tendency to elevate the status, e.g. an unskilled labourer may describe himself in terms suggesting special skill. Some people describe themselves as working in a supervisory capacity when they have no such responsibility; (2) a man who has been out of work for some time or who has been forced to temporarily change his occupation may quote his former occupation if he is likely to return to it, or his temporary occupation if it is likely in his opinion to become the permanent means of livelihood. At a time of widespread unemployment as in 1931 this could seriously distort the normal industrial pattern; (3) some of the older unoccupied or retired persons, especially those who would have preferred, and still hope to continue work, return themselves as engaged in their old occupations.

2.36 Occupations are primarily classified at the census according to the material in which the man works. There is a separate industrial classification according to the function performed by the employer so that workers of different types from welders to clerks might be grouped together if they combined to give the same main service, e.g. transport or engineering. Where labour is very mobile as in America the classification of occupation according to material processed may not be sufficiently stable; it is possible for a man to learn a step in production common to many materials and to make frequent changes of product. Changes in processes may take place without necessarily involving changes in the terms used to describe them and so from census to census it is possible that there are subtle changes in the content of a particular occupational class. The use of census statistics for making an assessment of differential mortality or fertility among occupations should not be attempted without a close study of the actual occupations covered by the classes under review.

2.37 A fuller discussion of census errors has been given elsewhere (Benjamin, 1955).

Migration records

2.38 (*a*) *National*. Movements (other than those of transient population) across the boundaries of a national state, whether from political considerations or from economic pressure, are of serious concern to the Government, and it is usual to keep detailed records. Under the Merchant Shipping Act 1906 details of names, ages, profession, last address and future permanent residence were obtained from the master of every ship, British or foreign, carrying any passengers to or from the United Kingdom by long sea routes. This requirement was abolished in 1964. Aliens are required to register with the local police.

2.39 The Board of Trade began to issue special reports in 1873 (with retrospective figures to 1815) and as from 1913 gave periodical statements in the *Board of Trade Journal.*

2.40 Table S of the Registrar General's Annual Statistical Review (Part II Tables Population) gives information of migration over a period of years.

Part (*a*) shows the balance of civilian passenger movement into and out from the United Kingdom, e.g.

Period	Between the United Kingdom and non-European countries
	Persons
1921–25	−753,500
1926–30	−599,000
1931–35	+140,300
. . .	
1958	−43,900
1959	−9,500
1960	+31,800
1961	+56,800
1962	+10,700
1963	−57,100
1964	−77,400

Part (*b*) shows the net intercensal population gain or loss by migration.

Part (*c*) shows migration between the United Kingdom and countries overseas during the year under review by country of last or intended future residence. This is based on a continuing small sample International Passenger Survey carried out by the Social Survey.

Part (*d*) shows migration into and out from the United Kingdom during the year by sex, citizenship, and route travelled.

Part (*e*) shows migration for the year by sex, age and citizenship.

Part (*f*) shows migration for the year by sex, age and marital condition.

Part (*g*) deals with the occupations of migrants, and

Part (*h*) with separate components of the United Kingdom.

2.41 In these tables Permanent migration means a declared intention by the passenger to reside for more than a year in the country of destination.

2.42 The growth of air travel has considerably diversified the routing of migration. The International Travel Survey, referred to above, is based on a very small sample and information of permanent migration to and from the United Kingdom is still scanty.

2.43 A measure of the accumulated volume of immigration is provided at the census by the question on the schedule asking for the birthplace of persons enumerated. The census tabulations show comparisons of distributions by birthplace and by residence, and in particular for local areas from large urban districts upwards, the numbers of males and females born in various countries.

2.44 (*b*) *Local migration.* In the planning of housing or industrial development, in attempting to design on the one hand an efficient agricultural economy and, on the other, the optimum location and size of industrial and commercial resources, much depends on a knowledge of internal distribution of population and of the factors which may influence the pace and direction of changes in that distribution.

2.45 Prior to 1939 very little information was available of local movements. The volume of net intercensal migration into an area could be estimated by comparing the intercensal changes in population with the natural increase. During and since the 1939–45 war National Registration provided useful data to the Government on movement between local areas. The actual wartime figures, though essential to the proper conduct of food rationing, would not represent normal movement since they were distorted by recruitment to the Forces, industrial mobilization and evacuation from bombed areas; peacetime figures have been reviewed in a special study of National Registration data (Newton and Jeffrey, 1951).

2.46 The impressions from this necessarily limited study are succinctly stated in a single paragraph: 'Although the evidence consists only of partial information about supposed characteristics so that general inferences must be speculative, when it is taken as a whole, a picture begins to emerge. It depicts people as being specially mobile at early adult ages before they have become settled in their trades and professions (though not before they have developed leanings to particular occupations) and in many cases before they have got married or started to rear families. It suggests movement inspired by prospects of better jobs elsewhere in chosen occupations. . . . The evidence also suggests changes of homes without changes of jobs in decongestion movements, in suburban expansions, and in movements along the lines of daily journeys to work.'

2.47 In the 1961 Census of Great Britain a question was asked on a sample basis about changes of address in the previous year. This has yielded information about the main streams of migration within the country and about the characteristics of the people who moved. A similar question has been asked at recent censuses in the U.S.A.

Population growth

2.48 The growth of the population from census to census is the product of the excess of births over deaths ('natural increase') and the excess of immigration over emigration. The rate of natural increase for a given period is the difference between the birth and death rates for that period.

2.49 Table 2.1 shows the intercensal increases in the population of England and Wales over the past hundred years:

TABLE 2.1   *England and Wales—Intercensal Increases in Population—annual rates per cent*

Intercensal period	Natural increase i.e. excess of births over deaths	Actual increase	Migration Balance (actual less natural increase)
1861–71	1·29	1·25	− 0·04
1871–81	1·41	1·37	− 0·04
1881–91	1·32	1·11	− 0·21
1891–1901	1·18	1·16	− 0·02
1901–11	1·18	1·04	− 0·14
1911–21	0·79	0·48	− 0·31
1921–31	0·57	0·53	− 0·04
1931–51*	0·39	0·46	+ 0·07
1951–61	0·44	0·52	+ 0·08

* Note that this is a twenty-year period.

2.50 It is clear from these figures that up to 1931 there was a substantial net emigration from England and Wales associated with export trading and the development of overseas territories. The emigrants consisted of adolescents or young adults with an excess of males over females, except in the period 1911–21. The flow was irregular in quantity, in particular there was a severe falling off in emigration between 1891 and 1901. The world wide economic depression of 1930, and movement of political refugees from Central Europe, reversed this flow after 1930. More recently full employment in Britain encouraged a large influx of immigrants from the Commonwealth and in 1960 it was considered necessary to impose legislative control mainly on the basis that the immigrant had to have proof of having secured employment in Britain before leaving their country of origin.

2.51 Similar figures cannot be given for the USA owing to past experience of defective birth registration in many States and to a less degree of defective death registration in a smaller number of States. The population in 1790 (excluding outlying possessions) was 3,929,214 and it increased by approximately one-third in each decade up to 1860 when it was 31,443,321. From 1860 the intercensal increase diminished somewhat irregularly in successive decades; in 1860–70 it was 23 per cent; in 1910–20 only 15 per cent; in 1920–30 16 per cent; in 1930–40 7 per cent; in 1940–50 15 per cent; and in 1950–60 16 per cent.

2.52 Table 2.2 shows the proportion of the total population which was coloured at recent censuses.

TABLE 2.2   *United States of America—Proportion of Population Coloured*

Year	Coloured* population per cent of total
1900	12·1
1910	11·1
1920	10·3
1930	10·2
1940	10·2
1950	10·0
1960	11·4

* I.e. Negro, Indian, Chinese, Japanese, etc. (mostly Negro).

2.53 The higher fertility of negroes is partly compensated by their excessive mortality especially in infancy; but the greater proportion of whites in earlier years was largely due to immigration from other countries. More recently there has been stricter control and limitation of immigration.

Royal Commission on Population

2.54 Concern at the apparently low level of fertility in the nineteen-thirties and its possible consequences for the economic future of Great Britain, at a time when the problems of post-war rehabilitation of the economy and of the Commonwealth were looming nearer, led to the appointment of a Royal Commission on Population in 1944 'to examine facts relating to the present population trends in Great Britain; to investigate the causes of these trends and to consider their probable consequences; to consider what measures, if any, should be taken in the national interest to influence the upward trend of population, and to make recommendations'.

2.55 In the last half a century the rate of growth of the population had sharply declined. These changes had been experienced by many other countries, particularly those with highly developed industrial systems. The national statistics furnished annually by the Registrars General had indicated that since the middle of the nineteenth century mortality had been steadily declining, that the expectation of life at birth had increased from 43 years in 1870 to 65 or more in 1944, but that the birth rate declined continuously from a peak of about 35 per thousand in the decade 1865 to 1875, to about 14.4 in the immediate pre-war years. The natural increase of population had been declining rapidly in this century from 4,587,000 in 1901 to 1911, to 1,160,000 in 1931 to 1941. The census tabulations with all their invaluable detailed pictures of the instantaneous sex, age and social distribution of the population, did little more in the present context than to reflect the results of these changes, together with the effect of a swing in migration. They did not show how or why these movements developed. It was known that an expanding industrial economy both encouraged and was encouraged by an expanding population, that the social and environmental conditions had reacted powerfully upon health and mortality. The broad picture had been clear but broad movements over the longer term were not sufficient for the short-term problem of deciding in what way and how fast the population was changing and whether it was possible to take any action to change the direction or the pace. A great deal more detail was needed by the Commission. A closer study was necessary of the interaction between social conditions and family building and certain special studies were undertaken.

2.56 Of fresh studies initiated on behalf of the Commission two were made necessary by a new factor in our demographic history—perhaps not a new factor, but a factor which, comparatively suddenly, had become more powerful—the practice of family limitation. To a greater degree than ever before there existed a distinction between fecundity, the potentiality of child-bearing, and fertility, the actuality of childbearing. Birth control first depended upon educational and economic advantage and contributed at least a part of the difference in the fertility of the various social strata. To investigate the present role of this factor a special enquiry was conducted into the practice of family limitation in Great Britain and its influence on fertility. (Lewis Faning, 1949.)

2.57 The Commission summarized the situation by saying that '(1) the great majority of married couples nowadays practise some form of birth control in order to limit their families, and (2) that they are successful not in the sense that birth control never fails, but in the sense that it reduces the number of conceptions considerably below the number that would otherwise take place'.

2.58 A second special study established the relative importance of the various financial strains of maternity and has measured the economic handicap of the large family (Joint Committee of Royal Coll. Obstet. and Pop. Invest. Committee, 1948). This investigation attempted to answer the following questions: what services are available to women bearing children, how far are they used, and what are the factors affecting and how do they help women to regard childbirth as a normal process; how far do they prevent premature birth and infant death and promote the health of mothers and infants; finally, what do parents spend on pregnancy and childbirth? The general conclusion of the Commission was that 'social developments over the past seventy or eighty years have tended to accentuate the relative economic and other handicaps of parenthood, and that despite recent amelioration these handicaps at nearly all income levels are still substantial. In the process of social advance until recently the family has been overlooked or given only a minor place in social policy. On the economic side the most important effect is that for most families the addition of children involves a substantial reduction of the family's standard of living; on the non-economic side the worst effect is felt by mothers who have shared little, if at all, in the great growth of leisure in modern times; and the overall effect has been to lower the status of the family in the national life.'

2.59 The last remaining section of original data, made available to the Commission, was the Family Census. Throughout their Report the Commission stressed the importance of family size as an index of population growth as distinct from other measures such as the birth rate or the so called 'reproduction' rates. The purpose of this census, which was taken on a sampling basis in 1946, was to obtain a picture of the building of families by persons married at specified ages in specified years, and belonging to specified social classes, throughout each stage of their fertile married life. (See p. 67.)

2.60 The Report reviewed succinctly the principal factors determining population growth, namely (1) migration, (2) mortality, (3) marriage and

(4) family size. Between 1871 and 1931 Great Britain sustained a continuous net loss by migration. This was reversed at the time of and after the depression of 1931. The effect of this reversal was to artificially sustain the growth of total numbers in the population and to affect the age and sex distribution of the population. The most striking effect was an increase in the proportion of men to women. The Report reviewed the decline in mortality over the last century and discussed the causes. It reached the conclusion that 'most of the wastage of human life which formerly took place at young and middle ages has now been cut out. Only among the old could further reductions in mortality have really considerable effects on numbers.' With regard to marriage the Commission distinguished between the proportion of people who married and the age at which they married; the latter was disposed to vary a great deal more than the former. It was noted that in the most recent generations (i.e. born since 1914) the proportion married in the age group 20–24 had been unprecedently high, reflecting a considerable reduction in the age at marriage. This had a powerful short-term effect on the number of marriages and annual births. The Commission reviewed the decline in family size and of the differential fall in social classes.

2.61 The significant result of these considerations was the conclusion that in Great Britain, allowing for further reduction in mortality, the average size of family was in 1949 only 6 per cent below replacement value.

2.62 These conclusions were soon overtaken by events. In 1955 a sharp rise in the flow of births occurred. This was partly due to the continued decline in the average age of marriage, partly to a shortening of birth spacing i.e. a tendency on the part of married couples to complete their families earlier in married life and to a less extent to a real increase in average family size. Commonwealth immigration has been a factor operating to increase average family size for the population as a whole. Most of this rise in flow represented a borrowing of births from the future and for this reason was expected eventually to exhaust its effect on the flow of births. Before this stage was reached, however, the post-war peak generation of 1947 had reached the reproductive ages and this, together with the real rise in fertility, ironed out the subsequent diminution in the flow of births which might otherwise have occurred. It is estimated that though earlier generations failed to achieve replacement, those born in 1943–48 will do so and more recent generations may more than achieve replacement.

Intercensal estimates

2.63 The population is only counted at census years and if it is desired to estimate the population appropriate to an intercensal year some assumption must be made as to the rate of growth of the population during the intercensal period.

2.64 (1) If migration data are available then they may be combined with the natural increase to compute the population in any given year. If the information is available this is the safest method particularly if the intercensal period comprises, for example, a sudden fluctuation due to war or economic causes, and does not follow the stable trend exhibited in the last preceding intercensal period.

(2) Failing information as to migration it may be assumed that intercensal growth is either in

(a) arithmetical progression, i.e. a constant *absolute* annual increase in population. If the population in 1921 is 154,000 and in 1931 is 160,000 it is assumed that the population is increasing by

$\dfrac{160,000 - 154,000}{10} = 600$ per year, and hence that the population in 1925 may

be estimated as $154,000 + 4(600) = 156,400$ or

(b) geometrical progression, i.e. a constant percentage of its *attained* size each year. This takes account of the fact that accession of population means more parents producing children and a proportionate increase in the size of the succeeding absolute increment. The difference between (a) and (b) is the difference between simple and compound interest. If R = annual rate of increase, then for the same example,

$$160,000 = 154,000 \ R^{10}$$

$$\text{or } \log_{10}R = \frac{1}{10}\ (\log_{10} 160,000 - \log_{10} 154,000)$$

$$= \cdot 00166 \text{ or } R = 1 \cdot 004$$

Hence population in 1925 is

$$\log_{10}{}^{-1}\ [5 \cdot 18752 + 4(0 \cdot 00166)] \text{ or } 156,370$$

Such estimates as these may be erroneous when applied to the entire country, and are still more likely to be in error for a local area such as a town which may in an industrial boom gain a rapid increase of working people with many children in a short time followed immediately by a period of stability as the boom passes with migration balancing natural increase.

(3) Even if data on migration are lacking, other sources of information may be drawn upon to indicate the direction and pace of growth, such as the list of Parliamentary electors (rated up by their proportion to the entire population at the last census) or local registers of the number of rateable dwellings (multiplied by the average number of inhabitants in each house).

(4) Estimates and projections by sex and age are discussed later (p. 37).

Nationality, race

2.65 Immigrants to a population may bring with them greater or less susceptibility to disease. They may bring with them some immunity to diseases which are endemic in their country of origin but have no protection to disease peculiar to the country to which they migrate. People brought up in countries where the struggle for existence is extremely hard may be subject to selective forces such that only a very strong stock survives. Nationality and race (so far as these qualities can be defined in a world where intermingling becomes increasingly extensive) are important elements therefore in describing a population. Their importance may sometimes lie in economic rather than genetic influences; for example, coloured peoples living in a predominantly white community may be forced to live in less salubrious areas and to accept occupations of a low social order. It is difficult also in making international comparisons to separate from inherent vitality not only social influences but the contribution of climate.

2.66 The census schedule normally includes questions as to birthplace and nationality. The information in Table 2.3 has been taken from the General Report of the 1931 Census and extended by reference to the General Tables of the 1951 and 1961 Censuses.

TABLE 2.3 *England and Wales 1851–1961—Persons at the Census returned as Born Abroad per 1,000 of Total Population*

| | *British subjects* | | |
| | *Born in Commonwealth countries, Colonies,* | | |
Census	*etc., outside U.K.*	*Born abroad**	*Foreigners*
1851	1·9	0·6	2·8
1861	2·6	0·9	4·2
1871	3·1	1·7	4·4
1881	3·6	2·2	4·5
1891	3·9	1·2	6·8
1901	4·2	2·8	7·6
1911	4·5	2·5	7·9
1921	5·4	2·6	6·0
1931	5·7	3·2	4·6
1951	7·7	6·0	8·7
1961	9·6	6·3	9·2

* Born in foreign countries (not British Dominions or Colonies) and British by birth or naturalization.

Migration to U. S.A.

2.67 America represents perhaps the greatest and most rapidly developed commingling of nationalities in the world's history. Between 1860 and 1920 the proportion of foreign born white people in the total population of the United States remained fairly stable at between 13 and 15 per cent, but thereafter the proportion fell to 11.4 per cent in 1930, 8·7 per cent in 1940, 6.7 per cent in 1950, and 5·2 per cent in 1960. The proportion was, as might be expected, higher in urban areas. The non-white (almost wholly negro) population was 14·4 per cent of the total in 1860, but the proportion gradually fell to 10·3 per cent in 1920 and it has remained stabilized at about that level. In 1950 the proportion was 10·5 per cent (14·5 per cent in rural farm areas).

2.68 In 1960 the distribution by country of birth of the foreign born white population of the U.S.A. was as in Table 2.4 (p. 32).

Sex

2.69 There are important reasons for requiring information of the sex distribution of populations both national and local. Fertility can only be properly assessed by taking account of the number of women of childbearing age and also of the relative supply of males and females as affecting directly the marriage potential and indirectly fertility. There are important sex differences in mortality (Martin, 1951) (see p. 73).

Sex ratios

2.70 In successive census years the number of females in the population has exceeded the number of males. The number of females for every 1,000

TABLE 2.4   *United States of America—Birthplaces of Foreign Born Whites*

Country of Birth	per cent
United Kingdom	8·9
Norway, Sweden, Denmark	4·8
Netherlands, Switzerland, France	3·2
Germany	10·6
Poland	8·1
Czechoslovakia	2·4
Austria	3·3
Hungary	2·6
Yugoslavia	1·8
U.S.S.R.	8·7
Italy	13·5
Other Europe	9·6
Asia	2·2
Canada	10·1
Mexico	6·2
Other America	2·5
Other or not known	1·5
	100·0

males* has varied from 1,057 in 1801, to 1,068 in 1911, 1,096 in 1921, 1,088 in 1931 and 1,067 in 1961. At birth the excess is in the reverse direction; in all countries for which records exist more male than female babies are born. In England and Wales during 1961 on the average 1,062 male births occurred to every 1,000 female births. The proportion has varied at different times and in different parts of the country. During the sixty years preceding 1918 the sex ratio varied between 1,032 and 1,049. In 1919 a ratio of 1,060 was recorded and in the two following years the ratio exceeded the pre-war level with values of 1,052 and 1,051. The ratio declined to 1,041 in 1926 and then rose steadily and between 1934 and 1938 high values varying from 1,051 to 1,056 were recorded. Still higher values were recorded during the 1939–45 war and after, as follows:

1939	1,056		1946	1,060
1940	1,053		1947	1,061
1941	1,053		1948	1,061
1942	1,063		1949	1,061
1943	1,064		1950	1,060
1944	1,065		1951	1,060
1945	1,061			

2.71 Crew (1937) has suggested that since the sex ratio (male to female) in stillbirths and abortions is higher than in live births, then changes in economic or hygienic factors which influence foetal mortality and affect the chance of a live birth will be reflected by changes in the sex ratio at birth. Martin (1948) has investigated this suggestion, but has found insufficient evidence to support it. He found correlation between the marriage rate and sex ratio in the same year $(0 \cdot 423 \pm 0 \cdot 082)$ and attempted to discover whether this was due to the effect of the marriage rate on average maternal age at confinement and parity distribution of births. It was true that the sustained high marriage rates of wartime years lowered the average age at marriage

* One may either speak of males per 1,000 females (masculinity ratio) or females per 1,000 males (femininity). It is customary to use whichever measure is greater than 1,000 and the reader must be on guard against a change from one to the other.

and the average parity order of the births (owing to there being a greater weighting of first births). Whilst there were suggestions of such effects (although it was likely that they were not the only factors involved) the data available were insufficient to produce conclusive findings.

2.72 Secular changes in the sex ratio at birth and differential mortality (see p. 73) have had consequent effects on the sex structure of the population. The better survival of females gives rise to their preponderance at all except early ages, but this preponderance is slightly abated after periods of high masculinity of births.

2.73 The lighter mortality of females exerts continuous influence up the age scale so that with advancing age the excess of females becomes relatively greater. In 1961, in England and Wales, there was at birth a male excess, at age 19 approximate equality; at age 40 the female to male ratio was $1 \cdot 02$, at age 70, $1 \cdot 53$, and over age 85 there were two females to every male.

2.74 In 1820, in the United States of America, there were 1,033 males to every 1,000 females in the population; in 1910 the proportion was 1,060 to 1,000, showing an increased preponderance of males, but thereafter the ratio declined. In 1920 it was 1,040; in 1930, 1,025; in 1940, 1,007. In 1950 the proportion was 986 so that there was actually a slight excess of females. In 1960 the ratio had further declined to 971. The earlier excess of males was undoubtedly due to immigration. In the negro population which has not been so affected by migration there were in 1910, only 989 males to 1,000 females, and in 1960 the ratio was 933. For the total population the sex ratio (males per 1,000 females) at birth in 1960 was 1,049, at 10–14 it was 1,033, at ages 40–44, 958, at ages 60–64, 913, and at ages 85 and over, 650, i.e. 20 females for every 13 males.

Age distribution—England and Wales

2.75 The age distribution of the population at any one time is the product of antecedent changes in fertility, mortality and migration. In England and Wales the decline in the birth rate after 1877 and reductions in mortality, more effectively at early ages, have resulted in a process of ageing of the population which prior to 1931 was accelerated to a small extent by the emigration of young persons, but has subsequently been little affected by migration.

2.76 Table 2.5 shows the proportion of the total population (per 10,000) in each age group at the censuses of 1871, 1901, 1931, and 1961:

TABLE 2.5   *England and Wales—Population of Persons by Ages per 10,000 at all Ages in 1871, 1901, 1931, 1961*

Age	1871	1901	1931	1961
0—	1,352	1,143	749	780
5—	2,259	2,099	1,635	1,516
15—	1,843	1,958	1,734	1,318
25—	1,471	1,616	1,605	1,265
35—	1,132	1,228	1,368	1,362
45—	879	892	1,235	1,399
55—	590	597	932	1,168
65—	337	331	536	764
75—	120	121	182	363
85 and over	17	15	24	65
All ages	10,000	10,000	10,000	10,000

B

2.77 These figures indicate that the high fertility of the latter part of the nineteenth century had produced in 1901 an abnormally youthful age structure with 32·4 per cent under age 15, 48·0 per cent aged 15–44, 14·9 per cent aged 45–64 and only 4·7 per cent aged 65 and over. The rapid transition from the higher fertility of the previous century to the lower fertility of the current century produced a discontinuity in the age structure as the supply of births was restricted and fewer children were moving up into the adult age groups to replace those dying at older ages. A bulge began to move up through the age range. By 1931 this bulge had expressed itself in a large increase in the proportion aged 45–64, from 14·9 to 21·7 per cent, and a smaller increase in the proportion aged 65 and over, from 4·7 to 7·4 per cent; and a reduction at younger ages, the proportion aged under 15 declining from 32·4 to 23·8 per cent. In 1961 the bulge had moved up to higher ages. The proportion aged 45–64 had increased only a little to 25·7 per cent, but the proportion aged 65 and over had swollen to 10·9 per cent.

2.78 The situation is better illustrated by fig. 2.1 which shows the age structure of the population of England and Wales in pyramid form for 1901 and 1951 together with a stable 'life table' population which would be built up from a constant annual number of births (and sex ratio) and subject to constant mortality at the 1953 level. It can be seen that as compared with the 'life table' structure (hatched area) the population in 1901 had an excess number of younger persons representing the higher fertility of the preceding years. In 1951 this 'bulge' (referred to above) can be seen to have moved up to older adult ages. The bulge represents the difference between the 1901 (dotted line) and 1951 areas (continuous line) above the point at which their boundaries cross, i.e. from 35 upwards. When this has passed right out of the top of the pyramid and provided there are no substantial changes in the level of fertility the population will assume the age structure of a stable population toward the end of the present century. The provision is important. There have been changes in fertility since 1955 the full effect of which cannot yet be assessed. (See para. 2.62.)

2.79 Other features of interest in the pyramid are (i) the abnormally large numbers aged 0–4 in 1951 as a result of the baby boom of the years following the 1939–45 war—largely representing births 'postponed' by war separation, (ii) the male deficiency at ages 50–70 as a result of the relatively heavy war losses in the war of 1914–18 and (iii) the preponderance of females at older ages due to the greater improvement in the mortality of females as compared with that of men.

Local variation

2.80 The age distribution of the population varies considerably from locality to locality. As compared with urban areas, rural areas have higher proportions of young children and old people, partly a product of higher fertility and partly of migration from the country to the town at employment ages, with an outward movement at retiring ages. As an exception it was noted in 1931 that the South West Counties though largely rural in character returned exceptionally low proportions of children with apparently little surplus for migration elsewhere at employment ages; on the other hand its favourable climatic and residential features attracted the elderly and out-standingly high proportions at ages after 60 were recorded.

Proportions at { 1953 Life Table
1901 Census
1951 Census

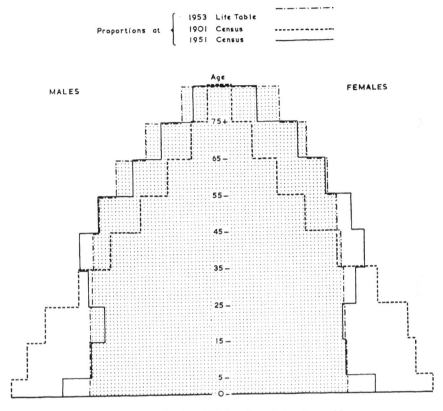

Fig. 2.1   England and Wales—Population Pyramid.

Local estimates by age

2.81 For England and Wales the numbers of males and females are given in age groups in the census tabulations for counties and larger administrative areas. In intercensal years the Registrar General has furnished national estimates in the *Annual Statistical Review*. Local estimates may be made either by assuming (if conditions are stable) that the estimated total population can be distributed on the basis of the last census, or since this assumption of stability can rarely be made, by working from census figures (after first adjusting for differences between the enumerated and the resident population [see p. 21]) and births since the census date and allowing for mortality. For the County of London the working sheet for the calculation of age group populations in the middle of 1952 for males might be as in Table 2.6 (all figures in thousands).

2.82 This calculation takes no account of migration. The Registrar General will have estimated the total migration in the locality in arriving at

TABLE 2.6 *Males—Calculation of Age Estimates*

Age last birthday	Estimated resident population 1951 Census	Deaths (a) 1951–52	Age Transfers (b)	Births (c) 1951–52	Estimated population mid-1952
0— 4	138·8	1·1	39·3	32·7	131·1
5—14	196·4	0·2	22·1		213·4
15—24	187·1	0·2	28·9		180·1
25—44	536·7	1·5	30·3		533·8
45—64	359·5	7·6	15·9		366·3
65—74	100·3	8·0	8·0		100·2
75+	41·2	8·2	—		41·0
Total	**1,560·0**	**26·8**			**1,565·9**

(a) Census date to mid-1952 within the age group—estimated by taking $\frac{3}{4}(1951) + \frac{1}{4}(1952)$ years.

(b) Estimated number moving up to next age group, i.e. terminal $1\frac{1}{4}$ years of group less allowance for deaths calculated on $\frac{5}{8}$ths of year at age specific death rate.

(c) Less $\frac{5}{8}$th of a year's infant deaths since these infants will have survived varying periods from 0 to $1\frac{1}{4}$ years and *on the average* $\frac{5}{8}$ths of a year, i.e. if the current male infant mortality rate under 1 year per 1,000 live births is 28 we have total male births $33,300 \times (1 - \frac{5}{8}[0·028]) = 32,700$.

estimates of total population published in the *Annual Statistics Review*, and this may be roughly distributed over all age groups in proportion to the total population in each age group by the simple expedient of rating down the crude age figures for both sexes to the published total, or advantage may be taken of information from housing authorities of the approximate age distribution of the balance of movement of families, e.g. in opening a new housing estate the authority will have some knowledge of the ages of the families applying for accommodation; or there may be other general knowledge of the character of migration. For London at mid-1952 the Registrar General gave an estimate of total population of 3,363,000, an increase of 10,000 as compared with the estimated resident population of 3,353,000 at census date and since the excess of births over deaths was 12,000 it is estimated that there was a net loss of 2,000 in the period (i.e. a gain of 1,000 males and a loss of 3,000 females). This loss is not true migration, but is simply a balance, i.e. the difference between the natural increase and the change from census total to the 1952 total estimate. Statistics of school attendance suggest that there was an emigration of some 15,000 children of ages 5–14 together with the corresponding adults represented by their families, say 45,000 in total; and general knowledge leads to the expectation that this would be partially offset by immigration of an almost equal number of adults of which perhaps 3,000 males and 15,000 females would be 15–24. Considering males only, therefore, we need to deduct 7·5 thousand at ages 5–14, add 3 thousand at ages 15–24, and allow for a loss at ages 25–44. The latter could be made of sufficient size to make the total agree with the official estimated total, after first adding to ages 45 and over a due proportion of the adult immigration. The resulting estimates by age may be compared with official estimates made by the Registrar General, in Table 2.7. Disagreement with this official estimate is trivial and arises from the fact that the latter was derived as part of a larger scheme embracing Greater London.

36

Details of the methods used in the General Register Office are given in Part III of the Statistical Review for 1964.

2.83 One important point should not be overlooked. If there are appreciable (net) numbers of men absent from the area on service with the Armed Forces these should be estimated and added to the census age group figures before the calculations are made and then subtracted again at the end. If this precaution is not taken, the gap on account of this service absence will be gradually moved higher up the age range instead of remaining at the same age as it should (mainly at 15–24). Conversely, if the area is one subject to an influx of servicemen the reverse operation should be carried out.

TABLE 2.7 *London County—Males (thousands)*

Age	Estimated population as described above			Official estimates of Registrar General
	Unadjusted	Migration adjustment	Adjusted	
0— 4	131		131	131
5—14	213	—7	206	204
15—24	180	+3	183	182
25—44	534	—1	533	534
45—64	367	+4	371	372
65—74	100	+1	101	101
75+	41	+1	42	43
Total	**1,566**	+1	**1,567**	**1,567**

2.84 The method of paragraph 2.81 can be applied not only to produce intercensal estimates but also to produce projections into the future of the effect of the continuation of existing trends in fertility, mortality and migration. The method is the same whether national or local populations are to be projected, but in the latter event figures appropriate to the locality must be used throughout. Now that computers are available to handle large repetitive calculations, it is usual to carry out the calculation by individual integral ages and to move forward from one calendar year to another even though a projection many years ahead may be required. For any year y (i.e. mid-year) the population aged x last birthday, denoted by yPx will consist of the survivors of $_{y-1}P_{x-1}$, of year $y-1$, together with the survivors of net immigrants during the year mid $y-1$ to mid y, who will be aged x at mid y. To obtain the survivors of $_{y-1}P_{x-1}$, this number is multiplied by a survival factor $(1-q_x)$ where q_x is the average death rate of the year of age $x - \frac{1}{2}$ to $x + \frac{1}{2}$ (note that x last birthday is equivalent to an average age of $x + \frac{1}{2}$). The net immigrants are usually estimated as at the mid-year i.e. as a surviving element but if counted as they enter then, on the average, a half year's mortality must be allowed for at the appropriate average age $(x + \frac{1}{2})$. At age 0 we take the surviving births of the period mid $y-1$ to mid y; subtracting from the births one half year's infant mortality.

2.85 To produce the figures of live births to be used in the calculation two alternative procedures can be adopted.

(1) It would be possible to carry out the calculations of projections separately for married women. The elements of marriage and divorce would have to be introduced and a further axis of classification ought to be introduced viz. duration of marriage. The mortality and migration elements would

37

also have to be appropriate to married women. Though a very detailed calculation it is feasible to consider a population of married women aged x and of marriage duration z (i.e. marriage age $x - z$) and to move this forward to become a population aged $x + 1$ and marriage duration $z + 1$ in the following year. To these populations, fertility rates specific for marriage age and duration of marriage might then be applied to generate the births over the period from mid-year to mid-year; an allowance would have to be made for illegitimate births.

(2) A simpler method is make a more general appraisal of the likely changes in size and constitution of the population of married women and the trend of changes in fertility rates, and thence to construct directly a trend curve of annual numbers of births; an informed and intelligent extrapolation of the recent trend. In making this projection it is advisable to study the implications for changes in average family size which experience has shown to be a measure which tends to change very slowly and is therefore a stable guide. This second method is usually sufficient for the purpose especially when projections are, as in most cases, regularly updated after checks against emerging experience.

Age distribution. United States of America

2.86 Table 2.8 shows the percentage age distribution of the population of the United States of America in 1880, 1900, 1920, 1950 and 1960:

TABLE 2.8   *Age Distribution Per Cent of U.S.A. Population*
(Coloured and White Combined)

	Census of				
Age	1880	1900	1920	1950	1960
0— 4	13·8	12·1	10·9	10·7	11·3
5—14	24·4	22·2	20·8	16·2	19·8
15—24	20·1	19·6	17·7	14·6	13·4
25—34	14·8	15·9	16·2	15·7	12·7
35—44	10·9	12·1	13·4	14·3	13·5
45—54	7·9	8·4	10·0	11·5	11·4
55—64	4·7	5·3	6·2	8·8	8·7
65—74	2·4	2·9	3·3	5·6	6·1
75+	1·0	1·2	1·4	2·6	3·1
Not reported	—	0·3	0·1	—	—
Total	100·0	100·0	100·0	100·0	100·0

2.87 The age structure of 1880 is typically that of a young population sustained by immigration of younger people and by the high fertility associated with a vigorously developing industrial economy. By 1900 a certain degree of ageing had taken place as those in the younger age groups had grown older. This process has continued throughout the years as fertility has fallen and the original flood of immigration has been reduced to a controlled stream of very much diminished proportions. In 1880, 38·2 per cent of the population were under age 15 and only 3·4 per cent age 65 and over; in 1950 the percentage under age 15 had fallen to 26·9 and the percentage aged 65 and over had risen to 8·2. This age structure in 1950 was still, it will be noticed, more youthful than that of England and Wales. In 1960 the effect of a rise in the flow of births can be seen in higher proportions below age 15.

REFERENCES

BENJAMIN, B. (1955) *Population Studies*, 8.288.
BENJAMIN, B. (1967) 'The Census as a source of social statistics' in *Society, Problems and Methods of Study*, ed. by A. T. Welford *et al.* Routledge, Kegan Paul. London.
CREW, F. A. E. (1937) *Report of British Association* 1937 (Nottingham), p. 95.
Interdepartmental Committee on Social and Economic Research (1951) Guides to Official Sources No. 2. *Census Reports of Great Britain 1801–1931*.
Joint Committee of Royal College of Obstetricians and Gynaecologists and the Population Investigation Committee (1948). *Maternity in Great Britain*, Oxford University Press. London 1948.
LEWIS FANING, E. (1949) 'Report on an Enquiry into Family Limitation'. *Papers of Royal Commission on Population*. Vol. 1. H.M.S.O.
MARTIN, W. J. (1948) *Medical Officer*, 79.153.
MARTIN, W. J. (1951) *J. Roy. Stat. Soc. Series A.*, 114.287.
NEWTON, M. P., and JEFFERY, J. R. (1951) Internal Migration. General Register Office. *Studies on Medical and Population Subjects* No. 5. H.M.S.O.
Royal Commission on Population (1949) Report Cmd. 7695. H.M.S.O.
United Nations *Demographic Year Book*. Statistical Office of U.N. Department of Economic Affairs, New York.

APPENDIX I

NATIONAL CENSUSES

The published reports of national censuses in most countries contain much of methodological interest as well as providing source material on a wide range of demographic topics. In England and Wales the results are published in a series of volumes by the General Register Office in London and in the United States the results are published by the U.S. Bureau of the Census in Washington. Applications should be made to these departments for details of current and past publications.

APPENDIX II

Registration districts

Vital registration services are *local* services and naturally related to the organization of local government administration. Thus in England and Wales the Registrar General has responsibility for the enforcement and operation of the various statutes relating to marriage, birth and death registration, but the local registrars are appointed, and their office premises provided, by local authorities (counties, county boroughs and London boroughs). The Registrar General prescribes the duties and inspects the work of registrars; he has powers of dismissal. There are some five hundred Registration Districts in England and Wales for each of which there is a Superintendent Registrar (who has special duties in relation to marriages, i.e. marriages may be solemnized in his presence without a religious ceremony); these districts are divided into 1,200 or so sub-districts each of which is in charge of a Registrar of Births and Deaths. For each district one or more registrars of births and deaths may also act as Registrar of Marriages. For the births and deaths the basic unit is the sub-district. Any county, county borough or London borough is of course identifiable with a whole number of registration districts (and of sub-districts). In the determination of the extent of sub-districts population distribution and transport communications are more important than total population size. In the administrative counties municipal boroughs and urban and rural districts are often split between registration sub-districts. Assignment of registration records to areas of residence is achieved by specific area coding, by reference to address of usual residence, during the data processing.

The system in Scotland is similar. There are no Superintendent Registrars. Registrars are appointed by the Town Councils of Burghs or the County Council outside the Burghs and are subject to prescription of duties and inspection by the Registrar General for Scotland.

In the United States of America registration is a State function and the National Office of Vital Statistics obtains uniformity in State procedure solely by advice and co-operation. Each State maintains a central division of vital statistics within its department of health. The States are divided into registration districts. Each city, incorporated town, or other primary political unit (township, civil district, etc.) usually constitutes a registration district; in some instances several political units may be combined to form a single district. A local registrar is appointed for every registration district and he transmits records first to county or city health departments and thence to the State Department of Health. (The latter send copies to the National Office of Vital Statistics.)

Census areas

In Great Britain the Registrars General are responsible for the population census enumeration and the local registrars play an important part in this operation. Full advantage is taken of their knowledge of local conditions and the existing organization of the registration service forms a natural framework for the census. Each registration sub-district is split up into an integral number of Ordinary Enumeration Districts (the term 'ordinary' is used in distinction from the special enumeration districts created where an institution was large enough to constitute an enumeration unit in itself). The content of an ordinary enumeration district in 1961 was of the order of 700–800 persons. Any local government area could be built up by putting together a whole number of enumeration districts; a sample population representative of a local government area could be obtained by choosing a sample of enumeration districts. If during the intercensal period local government boundaries change the enumeration districts at the next census are adjusted to retain this correspondence.

In the United States there are also enumeration districts defined in terms of an enumerator's work load and planned that they could be added together to form political areas (minor civil divisions, and in turn counties). In 1950 the census statistics were presented for 'urbanised areas' which reached beyond the larger cities to the closely settled urban fringes around them. Apart from and outside these urbanized areas the United States Bureau of the Census also recognized 2,400 certain unincorporated places, i.e. a definite nucleus of residences with its surrounding closely settled area, and statistics were provided for 1,430 of them with 1,000 or more inhabitants. In the larger cities small permanent statistical areas or census tracts as they are called have been established. These are not so closely tied to local authority boundaries. They are drawn in such a way as to secure a greater degree of homogeneity in relation to urban development and racial economic and social characteristics. Their high degree of permanence facilitates intercensal comparisons.

Local government areas

Population and vital statistics primarily serve administrative purposes and so, the world over, the basic unit for tabulation purposes is the area served by a district local authority. The following table shows the principal units involved in published tables; for England and Wales, Scotland, and the United States.

Urban and rural areas

There are no entirely satisfactory definitions of 'urban' or 'rural' areas. Sociologists and vital statisticians differ a little in their approaches, the former thinking in terms of different ways of living together and social attitudes, while the latter tend to pay more attention to material factors such as population density and street formation. For population census purposes the most practicable method (involving considerable cartographic analysis) would be to define 'urbanized land' as a piece of land covered by buildings sited in a recognizable street pattern or as two or more such pieces separated from each other by (say) less than a mile, and the whole containing a population of (say) 5,000 persons or more. The arbitrary limits of one mile and 5,000 persons are suitable for England and Wales but would not necessarily be suitable in other countries. In Scotland a minimum figure of 1,000 has been used in this type of analysis.

40

POPULATION

For mortality purposes, the General Register Office of England and Wales have identified certain rural districts as 'truly rural', the criteria for selections being (*a*) not more than one per cent of the total rateable value of the district should be assessed as industrial property, (*b*) the rural district should not be contiguous with any urban district with a population of 25,000 or over or with a group of urban districts where the population is 25,000 or over, (*c*) the density of population within the district does not exceed one person per four acres.

England and Wales

The country is split into 58 *Administrative Counties* and the area of the Greater London Council which subsumes the areas of the former counties of London and Middlesex. Within these Administrative Counties there are 82 *County Boroughs* of the same general status as the counties; their populations normally form entirely separate statistical units except that in certain census tabulations the 'administrative counties and their associated county boroughs' are used as divisions of the total populations.

Within Greater London there are 32 *London Boroughs and the City of London*. Within the administrative counties there are (1) 270 *Municipal Boroughs*; (2) 535 *Urban Districts*; Some urban areas are divided into wards for local electoral purposes. (3) 473 *Rural Districts*. (4) Within Rural districts, the 11,162 *Civil Parishes*. These areas appear in some census tables but do not appear in the normal tabulations of vital statistics.

Aggregates. For summary purposes the country has been divided into 9 Standard Regions each comprising several couny ties or parts of counties including associated county boroughs. This enables a broad examination to be

Scotland

There are 33 *Counties.* Within these Counties there are (1) 4 Counties of cities (Aberdeen, Dundee, Glasgow, Edinburgh); these like the county boroughs in England and Wales have the same status as counties; (2) 20 Large Burghs (similar to municipal boroughs in England and Wales). (3) 176 Small Burghs (equivalent to urban district councils in England and Wales); (4) 198 Non-burghal towns and villages. These have no legally defined areas and are identified only in census tabulations. Some of these towns have populations greater than that of many of the Burghs, and many occur within the central industrial belt of the country. It has been customary to regard those with a population of 1,000 or more as urban but this is an arbitrary distinction; (5) 869 Civil Parishes. As in England and Wales these do not figure in the normal tabulations of vital statistics though their populations are given in census tables.

United States

Within each State, there are the following types of area

(1) *Counties* sub-divided into

(i) *Metropolitan Counties.*

(ii) *Non-metropolitan Counties* according to criteria laid down by the U.S. Bureau of the Census. A metropolitan county must have at least one city with a population of 50,000 or more, or be contiguous to a metropolitan county so defined and with its population integrated socially and economically with the central city of the area.

(2) *County districts, cities and villages.* These are normally classified into urban and non-urban. A district is a city of 10,000 or more population, a village of 2,500 or more forming 50 per cent or more of the population of a town, or a place of population 10,000 or more having a density of 1,000 or more persons per square mile.

B*

41

England and Wales	*Scotland*	*United States*

made of geographical differentials and of the influence of the higher industrialization of the northern areas, and of the more agricultural and rural character of Eastern and South-Western areas.
 	
For the study of urban and population density effects, the local authority units are aggregated as:
Conurbations
Outside conurbations
  Urban areas with populations of 100,000 or more
  Urban areas with populations of 50,000 and under 100,000
  Urban areas with populations under 50,000.
  Rural districts.		

CHAPTER 3

REGISTRATION OF BIRTHS, DEATHS AND MARRIAGES

3.1 Registration of baptisms, marriages and deaths in England and Wales dates back to 1538 in the reign of Henry VIII when the clergy in every parish were required to keep a weekly record of these events. This emerged from the early recognition that it was in the interests of individuals, for legal and other purposes, that there should be permanent, formal, personal recording of these matters to provide proof of age, where necessary, to detect bigamy and to guard against destruction of infants. Except for a brief period from 1653 to the Restoration this recognition did not become statutory until the passage of the Births and Deaths Registration Act, 1836, which established the General Register Office, divided up the country into registration districts (there are now over 500 in England and Wales) and provided for the registration of births and deaths, though no penalty was imposed in the event of refusal to register (Dr Farr estimated deficient registration at the time at 5 per cent). After a short delay the Act became effective from July 1, 1837. A penalty was applied by the Births and Deaths Registration Act, 1874, and registration became progressively more complete; failure to register is today extremely rare. Legislation has been consolidated in the Births and Deaths Registration Act, 1953, the Marriage Act, 1949, and the Registration Service Act, 1953.

Births—England and Wales

3.2 Under the Act of 1953 it is required that the father and mother of every child born alive or in their default by death or inability 'the occupier of the house in which a child was to the knowledge of that occupier born', or 'any person present at the birth', or 'any person having charge of the child' shall give to the Registrar within forty-two days from the date of the birth, information of the particulars required to be registered. These particulars which are separately prescribed by regulations made under the Act are—

(1) Date and place of birth
(2) Name, if any
(3) Sex
(4) Name and surname of father
(5) Name and maiden surname of mother
(6) Father's occupation
(7) Signature, description and residence of informant.

3.3 The putative father is not required to furnish any particulars concerning the birth of his illegitimate child and his name is not to be entered in the Register except at the joint request of himself and of the mother, in which case both must sign the Register. The Registrar may require the attendance of any of the persons described above to give him information for the registration but Registrars are instructed not to call upon medical practitioners or other persons present at the birth except as a last resort.

3.4 An Act of 1926 had instituted the compulsory registration of stillbirths (over 28 weeks gestation) and this is consolidated in the 1953 Act. Similar information is recorded as for live births and in addition the nature of the evidence showing the child to have been stillborn which must be either a certificate signed by a medical practitioner or midwife that the child was not born alive or a declaration by the informant in a prescribed form that no medical practitioner or midwife has attended or examined the baby or that no certificate can be obtained and that the child was not born alive. Since 1960 the cause of stillbirth, as given on a doctor's or midwife's certificate has been recorded. (Population (Statistics) Act 1960.)

3.5 Apart from the main legislation relating to compulsory registration an important step forward in the provision of statistical knowledge was taken by the passage of the Population (Statistics) Act 1938. It had for some time been recognized that the existing registration details did not provide an adequate basis for deciding what were the important factors affecting the variation of fertility. The matter became more pressing as the decline in the birth rate persisted and facts were needed in order to frame a policy which might meet the general concern about the population trend. Under this Act additional information could be sought upon registration; these additional details were for statistical purposes only, were therefore treated as confidential and were not entered in any public register. The details were—

On registration of live or stillbirth
  (1) Age of mother and (if the parents are married to each other) the
  (2) Date of marriage
  (3) Number of children by present husband, and how many still living
  (4) Number of children by any former husband, and how many still living.

The Population (Statistics) Act 1960 substituted the following particulars for those previously required under the 1938 Act, at the registration of a live or stillbirth:

  (1) In all cases the age of the mother
  (2) Where the name of any person is to be entered in the register of births as father of the child, the age of that person
  (3) Except where the birth is of an illegitimate child—
      (i) the date of the parents' marriage
      (ii) whether the mother has been married before her marriage to the father of the child
      (iii) the number of children of the mother by her previous husband and by any former husband, and how many of them were born alive or were stillborn.

3.6 Under the 1960 Act certain additional particulars are also obtained at death registration (see p. 49).

Possible developments in birth registration

3.7 At the present time no attempt is made to record at birth registration either the birth weight or the gestation period. These are factors affecting infant mortality which are of as much if not more importance than the occupation of the father. Indeed while the father's occupation only indirectly affects mortality by conditioning the environment (nutrition, warmth, protection from infection, and general parental care) these other factors (neither of which is independent of the other) directly determine the resources for sustaining life. In prematurely born infants such resources are commonly inadequate to meet the risks of infection or the respiratory need of extra-uterine existence and mortality is high; only in this sense can prematurity be regarded as a mortality risk.

3.8 It has to be admitted that the estimation of gestation period is subject to wide margins of error in individual cases since menstrual information is not unequivocal, but the information is recorded by the midwife and doctor, and indeed has to be estimated for registration purposes in the event of the delivery of a dead foetus. The birth weight is also recorded and is furnished to the local health authority, on the postcard used for birth notification under the Public Health Act (see p. 46), in order that premature infants (officially distinguished by having a birth weight $5\frac{1}{2}$ pounds or less) can be given special attention by health visitors. A small measure of reciprocity between registration and health authorities might suffice to transfer this information to the birth register though, of course, for a large number of births, even one small additional detail can represent a heavy total work load, and cannot be lightly undertaken. Birth weight is recorded at registration in France.

Births—United States

3.9 Legally and historically, vital registration has developed in the United States as a function of State Governments. A National Division of Vital Statistics was established in the United States in 1850, (1) to compile and publish vital statistics and, (2) to promote uniform registration and statistics throughout the country. The National Office collected its data initially from census enumerations; it has compiled data from copies of State records since 1900. The national vital records and statistics system of the United States is best described as a confederation of about 56 autonomous areas and the National Division of Vital Statistics. Uniformity has been promoted and primarily achieved through the use of a Model State Vital Statistics Act, Standard Certificate Forms, Rules of Statistical Practice, and close co-operation by joint committees of State and Federal officials. The National Office also provides technical assistance and advice to State offices upon their request. Completeness and uniformity of registration and statistics have been promoted also by establishing Registration Areas for the several types of vital events. To be eligible for admission to these Areas, a State has to conform with the Model Law, Standard Certificate Form, have a central State File, attain an acceptable degree of registration completeness, and furnish data to the National Office.

3.10 The particulars registered at birth in America normally follow a standard approved by the United States Public Health Service and revised decennially; they include:

(1) Place and date of birth
(2) Usual residence of mother
(3) Child's name
(4) Sex
(5) Name, colour, age, birthplace, occupation and industry of father
(6) Maiden name, race, age, birthplace, education, previous births of mother
(7) Gestation period
(8) Birth weight
(9) Whether legitimate.

Provision is made for details of complications of pregnancy and confinement, and for birth injury or congenital malformation of child to be inserted in the space at the foot of the registration form.

3.11 As the great majority of births (over 90 per cent) occur in hospitals, the model law places responsibility upon the hospital administrator to prepare and file a record for each event occurring in his hospital. The physician is responsible, however, for certifying to the fact of birth and certain details.

3.12 Similar details are asked for in the case of a foetal death. The funeral director or person in charge of the disposition of the foetus is responsible for obtaining the personal particulars and for filing the completed certificate with the local registrar of vital statistics (a deputy of the State registrar) but the physician is enjoined in the absence of a funeral director to report the foetal death.

Notification under the Public Health Acts

3.13 In England, apart from registration, it is required by the Public Health Act 1936 that the person in attendance on the birth, and the parent if residing at the place of birth, shall notify the local health authority (County or County Borough Council or London Borough) within 36 hours in order that Health Visitors may make early visits for welfare purposes. This applies equally to live or stillbirths. Statistical aspects of the Health Visitors' work are dealt with on p. 214 but it may be mentioned here that it is customary for local registrars and local health officers to compare their lists of registrations and notifications and the reciprocal reporting of discrepancies over a period of time in order to allow for the lag between notification and registration, leads to a high degree of accuracy in records. (Under the Public Health (Notification of Births) Act 1965 some notifications may be sent to Medical officers of municipal boroughs or urban or rural districts.) The details furnished on birth notification (by postcard to the local health authority) include name, address, date and place of birth, live or stillborn, and birth weight.

Distinction between live and stillbirth

3.14 The distinction between live and stillbirth and in particular the definition of the latter has been the subject of international discussion to ensure comparability between national statistics. While in England the foetus must be of twenty-eight weeks gestation for the death to be registered as a stillbirth, in the United States the general rule is that foetal deaths after *twenty* weeks' gestation are registered as stillbirths, though in some States the period is as short as four months and in some, all products of conception are registered. This alone creates a large difference in the reported stillbirth rates in the two countries.

3.15 The WHO in 1947 indicated some concern at the lack of any international definition of a stillbirth. There was no agreement between countries as to the boundaries to be fixed between live and stillbirth or between stillbirth and abortion. In some countries an infant who died before registration of birth had been carried out was not counted as a live birth or a death. The argument adduced for the short gestation period adopted for defining a stillbirth in the USA was that a small proportion of infants born before twenty-eight weeks showed signs of life and might even survive. Against this it was argued that 'there was no real reason why the dividing line between abortion and stillbirth need be fixed at a duration of gestation below which signs of life *never* occurred. What was needed was the choice of a duration of gestation at which it could be said that there ought to have been signs of life and if there were not then there was something wrong.' Much evidence was laid before the Expert Committee on Health Statistics to examine with a view to international agreement. The view was pressed that the term stillbirth should be abandoned but it was agreed that it could not be made a condition of international agreement that the term should be abandoned in countries where the term was employed in legislative usage.

3.16 The Committee concentrating on the need for information of total foetal wastage which could not be secured under any of the current definitions of stillbirth, concluded that 'foetal death' rather than stillbirth should be defined and proposed the following definition (as the reverse of a definition of a live birth)—

'Foetal death is death prior to the complete expulsion or extraction from its mother of a product of conception, irrespective of the duration of pregnancy; the death is indicated by the fact that after such separation the foetus does not breathe or show any other evidence of life, such as beating of the heart, pulsation of the umbilical cord or definite movement of voluntary muscles.'

3.17 The Committee also recommended that all live births and foetal deaths should be tabulated according to the following periods of gestation:

Less than 20 completed weeks of gestation	Group I
20 completed weeks of gestation but less than 28	Group II
28 completed weeks of gestation and over	Group III
Gestation period not classifiable in Groups I, II, III	Group IV

3.18 Groups I and II have hitherto been referred to as abortions, and Group III as stillbirths. Group III is regarded as the minimum attainment of registration.

3.19 Whilst there has been some trend towards adherence to these definitions, adoption is as yet far from complete. In many countries there are legal difficulties in making a change in the juridical definition of a stillbirth.

Correction for residence

3.20 In England while births are required to be registered in the area of *occurrence* they are reallocated by the General Register Office for statistical purposes to the area of *residence* of the mother. This prevents a local birth rate from being inflated by the presence of large maternity hospitals. Local health authorities take steps to similarly transfer notifications of non-resident births. In America a similar procedure of correcting registrations is followed.

Registration of deaths—England and Wales

3.21 Like that of births, registration of deaths dates from the Act of 1836, but it did not become subject to penalty until 1874. Accurate analysis of deaths by cause was not made possible until the Act of 1874 introduced a certificate of cause of death to be signed by a medical practitioner.

3.22 Every medical practitioner attending the deceased in his last illness is required to furnish a certificate stating the cause of death to the best of his knowledge and belief and to deliver it forthwith to the Registrar. The Registrar cannot give a certificate authorizing the disposal of the body until this has been done and he is satisfied that if the case is one which should be reported to the Coroner, the Coroner has completed his investigations. The Registrar himself may report any death to the Coroner where it appears unnatural (see 5.18).

3.23 Unless the death has been reported to the Coroner, information for the registration of every death has to be delivered to the Registrar of the district normally within five days of its occurrence by any relative of the deceased present at the death or in attendance at the last illness; or failing these by any other relative of the deceased dwelling or being in the same district as the deceased; or such person present at the death; or the occupier of the house or each inmate of the house; or the person causing the body of the deceased to be buried. If the deceased did not die in a house a similar chain of responsibility is enacted.

3.24 The cause of death is entered in the register from the medical or Coroner's certificate but in the very rare cases where there is no such certificate it is entered on the best information available. In 1963, 82·6 per cent of all deaths were certified by medical practitioners and 17·2 per cent were certified as the result of inquest, or Coroner's postmortem without inquest (0·2 per cent uncertified).

3.25 Deaths are reallocated to place of residence in the same way as are births.

3.26 The information required by regulation under the Births and Deaths Registration Act 1953 to be registered for deaths is as follows—

(1) Date and place of death
(2) Name, surname
(3) Sex
(4) Age
(5) Occupation (father's occupation for children under 15, or for a spinster or divorced woman; husband's or former husband's occupation for married women or widows)
(6) Cause of death
(7) Signature, description and residence of informant

3.27 Additional particulars recorded at death registration under the Population (Statistics) Act 1960 are:

(1) Whether the deceased was single, married, widowed or divorced
(2) the age of the surviving spouse, if any, of the deceased.

Registration of deaths in United States

3.28 The physician's principal responsibility in death registration is to prepare the medical part of the death certificate. The funeral director, or other person in charge of interment, is responsible for completing those parts of the death certificate that call for personal information about the deceased and for filing the certificate with the local Registrar of the district in which the death occurred. Each State prescribes the time within which the death certificate must be filed with the local Registrar.

3.29 In general, the duties of the physician are to:

(1) Prepare and sign the medical certification section of the death certificate, and enter the date of death.

(2) Return the signed death certificate to the funeral director promptly, so that the funeral director can file it with the local Registrar within the prescribed time.

(3) Know the State and local regulations regarding responsibility for medical certification when death was due to external causes or occurred without medical attendance.

(a) When death is the result of an accident, homicide, or suicide the law usually requires that the medical examiner or coroner for the district in which the death occurred investigate the case and certify to the cause of death. Hence, it may be the physician's duty to report the case to the medical examiner or coroner.

(b) Similarly, if death occurred from natural causes without medical attendance, the law usually requires that the medical examiner, coroner, or health officer, shall complete the medical certification.

(4) Co-operate with the local or State Registrar by prompt reply to his queries concerning any entries on the medical certification.

3.30 The details required include place of death, usual residence, name, date of death, sex, race, marital status, date of birth, occupation, birthplace, citizenship, parents' names, social security number, cause of death, disposal of body.

Marriages

3.31 In England the information recorded at civil marriages, or by the person solemnizing a religious marriage and transmitted to the Registrar, comprises—

(1) Date of marriage
(2) Names and surnames
(3) Ages
(4) Marital conditions
(5) Occupations
(6) Residences at time of marriage

(7) Fathers' names and surnames

(8) Occupations of fathers together with the precise place of marriage and form of ceremony

3.32 Similar information is recorded in America. Individual States vary in their practice though they aim at the Standard Record of Marriage which includes items 1–6 above and also the number of previous marriages. Some States show items of parentage but rarely occupation of father.

Publications of the Registrar General in England and Wales

3.33 The principal vital statistics for each calendar year for individual districts are supplied regularly to local medical officers of health as soon as possible after the end of the year, i.e. in April or May, under normal conditions.

3.34 The figures include estimates of population, numbers of births by sex and legitimacy, numbers of deaths by sex classified to the thirty-six groups of the abridged list of causes used in the *Registrar General's Statistical Review* and to certain special individual causes, numbers of deaths of children under one year of age by sex and legitimacy, and a summary of the principal rates in England and Wales as a whole.

3.35 In addition, the medical officers of health for counties, county boroughs and the London Boroughs are supplied with the age distribution of the deaths classified to the thirty-six headings of the abridged list.

3.36 *The Registrar General's Weekly Return.* The Return, which is published on the Saturday following the week to which it relates, contains—

(i) A record of the number of births, stillbirths, deaths, infant deaths and deaths from some of the principal epidemic diseases registered in the preceding week in England and Wales, Greater London, and the Counties (including associated County Boroughs).

(ii) A serial record of these figures and of notifications of certain infectious diseases for the current and preceding weeks, with cumulative totals up to date and corresponding figures for recent years for (*a*) England and Wales (*b*) Greater London.

(iii) A record of the deaths by age and from the principal causes in Greater London.

(iv) A record of the numbers of cases of infectious disease notified in each local government area.

(v) A record of the numbers of new claims to sickness benefit made under the National Insurance Act in the current week and three preceding weeks, together with weekly averages for earlier periods, for England and Wales and the Standard Regions. (These statistics are supplied by the Ministry of Social Security.)

(vi) Values of air temperature, rainfall and sunshine in certain large towns and meteorological observations taken at Kew Observatory, Richmond, supplied by the Meteorological Office.

3.37 *The Registrar General's Quarterly Return.* This publication contains:

(i) A serial record of the principal quarterly and annual figures of births, stillbirths, marriages, deaths, infant deaths, deaths under four weeks, and perinatal deaths; and rates. Figures are given for England, Wales and for standard and Hospital Regions.

(ii) Records of the numbers of notified cases of infectious disease compiled from the special quarterly returns from Medical Officers of Health.

(iii) A record of the number of births and deaths in certain cities abroad, and infant mortality by quarters over the last few years in several countries other than England and Wales, compiled from special returns sent by them.

(iv) A table showing the numbers of deaths from the principal causes, distinguishing sex, registered in England and Wales in each of the last nine available quarters. The latest quarter available is generally that preceding the one to which the return relates.

(v) An analysis of migration statistics.

(vi) A table showing the numbers of insured persons absent from work owing to certified sickness or industrial injury (or prescribed disease) on specific days in three consecutive months in England and Wales and in the Standard Regions. These figures are supplied by the Ministry of Social Security.

(vii) Values of air temperature, rainfall and sunshine in districts of England and Wales in each month of the calendar quarter, supplied by the Meteorological Office.

3.38 Certain non-quarterly information is included in the issues for certain quarters of the year, e.g. the March Return contains a detailed analysis of deaths assigned to Greater London, by cause and age, and information on population, births and deaths in England and Wales and within the administrative counties during the preceding year; the December Return contains some annual vital statistics and textual summary relating to the experience of the country as a whole in the year then ended; and also population projections.

3.39 *The Registrar General's Statistical Review (Annual)*. In normal years this Review appears in three volumes, two containing statistical tables (Part I, Medical, and Part II, Population) and the third (Part III) a Commentary with additional tables.

3.40 The Review contains all the detailed vital statistics compiled in the processes described above, and also contains those derived from the morbidity data which have become available. Part I deals, therefore, mainly with mortality statistics and statistics of the notifiable infectious diseases. Part II contains statistics of births, marriages and population, and since 1938 of fertility also. The Commentary contains a critical review of the principal features of the figures published in the volumes of tables together with special analyses and tabulations. From time to time in the medical section a few diseases are selected for fairly exhaustive examination of trends and over the course of the years the Commentary provides a complete analysis of the major trends in vital statistics such as is not to be found in any other source. Similarly, the population section of the Commentary provides detailed examination of modern measures of population replacement, of divorce statistics and of such matters as population estimates.

51

3.41 *Studies on medical and population subjects.* This comprises a series of occasional publications designed to provide in convenient form a more extensive treatment of important subjects than is practicable within the limits of the annual *Statistical Review.* Topics so far covered include cancer registration, morbidity measurement, hospital in-patient records, general practitioner statistics and internal and external migration.

Publications in Scotland

3.42 The General Register Office in Scotland publishes—

(1) A weekly return containing the births and deaths and marriages and related rates in principal towns; a classification of deaths showing those due to epidemic disease, tuberculosis, respiratory disease, violence, those under one year and those over sixty-five years of age; certain meteorological details.

(2) A quarterly return giving similar information as in the weekly return for Scotland and local areas with figures for the quarters of previous years; deaths in Scotland during the quarter by cause and age; deaths by cause in the counties and large burghs; meteorology.

(3) An Annual Report with detailed statistical tables and commentary both medical and civil.

Publications based on registrations in America

3.43 Copies of birth and death registration certificates filed in the States are sent to the National Office of Vital Statistics and also weekly reports on communicable disease. The National Office publishes the following current reports—

3.44 *Morbidity and Mortality Weekly Report.* Statistics of the reported incidence of certain communicable disease in each State. Total deaths registered in major cities for the current week, the previous week, with cumulative totals.

3.45 *Monthly Vital Statistics Report.* Monthly and cumulative data on births, marriages, deaths, and infant deaths for the States, certain cities, and the Territory of Hawaii. Death rates by cause of death, age, sex, and race, estimated from a 10 per cent sample of the death certificates filed in State and independent city vital statistics offices. Provisional divorce data are also presented for twenty-eight specified States, Hawaii and Virgin Islands.

3.46 *Vital Statistics of the United States, Annual Report, Volume I.* Marriage, divorce, natality, foetal mortality, infant mortality, and total mortality data for the United States, Alaska, Hawaii, Puerto Rico, and Virgin Islands. Figures on marriages for each reporting area by month; by age, race and previous marital status of bride and groom; and by number of present marriage. Divorces for each reporting area by month; by legal grounds for decree; by party to whom granted; by number of children affected by decree; and by duration of marriage in years. Live births by attendant; foetal deaths; total, infant and neonatal deaths; by race for each State and county; and for metropolitan and non-metropolitan counties. Detailed figures on live births, foetal deaths, and infant deaths for the United States and each State; for metropolitan and non-metropolitan counties in each State; and for the Territories and possessions. Live births by month, race, and sex; births by race, nativity of white parents, sex, age of parents, and birth order; births by weight at birth, race, period of gestation, attendant at birth; and plurality. Cases of plural births classified by the number of children born alive and born dead. Foetal deaths by age of mother, race, sex, and birth order; by attendant and gestation group; and by weight at birth, race, period of gestation, and plurality. Infant and neonatal deaths from selected causes by month, and by age, race, and sex. Total deaths from selected causes by age, race, and sex; by month; by minor civil divisions, for the Territories and possessions. Introductory text on classification and interpretation of vital statistics. Textual and summary tables including abridged life tables for each race-sex group.

3.47 *Vital Statistics of the United States, Annual Report, Volume II.* Mortality data: Statistics on deaths for the United States, each State and county; and for metropolitan and non-metropolitan counties. Deaths by month, age, race, and sex; deaths from each cause by race and sex; deaths from selected causes by month, and by age, race, and sex; deaths by marital status.

3.48 In addition periodical reviews are issued covering several years and also life tables, National, Regional and State. The National Office of Vital Statistics also publishes summaries of International Vital Statistics.

CHAPTER 4

FERTILITY—MEASURES AND TRENDS

4.1 The population growth is the net result of gains from births (fertility); of losses from deaths (mortality) and of movements from or to countries outside the national boundaries (migration).

4.2 Fertility measures the rate at which a population adds to itself by births and is normally assessed by relating the number of births to the size of some section of the population, such as the number of married couples or the numbers of women of childbearing age, i.e. an appropriate yardstick, of potential fertility. Clearly the number of births though dependent upon intention and willingness is limited by the number of women exposed to the risk of pregnancy and in all consideration of fertility measures the choice of exposed-to-risk is all important.

The instability of fertility

4.3 Since over ninety per cent of all births in England and Wales are legitimate, the extent to which people marry at any time exercises a powerful influence on the subsequent flow of births. The number of couples who marry will depend upon the available numbers and the relative age distributions of men and women within the marriageable age period and these will depend upon antecedent births (and the marriage experience producing them); thus future fertility depends upon past fertility. Though there are thus these quantitative restraints on the variation of fertility, there is also an important element of unpredictable fluctuation due to human volition. Knowledge of contraception now extends to all classes of the community and births are by no means always the chance products of sexual impulses. It is realistic to speak of family planning with the implication that parents may with varying degrees of diligence endeavour to determine the size of their family and the intervals between births. The swings of economic fortune and the pressure of social attitude (e.g. general fears about the size of the population) may modify this 'planning' even in a short space of time, so that stable trends of fertility over long periods are not to be expected and long term forecasts of fertility are subject to wide margins of error.

Factors affecting fertility variation

4.4 The number of children produced by a group of women in a given year will depend upon their ages, whether they are married, how long they have been married and how many children they have already borne. It will depend also upon the economic resources, housing conditions and the educational facilities available. It may also depend upon where they live, e.g. whether in an urban or a rural environment. Immigrants may bring with them attitudes to family size typical of their country of origin. All these factors merit study

54

partly because knowledge of them enables more reliable forecasts to be made, for example, for local authorities who may want to know what nurseries or schools to build in the future, partly also because if any demographic policy, e.g. family allowances, is to be framed, then these factors determine the pattern of that policy, and finally in studying the effect of those factors upon fertility the Medical Officer of Health may also gain some clues to their effect upon health.

Birth rate

4.5 The crude birth rate is usually calculated by relating total live births in a year to the total population of all ages and expressing it as a rate per 1,000. The total population is not the proper population at risk so far as births to women are concerned since it contains males, and also females outside the childbearing ages. The crude birth rate is satisfactory only when the true exposed to risk is a fixed proportion of the total population, i.e. when it is used for the same community in a short series of years, or in comparing the birth rates of communities whose populations are known to be nearly, if not quite, equal in their age and sex composition and in marital condition, If, however, the number of women, especially of married women, of childbearing age changes in the one community studied or differs in the two populations compared the crude birth rate will vary from this cause apart from true fertility variations.

4.6 The *general fertility rate* is obtained by expressing the live births as a rate per 1,000 of women of childbearing age, taken as either 15–49 or 15–44. (It is possible also to calculate the similar index of males of fertile ages with a suitably older age limit especially where, as is sometimes the case, reproductivity is being studied in relation to the male population.) The difficulty is that although the general fertility rate takes into account the proper exposed to risk, it requires estimates of the female population by age and marital status in inter-censal years and for small local areas this may involve more error than would be entailed in using crude birth rates for comparison. It is possible to introduce some correction to birth rates for differences in population age structure. An area comparability factor may be calculated which represents the ratio of an 'expected' birth rate—obtained by applying standard (usually national) fertility rates by age to, the local population structure—to the actual rate recorded in the standard population. If this factor is above (below) unity it indicates that the local rate must be correspondingly reduced (increased) to allow for departure from standard population structure. If local birth rates in inter-censal years are multiplied by the appropriate census-based factors the rates thus adjusted are comparable. This is the method used by the Registrar General for England and Wales.

Area comparability factors

4.7 Area comparability factors for use with birth rates were introduced in 1949. The present series of ACF.s used by the Registrar General are effectively indirect standardizing factors (see p. 93) and are based on the sex and age composition of the population as determined by the 1951 Census.

4.8 Effectively if P_x is the number of women in the population aged x to $x + 4$; and P is the total population of all ages and both sexes: f_x is the group fertility rate for ages x to $x + 4$; and accents indicate local area figures, national figures being unaccented, we require as an indirect standardizing factor to adjust the crude local birth rate

$$\frac{\Sigma f_x \cdot P_x/P}{\Sigma f_x \cdot P'_x/P'}$$

which, as it should be, is greater than unity if the local age structure is such that P'_x/P_x is relatively lower at the younger ages where fertility rates are higher, i.e. if the local population is relatively deficient of women at child-bearing ages. But since $\Sigma f_x \cdot P_x/P$ is the persons of all ages rate R for England and Wales, then the expression may be written $\Sigma \dfrac{P'}{(f_x/R) \cdot P'_x}$, a form which facilitates computation. Thus in accordance with this expression the procedure is as follows:

4.9 The childbearing component of the population of England and Wales, taken for this purpose as women aged 15–44, is separated into six five-year age groups (viz. 15–19, 20–24, etc.). Group birth rates are then obtained by dividing the number of live births occurring to mothers in each age group during the triennium surrounding the last census by three times the corresponding census population. The group rates are then each divided by a rate for persons of all ages, calculated on a similar basis to the group rates but using total live births and total population, to give a series of group weighting factors. To obtain the ACF for any given area the census female population in each of the six age groups is multiplied by the appropriate weighting factor and the products accumulated. The total population of the area divided by the result gives the area comparability factor.

4.10 It should be kept in mind that the ACF for any given area relates to the population of the area as defined by the boundaries existing at the time of the census. Provided that in the meantime there are no changes in boundary or other population movement (e.g. special housing or New Town development) important enough to disturb appreciably the relative sex and age distribution of the population included, the ACF will remain applicable until a new series of factors can be calculated on the basis of the next census. Where an area is affected by the special changes referred to, the ACF is recalculated on the basis of the most up-to-date knowledge of the movements involved.

4.11 To overcome the difficulty of the comparison of crude birth rates between different areas an approximate adjustment may be made by multiplying these rates by the ACF. The nature of this correction has to be borne in mind when interpreting the adjusted rates. The ACF simply allows for the varying proportion of women of childbearing ages in the aggregate local population, but not for any other factors, e.g. the proportion of these women who are married. Adjustment for the latter is required if the object is to compare the fertility levels of married women in different areas (and it would be possible to incorporate such an adjustment into the ACF by simply making f_x and P_x but not P relate to married women). On the other hand, if the object is to compare the birth increment to local populations, the proportion married is separately examined, amongst other things, as a possible source of birth variation after such variation (adjusted for age and sex) has been ascertained.

Legitimacy

4.12 Where possible it is appropriate to sub-divide the general fertility rate into two components (1) the ratio of legitimate births to married women 15–49, (2) the ratio of illegitimate births to unmarried women 15–49. This secures a better relationship between births and exposed to risk but even so it is not a precise method. If a marriage takes place during pregnancy, the birth is registered as legitimate and this tends to reduce the true illegitimate fertility and to increase the legitimate component. If a married man dies before his child is born the birth is legitimate and appears in the numerator of (1) while the mother as a widow appears in the denominator of (2). Broadly, however, an accurate picture is obtained.

4.13 The various methods described above have been applied to measure legitimate and illegitimate fertility in two London Boroughs; Kensington and Stepney in 1921. These two Boroughs were then two areas of sharply different social status. In Kensington there was a high proportion of female unmarried domestics, who scarcely contributed to the birth rate; in Stepney relatively few. In Stepney there was probably little, and in Kensington much, practice of birth control.

TABLE 4.1   *Fertility in Kensington and Stepney—1921*

	Kensington	*Stepney*	*Stepney per cent of Kensington*
I. Legitimate			
A. Crude birth rate per 1,000 total population	18·1	24·2	133
B. General fertility rate per 1,000 women aged 15–49	49·0	88·9	181
C. General fertility rate per 1,000 *married* women aged 15–49	136·0	175·9	129
II. Illegitimate			
A. Crude birth rate per 1,000 total population	1·34	0·59	44
B. General fertility rate per 1,000 women aged 15–49	3·62	2·16	60
C. General fertility rate per 1,000 unmarried women aged 15–49	5·66	4·37	77

4.14 The legitimate birth rate by the most accurate method C was 29 per cent higher in Stepney and it will be noted that the crude birth rate reflected this difference more clearly than method B. On the other hand, the excess of illegitimacy in Kensington is greatly exaggerated by method A and to a less extent by method B.

4.15 It should be borne in mind that however misleading as a pure measure of fertility the crude birth rate does give the gross rate of increase of the population by births.

4.16 Illegitimacy is sometimes expressed by calculating illegitimate births as a *percentage of total live births*. Though satisfactory when applied to short term comparisons this method may be misleading over a long term for if the legitimate birth rate were declining and the illegitimate birth rate were constant, the percentage illegitimacy would show an increase. This increase would, from a public health point of view, be realistic as a measure of a rise in the relative supply of illegitimate as compared with legitimate infants (and this is indeed the context in which it is usually used) but it would not be an accurate trend of the rate of fertility in unmarried persons. The percentage illegitimacy may fluctuate considerably when war conditions disturb normal relationships as the figures in Table 4.2. show

TABLE 4.2   *Illegitimate births per cent of total live births—England and Wales*

1938	4·2	1945	9·3
1939	4·2	1946	6·6
1940	4·3	1947	5·3
1941	5·4	1948	5·4
1942	5·6	1949	5·1
1943	6·4	1950	5·1
1944	7·3		

Multiple births

4.17 Owing to the occurrence of twins, triplets and higher orders of multiple deliveries a distinction has to be drawn between the number of mothers confined in a particular period, usually referred to as the number of maternities* and the total births, live and still resulting therefrom. In England and Wales in 1950 the ratio of births to maternities was 1,013 births to every 1,000 mothers confined. The frequencies of occurrence of different degrees of multiplicity were, in England and Wales, in 1950

Type of multiple maternity	*Frequency per* 1,000 *maternities*
Twins	12·6
Triplets	0·14
Quadruplets	0·0014
Quintuplets	Nil

It is often found that approximately

$$\frac{\text{Twin maternities}}{\text{Single maternities}} = \frac{\text{triple maternities}}{\text{twin maternities}} = \frac{\text{quadruplet maternities}}{\text{triple maternities}}$$

Variation of fertility with age of mother and duration of marriage

4.18 It will be seen from Table 4.3 for England and Wales in 1954 that fertility rates (maternities as defined above per woman per year of risk) decline with advancing age of mother and with lengthening duration of marriage (excluding the first year of marriage in which the mothers are at risk of maternity for only three months, apart from premarital conceptions). At each duration the rates decline with increasing age of mother, and at each

---

* Strictly a maternity is defined in England and Wales as a pregnancy which has terminated in the birth of one or more live or stillborn child(ren).

age of mother, after rising to a maximum in the second year of marriage they decline with lengthening duration of marriage except in those under age twenty where, after the inflation of the first year by premarital conception, they rise.

TABLE 4.3 *Legitimate Maternity Rates for women married once only per year of risk in 1954—England and Wales*

Age of married women	All durations	Marriage duration in completed years													
		0	1	2	3	4	5	6	7	8	9	10–14	15–19	20–24	25 and over
All ages under 50	0·089	·282	·257	·222	·207	·185	·156	·131	·111	·093	·078	·047	·019	·006	·001
Under 20	0·423	·465	·330	·361	·430	—	—	—	—	—	—	—	—	—	—
20—	0·254	·272	·274	·245	·242	·299	·211	·209	·239	·352	—	—	—	—	—
25—	0·171	·237	·244	·216	·206	·192	·167	·146	·131	·119	·112	·122	—	—	—
30—	0·099	·233	·232	·198	·182	·168	·145	·128	·111	·096	·082	·066	·072	—	—
35—	0·049	·176	·185	·141	·136	·123	·106	·091	·083	·070	·061	·041	·035	·042	—
40—	0·015	·057	·066	·053	·054	·041	·040	·034	·031	·026	·022	·017	·012	·011	·011
45—	0·001	·003	·004	·003	·003	·003	·003	·002	·003	·002	·002	·001	·001	·001	·011

4.19 Clearly these two factors are of considerable importance in assessing fertility prospects for a particular population.

Other indices of fertility

4.20 The birth rate in a particular year is merely a short term measure of the flow of births and gives no guidance to the long term effects of contemporary variations in fertility. The important fact to be ascertained is whether or not the current level of fertility, if maintained, is such that in the long run the population will increase or decrease in size and as a corollary whether or not changes in age characteristics of the population are foreshadowed. From this problem there emerges the concept of population maintenance or replacement.

4.21 It might be thought that the natural increase was itself an adequate measure of population maintenance. The natural increase, however, though a correct arithmetical expression of the balance of births over total deaths, indicates only the population changes (aside from migration) in *one* year and not the trend. In any one year the total deaths depend upon the present age structure of the population which though affected by past fertility is not sensitive to current changes in fertility. If, as in England, past fluctuations in fertility and mortality have been such that a bulge in the curve of age distribution is working its way up through age groups (see p. 34) there will come a time when a large increase in the population at advanced ages will produce a sharp rise in the annual deaths. Thus it may be that even though fertility at that time may be rising the natural increase will be more affected by the change in the number of deaths than by changes in the flow of births. The two components of the natural increase are quite unrelated to each other and their coincidental balance though important cannot be expected to give any indication of the long term growth of the population.

4.22 The concept of replacement involves measurement of effects over a period of time and as will be seen shortly requires the focus of attention upon generations rather than on the addition of births within a short period of time.

Replacement

4.23 Suppose we consider the simplest measure of population maintenance. Assume that the current annual number of births continues indefinitely and calculate the size of population that would ultimately result when stationary conditions had been attained. Some assumption has also to be made as to future mortality and it is usual to accept current mortality rates. Life table survival factors based on these mortality rates are applied to these births to yield the ultimate stationary population. In England and Wales in 1936–40 the average annual number of live births was 608,330 and the deaths averaged 513,155. A population recruited from this supply of births and exposed to current mortality would number 42·64 millions. The actual average population in the same period was 41·28 millions. Thus the number of births in 1936–40 though considerably greater than the number of deaths in the period was only three per cent more than that (588,930) required to maintain the population. Table 4.4 provides a similar measure for each post-war year from 1946 to 1954.

TABLE 4.4 *Annual births expressed as a percentage of the number required to maintain the population of England and Wales during* 1936 *to* 1940

	per cent		per cent
1946	139	1951	115
1947	150	1952	114
1948	132	1953	116
1949	124	1954	114
1950	118		

4.24 The percentages, since they are all based on the same mortality assumptions, naturally vary in exact proportion to the total births and improve very little upon the latter figure so far as it may be used to indicate any trend, except to focus attention upon the sufficiency of the births to maintain the population.

4.25 It has, however, to be borne in mind that a large proportion of the population are not in the child producing age group and, therefore, the current births can hardly be related to them. If in fact the important proportion inside the childbearing age group is temporarily unduly high, the births will be high in relation to the total population and the percentage maintenance of the current population *of all ages* will give too optimistic a picture. We shall have no warning that when the temporary inflation of the childbearing age group passes, the flow of births may not suffice to maintain the population. We might, therefore, consider whether or not parents are maintaining the population of parents, calculated in exactly the same way as before except for the restriction of age.

4.26 Suppose we take the child producing age group as 15–49. The 1936–40 births (608,330 average per annum) would maintain a stationary population containing 20·15 million persons (both sexes combined) aged 15–49. The actual population in England and Wales in the age groups numbered 22·14 millions in 1936–40 (average). The extent of 'parental maintenance', as a percentage of 22·14 millions was 91. It would in fact have required 668,410 births a year for parental replacement compared with 588,930 required on the total population basis used above. Thus, owing to the 1936–40 age structure of the population (with a high proportion in the parental age group) the number of births required to produce parental replacement is more than sufficient to support the total population of all ages and an index of parental replacement would be lower in every year (by 12 per cent) than the total population indices shown in the above table.

Gross reproduction rate

4.27 Although we have taken account of the childbearing population as distinct from the total population we have not subdivided this population according to age in order to take account of differential fertility at different ages within the group. It is necessary to do this in order to obtain a clearer picture of possible variations such as may arise from unusual features of the age structure of the population even within the childbearing group. The first step is to calculate the fertility rate *at each age* of parents, that is the ratio of the births of mothers (or fathers) of a particular age to the number of mothers (or fathers) living at that age.

4.28 With age fertility rates available we may now consider whether if these rates are maintained the mothers (or fathers) will produce sufficient girl infants (or boy infants) during the reproductive part of their lives (assumed to be 15–49) to replace themselves before they pass out of the parental age group. If mortality is ignored we add together the age fertility rates (for births of a particular sex) to yield the expected number of girls (boys) produced by women (men) in their reproductive lives. This is known as the gross reproduction rate, and a value of unity might be held to indicate 'replacement' (though we shall see later that this is not valid).

4.29 The calculation proceeds as in Table 4.5 (for women)—

TABLE 4.5 *England and Wales—1954*

Age	Female population (1,000)	Total live births (females only)	Mean fertility rate
15–19	1,399	15,133	0·01082
20–24	1,422	94,155	0·06621
25–29	1,521	102,676	0·06751
30–34	1,756	72,490	0·04128
35–39	1,451	31,402	0·02164
40–44	1,689	10,640	0·00630
45–49	1,667	700*	0·00042
Total	**10,905**	**327,196**	**0·21418**

* Including 12 births to mothers aged 50 and over.

4.30 It may be assumed that the mean fertility rate can be applied at individual years of age so that the sum of the age rates over the period 15–19 will be five times the mean rate (since five individual years of age are involved). Thus the total fertility, i.e. total expected births to a woman passing through the age group 15–49 = 5 × 0·2142 or 1·071. Note that the total fertility rate is (for female births,) 327,196/10,905,000 or 0·0300 and that applying this at all ages would give a crude index of 0·0300 × 35 or 1·050.

4.31 The gross reproduction rate may be expressed symbolically by the formula

$$\sum_{x=0}^{x=\omega} {}^s i_x$$

where ${}^s i_x$ = fertility rate at age x, specific for sex, i.e. female births to females or male births to males and ω is the upper limit of age.

Net reproduction rate

4.32 The gross reproduction rate fails to take account of the mortality of infants before they themselves become the same age as that of the parents they are supposed to replace and of mortality among parents before the end of the childbearing period. In order to make allowance for the mortality of infants we need to apply to the estimated births in each age group, survivorship factors up to the present age of the parent. The formula becomes

$$\sum {}^s i_x \cdot {}_x p_0$$

Where ${}_x p_0$ is the chance of survival from birth to age x according to the currently applicable life table for the appropriate sex. The calculation proceeds as in Table 4.6.

TABLE 4.6 *England and Wales—1954*

Age group (1)	Fertility rate (female births) (2)	Survival factor (3)	(2)×(3) (4)
15–19	0·01082	0·9694	0·01049
20–24	0·06621	0·9668	0·06401
25–29	0·06751	0·9632	0·06503
30–34	0·04128	0·9584	0·03596
35–39	0·02164	0·9519	0·02060
40–44	0·00630	0·9424	0·00594
45–49	0·00042	0·9279	0·00039
Total			0·20602

Female net reproduction rate = 5 × 0·2060 or 1·030

4.33 If the rate is greater than unity it is assumed that the population is more than reproducing itself. Reading the formula forward it measures the extent to which mothers produce female infants who survive to replace them; reading the formula backwards it measures the extent to which a generation of girl babies survive to reproduce themselves as they pass through the childbearing age group.

4.34 It is important to bear in mind that for replacement to be attained a generation of women (or of men) must produce a replacement for every member of the generation. Thus the surviving adults of a generation must *on average* produce rather more than one replacement each, to allow for the fact that some children will fail to survive to adult life. Similarly a cohort of married couples (i.e. women married in the same year) must produce *on average* more than two children, since they must count on a double loss, namely from death and from failure to marry. These generations or cohorts may replace themselves at any time during the thirty years or so of female reproductive life. It does not matter very much in which years they produce their children and any one year is a small fraction of the total thirty years. Furthermore, the total birth experience of a single calendar year consists of the aggregate of the experiences of a number of generations or alternatively of a number of marriage cohorts. If each generation or cohort concerned has but few children in that year for some reason such as economic depression or danger from war or wartime separation, nothing could be more ridiculous than to hypothecate that some future generation will, at each age have the same low rates as those of the many generations concerned in the fertility of the year in question. The average addition to a family in a single year is thus a small part of the whole average family and calendar year reproduction rates (in any shape or form) are very imperfect measures of replacement. They are in fact nothing more than standardized calendar year birth rates on a scale which approaches unity at a replacement level. The value for a single year has no more significance than any other birth rate and only a persistent trend substantially above (below) unity might be an indication of a growing (declining) population.

Male and female indices

4.35 It will be obvious that, though female reproduction is commonly considered, a reproduction rate appropriate to the replacement of *male* babies may be calculated by using factors appropriate to that sex. Usually a higher rate is obtained. The difference arises partly from the inequality of the numbers of the two sexes in each age group, and in the proportions married at successive ages, which result in inherent inconsistency between male and female nuptiality assumptions based on current experience, and in the age incidence of fertility; the average length of a generation (difference in age between parent and child) in England and Wales is about three years longer for men than for women, so that for the same annual rate of natural increase, the rate for a generation interval would be larger.

4.36 The dilemma can be ignored and an arbitrary choice made of either the male or the female rate (usually the latter) as the working index—they are likely to have similar trends—or joint net reproduction rates may be calculated, i.e. taking the two sexes together as if no distinction existed between them.

Other factors

4.37 The net reproduction rate makes allowance only for abnormal age distribution. Other factors need to be considered. A sudden rise in the marriage rate would produce temporary increases in age fertility rates in subsequent years. For this reason reproduction rates are sometimes marriage-standardized, though this raised the problem of choice of marriage basis, and the index is no longer automatic. It must be reiterated that family building suffers temporary fluctuations too, for example, when war or economic crises cause postponement of births which are later made up by equally temporary high fertility. This last type of variation may only be a change in the timing of births within the individual families without affecting the ultimate size of the families when completed. Fertility rates in such a period would not reflect the current trend of size of family in the population.

Cohort or generation analysis

4.38 As we have remarked, quite sharp changes in duration fertility rates may arise from changes in the timing of family building within married life without necessarily implying any change in the ultimate size of family. It is not therefore surprising that the average size of family of completed fertility (number of live born children produced by a married woman by the end of her reproductive period of life) has been found to exhibit much more stability than do the specific fertility rates from year to year. As the estimation of completed family size of married couples (as a means of estimating replacement prospects) is in fact the primary object of fertility studies modern demography has turned its attention to this measure.

4.39 Statistically this involves following through a group of persons born in a particular year (a generation) or married in a particular year (usually called a marriage cohort) throughout their lifetimes and recording the number of children they produce.

4.40 Considering first the marriage cohort we can see that the women who contribute to the fertility rate for marriage duration 0— in 1950, will contribute to the fertility rate for marriage duration 1— in 1951, 2— in 1952 and so on. The cumulation of these rates for all durations will produce the ultimate or completed family size of women married within the same period. In this example, however, the period will overlap calendar years as the births at duration 0— in 1950 will include those of women married in 1949 as well as those married early in 1950. It is usually desirable to follow a group of women married in a particular calendar year. For this reason it is necessary to tabulate the births not only by year of marriage duration but also by calendar year of marriage. The tabulation is also carried out separately for different age groups at marriage as the marriage age has an important effect on the family size—women married for the first time at age 45, for example, will already be near the end of their reproductive life and will have no opportunity to produce a large family. The cohort is then specified by age at marriage and (usually) calendar year of marriage.

The relative stability of family size

4.41 We have said that mean ultimate family sizes exhibit more stability than annual fertility rates. This may be illustrated by the figures in Table 4.7 which have been extracted from the Fertility Report of the 1961 Census of England and Wales. For summary purposes all marriage ages (under 45) have been combined. This is reasonable for cohort comparisons as there was little change in the age structure of marriages from year to year over the period to which these figures relate.

Generation replacement rates

4.42 For the purpose of considering the extent to which the population is replacing itself the marriage cohort experience is not very satisfactory, mainly because it is necessary to make some notional allowance for a corresponding number of women who do not marry and are therefore not part

TABLE 4.7 *Women with uninterrupted first marriage. All marriage ages under 45*

Calendar year of marriage*	Mean family size (live born children per married woman)
1910	3·06
1911	2·96
1912	2·85
1913	2·81
1914	2·75
1915	2·50
1916	2·46
1917	2·47
1918	2·43
1919	2·50
1920	2·42

*These cohorts may be regarded as having completed their fertility.

of the marriage cohort but for whom replacements must be found among the total offspring considered to be produced by the cohort (with allowance for illegitimate fertility). Such women being outside the cohort are by the same token difficult to fit into the concept of cohort replacement. Moreover their numbers can hardly be assessed from the marriage experience of the year in question for we are concerned with making some allowance for a number of women 'corresponding' in some way to the cohort, who will reach the end of their reproductive period without being married, and the marriage experience of a single year may be a misleading guide; for example, economic conditions may produce some temporary postponement of marriages. In what way should these spinsters 'correspond' to the cohort which consists of a number of women married at many different ages, i.e. members of many different generations? We can only use current nuptiality based on a period of years as in Table 4.8.

TABLE 4.8 *England and Wales—Marriages of 1945*

Age at marriage	No. of spinster marriages (thousands)	Projected ultimate family size (a)	Combined chance of surviving and of marrying between ages 15 and 45 (b)	Replacement Index (assuming female births 0·4854 of all births)	
Under 20	56·9	2·75		Legitimate	
20–24	191·2	2·25		(2·129 × 0·8689 × 0·4854)	0·898
25–29	66·3	1·90		Illegitimate (add 4·7 per cent)	0·042
30–34	23·4	1·40			
35–39	11·1	0·73			0·940
40–44	5·8	0·26			
	354·7	Mean 2·129	0·8689		

(a) By simple extrapolation of family size (live born children) as shown for successive years of marriage duration year by year in Table PP of the Registrar General's *Statistical Review Part II*.

(b) According to a joint mortality and nuptiality table (with allowance for risk of marriage being broken before age 45). Strictly this factor should be varied according to the period of time over which the family is produced to allow for generation changes in mortality and marriage rates, but this has been ignored for simplicity.

C

65

4.43 The conceptual difficulty remains however and it is preferable to abandon year of marriage as the reference point in favour of year of birth, i.e. to calculate a replacement rate applicable to a single generation—those born in a particular calendar year. For this purpose we follow the generation throughout childhood, marriage and reproductive life subjecting it to the mortality, nuptiality and fertility actually recorded for that generation if it has reached the end of reproductive life, or forecast for it, if not.

4.44 The computation if performed correctly is complicated and laborious but not essentially difficult. The stages are as follows—

(i) A combined mortality and nuptiality table is constructed which shows at age x the number of women surviving to that age from 100,000 births (or some other convenient starting number, or radix as it is called), and among these the distribution by marital status. The table would also show the number of spinster marriages, widowhoods, divorces, remarriages and deaths, based on the rates of decrement assumed in the table. The married women of age x are divided according to the duration of their current marriage.

(ii) At each age and marriage duration the specific legitimate fertility rate appropriate to the age and duration and to the class of married woman (once-married or re-married) is applied to estimate the number of live births for that interval. At each age illegitimate fertility rates are applied to the unmarried women. The addition of these births when divided by the original radix of the nuptiality and mortality table gives the average family size for the generation. Application of the ratio of female to male births yields the number of female births to replace each original female birth, viz., the generation replacement rate. Full details of such a calculation will be found in Appendix 2 of Chapter 4 of the Fertility Report of the 1951 Census (General Register Office, 1958).

4.45 A close approximation to the rate may be obtained by using a procedure similar to that outlined above for the marriage cohort. The difference is that in the column headed 'number of spinster marriages' the actual numbers of marriages of the cohort are replaced by the numbers relating to a particular generation (derived from an abridged nuptiality table). As we are dealing with the marriage experience of the whole generation, there is no longer any need for the factor 0·8689 which allowed for replacement of unmarried females (this factor will be implicit in the relationship between the size of the generation (the radix of the nuptiality table) and the total number of marriages up to the end of the reproductive period). Otherwise the calculation follows the same procedure. It is worth noting from the 1951 Census Fertility Report already referred to that for the most recent generations for which current rates of marriage and fertility rates were adopted on a hypothetical basis the approximate replacement rate obtained by this method was only 0·34 per cent above that obtained by the full procedure.

Family distributions, 1911, 1946 and 1951

4.46 An attempt was made in the 1911 Census to obtain from living married women of all ages the number of children they had had at any time. This gave useful information of the trend of family size, though there were difficulties of interpretation arising from (1) rejection of schedules owing to evidently faulty or incomplete information; (2) probable omission of children who died at very early infantile ages many years before the census; (3) the selective nature of the data which was based only on the living (those women who died after marriage, and whose fertility might well have been different from the living, were omitted).

4.47 A similar enquiry was carried out for the Royal Commission on Population in 1946. A 10 per cent sample of the married women in Great Britain was drawn from food rationing records. Each woman was asked, by a personal interviewer, questions covering her age, details of her marriage(s), dates of birth of every live-born child she herself had had (whether or not they were alive at the census date); the occupation of her husband; and the number of her children under sixteen years of age who were still alive at the census date. It has to be borne in mind that the census was taken just before a post-war period of exceptionally large numbers of births, but the figures could nevertheless be projected forward by using the statistics of births by duration of marriage obtained by the Registrar General from birth registrations.

4.48 The main results (Glass and Grebenik 1954) summarized very briefly were: The number of live births per married woman declined from 5·8 for marriages of 1870–79 to 3·04 for marriages of 1910 and to 2·21 for marriages of 1925; the large family had been virtually eliminated—in the late nineteenth century families of five or more children constituted three-fifths of all families, the marriages of 1925 were dominated by one- and two-child families, and over the period childlessness had doubled in frequency; social differences remained—for women marrying in 1920–24 at 20–24 years of age the number of live births per woman varied from 2·02 in the professions and 1·90 for salaried employees to 2·96 for manual wage earners and 3·76 for labourers; for recent marriages forecasts of ultimate family size indicated a shortfall from replacement of from two to six per cent depending on the assumptions about marriage, illegitimacy and mortality.

4.49 At the population census of 1951, fertility questions were addressed to married women under the age of fifty (see p. 17). These questions referred to children born in marriage and asked for the total number of children born alive up to the date of the census (including any of a previous marriage and any that had died); and whether a child had been born alive during the twelve months immediately preceding the census. The results were published in a special Fertility Report (1958); they confirmed and carried forward the story told by the Family Census of 1946, viz. that soon after the middle of the nineteenth century there began a long decline in fertility due to the spread of family limitation, but within the last generation there had been a significant rise in fertility. There was every expectation that generations born just after the end of World War II would have families as large as those born in the early nineteen twenties.

4.50 There had been some change in the time pattern of family building. The figures in Table 4.9 (see page 68) show the proportion of the total family born in different periods of married life.

4.51 There had been a slight but unmistakable tendency for a higher proportion of the family building to be completed in the first ten years of married life. The effect of the war in postponing births can be seen for the 1940 cohort.

TABLE 4.9 *Proportion (per 1,000) of mean family size produced in different intervals of marriage duration*

Calendar year of marriage	Duration of marriage (years)					
	0–4	5–9	10–14	15–19	20+	Total
1920	546	252	127	58	17	1,000
1930	542	246	133	66	13	1,000
1940	474	339	120*	51*	16*	1,000
1950	551	272*	111*	49*	17*	1,000

* Projected on the basis of current fertility rates.

4.52 Generation replacement rates (female), calculated in the manner already indicated rose from 0·672 for the generation born in 1903–08 to 0·795 for those born in 1913–18 and were projected at 0·978 for the generation of 1938–43 and 1·014 for that of 1948–53. Of the increase of 51 per cent between the 1903–08 generation and the most recent generation examined (1948–53) about half was due to improved mortality, a quarter was due to the increase in family size, and the remaining quarter to the rise in marriage rates.

Differential fertility

4.53 Fertility varies not only with age and duration of marriage but also with occupation and social class, area of residence (e.g. rural or urban), religion and other factors. These factors are clearly of interest to those who may have to estimate the possible effect of steps taken by the community to influence fertility through any of them, e.g. family allowances; but they are also of interest to health authorities and hospitals in indicating the nature of the population with which the maternity services will have to deal.

4.54 Considerable examination of the effect of social class as indicated by occupation of the father was undertaken by Dr T. H. C. Stevenson from the results of the 1911 fertility inquiry. Some results are summarized in the table 4.10—

TABLE 4.10 *Standardized total fertility (according to date of marriage) for each social class per cent of the total for all occupied persons, England and Wales 1911 Census*

Date of marriage	Social Class							
	I Upper and middle classes	II Intermediate	III Skilled labourers	IV Intermediate	V Unskilled labourers	VI Textile workers	VII Miners	VIII Agricultural labourers
1906–09	80	92	98	102	114	87	120	114
1901–06	79	91	98	101	112	86	122	114
1896–1901	76	89	99	101	114	86	125	114
1891–96	74	88	99	101	113	88	127	115
1886–91	74	87	100	101	112	90	126	114
1881–86	76	89	100	101	110	92	124	114
1871–81	81	93	101	101	107	93	117	109
1861–71	88	96	101	100	104	94	113	104
1851–61	89	99	101	99	103	94	118	105

4.55 Features which have to be borne in mind are heterogeneity of occupational classes, differing average age of marriage (professional men may defer marriage until attainment of a certain status), changes in occupation between the ages of highest fertility and those at which the fertility is recorded.

4.56 The general impression gained from similar studies of differential fertility as revealed (a) by using occupational classification of the population at the Censuses of 1921 and 1931, and related birth registrations to calculate differential fertility rates (b) by the results of the Family Census 1946 and the Censuses of 1951 and 1961, is that the proportionate differences between social classes have tended to narrow but are still substantial.

4.57 The figures in Table 4.11 are taken from the Fertility Tables of the 1961 Census. They show a continuing range of variation as wide as that found in 1911—

TABLE 4.11 Ratio (per cent) of mean family size to that for all women married once only (standardized for age at marriage)

Socio-economic group of husband	Duration of marriage		
	10–14	15–19	20–24
Employers and managers			
Large establishments	95	92	92
Small establishments	93	91	91
Professional workers			
Self employed	114	115	109
Employees	96	94	96
Intermediate non-manual workers	92	90	91
Junior non-manual workers	88	89	90
Personal services workers	103	103	95
Foremen and supervisors manual	97	95	95
Skilled manual workers	100	101	101
Semi-skilled manual workers	104	104	106
Unskilled manual workers	120	120	118
Own account workers (other than professional)	98	97	93
Farmers			
Employers and managers	117	117	120
Own account	109	109	110
Agricultural workers	106	112	117
Armed Forces	119	120	115

Marriage rates

4.58 It will be obvious from the previous discussion of fertility measures that it is impossible to separate legitimate fertility rates from the age and marriage duration structure of the population of married women which support these rates. The fertility rates must not be considered in isolation but must always be considered against the marriage experience which permits them.

4.59 As for all other vital rates, marriages must be related to the population at risk, viz. first marriages of females to the spinster population; remarriages to the numbers of widowed or divorced. The likelihood of marriage varies very much not only with the age of the prospective bride (or bridegroom) but also with the relative supply of spinsters and bachelors at any particular combination of ages (not so much at the *same* age, for bachelors tend to marry spinsters who are their juniors by a year or two).

4.60 It is usual therefore to calculate age specific marriage rates as below for example:

TABLE 4.12 *England and Wales, 1955—Annual marriage rates per 1,000 bachelors, widowers and divorced men, spinsters, widows and divorced women by age*

Age	Bachelors	Widowers and divorced men	Spinsters	Widows and divorced women
15—	8·2	—	50·5	—
20—	146·3	92·0	255·3	433·7
25—	181·1	411·0	164·4	445·3
30—	108·5	284·9	79·4	199·5
35—	48·5	183·9	30·8	82·8
45—	17·6	116·4	10·7	30·5
55 and over	5·1	20·2	2·1	3·1

4.61 In England and Wales, as in many other countries, the period since World War II had been characterized by high marriage rates and earlier marriage ages. This has contributed to a temporary rise in the flow of births but the permanent effect upon fertility had been reduced by the growing tendency (common to most communities where family limitation is practised) for family building to be completed relatively early in married life and not to be proportionately extended by any increase in the length of married life falling within the reproductive age period.

4.62 What is important for fertility prospects is the proportion of women who reach the end of the reproductive age period without getting married. This proportion has been falling in recent years as a result of high marriage rates.

TABLE 4.13 *Proportion of spinsters in female population aged 45–49 in England and Wales: per 1,000*

1921 Census	168
1931 Census	168
1951 Census	152
1961 Census	105

4.63 It has been estimated (General Register Office, 1958) that if present trends continue, this proportion will eventually fall to about fifty-five per thousand, i.e. about as low as is possible when it is borne in mind that a small proportion of women will always be physically or psychologically unsuited to marriage. Hocking (1953) has written of the 'decline in spinsterhood' and has drawn attention to the progressive depletion of the reservoir of marriageable spinsters by the continued high marriage rates. At all but the very youngest ages marriages have outnumbered the new accessions each year into the age group. The bachelor population has been subjected to the same influences though to a smaller extent. For this and other reasons couples have tended to get married at younger ages.

4.64 Reference has already been made (p. 66) to the use of a net nuptiality table, viz. a table showing, out of a given generation of births, the proportion still alive and (*a*) unmarried or (*b*) married, at any particular age. Such a table is derived from a combination of marriage rates and mortality rates.

4.65 A practical procedure is as follows:

x	Number of spinsters living at exact age x	Central rates of death dm_x	first marriage mm_x	Probability of death or marriage $\dfrac{2(dm_x+mm_x)}{2+(dm_x+mm_x)}$	Deaths x to $x+1$	Marriages x to $x+1$
0	10,000					
15	9,661*	0·00052	—	0·00052	5	—
16	9,656	0·00058	0·00657	0·00712	6	63
17	9,587	0·00064	0·02599	0·02628	6	246
etc.						

* By ordinary life table processes (see p. 101 and also the line for age 15). For age 17 we have, total decrement = 9,587 × 0·02628 = 252 of which deaths = mean population × central death rate = [9,587 − ½(252)] × 0·00064 = 6 and marriages = 252 − 6 = 246.

4.66 A full table and a discussion of the methodology will be found in the Fertility Report of the 1951 Census (*loc. cit.*).

REFERENCES

General Register Office (1917) Census of England and Wales 1911, Vol. XIII, *Fertility of Marriage*.
General Register Office (1958) Census of England and Wales 1951, *Fertility Report*.
General Register Office (1966) Census of England and Wales. *Fertility Tables*.
Royal Commission on Population (1949) Report Cmd. 7695.
Royal Commission on Population (1950) Papers of Statistics Committee, Vol. II.
Royal Commission on Population (1954) Papers Vol. VI, "The Trend and Pattern of Fertility in Great Britain" by D. V. GLASS, and E. GREBENIK
HOCKING, W. S. (1950) *J. of Inst. Act. Stud., Soc.* 10.24.
HOCKING, W. S. (1953) *J. of Inst. Act. Stud., Soc.* 12.119.
MEADE, J. E., and PARKES, A. S. (ed.) Genetic and Environmental Factors in Human Ability, pp. 177–184. Oliver and Boyd, London, 1966.

CHAPTER 5

MORTALITY—DEATH RATES AND CAUSES

5.1 The risk of dying varies with a number of factors—sex and age and those factors which either influence the physical constitution or the environment of the people, such as birthplace, geographical locality of residence, occupation, marital condition. Methods of measurement have therefore to be designed to differentiate the influence of these factors as well as to distinguish the contribution of different medical causes of death (types of disease or injury).

5.2 Death rates measure the relative frequency of death in a particular population in a specified interval, i.e. the rates proportion the deaths to a population of a standard size. For example 5,128 deaths in a population of 216,342 persons may be expressed as 2,370 deaths per 100,000 or 24 deaths per 1,000 according to whichever is the convenient unit. Such rates may be classified as general or specific, the first relating to all causes of death and to the general population, the second to special causes of death or to deaths in particular sections of the population, or both.

5.3 Whether general or specific death rates are under consideration it is important to be sure that the population used in the calculation is precisely that which produced the deaths also used in the calculation; conversely the deaths must comprise all those occurring in this population and no others. The denominator of the rate (of which the numerator is the relevant number of deaths) is commonly referred to as 'the population at risk' or the 'exposed to risk'. Adherence to this rule underlies the practice observed in Great Britain and in many other countries of transferring records of deaths from place of death to administrative area of place of residence if different. This avoids the difficult task of attempting to allocate deaths to the place where the fatal disease was contracted. It conforms with the recommendation of the United Nations in their published 'principles for a vital statistics system' (1953).

5.4 A general death rate must relate to a specified unit of time, e.g. year, quarter, etc., and is the total number of deaths occurring in that interval of time calculated as a ratio to the population at risk, and expressed in terms of some unit population size, e.g. 1,000, 100,000 or 1,000,000. There is no hard and fast rule; some prefer to decide upon the maximum number of digits that will be used in the rates and to use such a unit as avoids the employment of decimal places (i.e. use 2,678 per 1,000,000 instead of $2 \cdot 678$ per 1,000) while others prefer to use the smallest unit which allows the smallest rate to be not less than $0 \cdot 1$, (i.e. they would use $0 \cdot 15$ per 1,000 but not $0 \cdot 015$ which would be expressed as 15 per million). Often comparability with already published tables forbids any choice.

5.5 The population at risk in most vital statistical calculations is the mean

72

population of the area (or class of person considered) over the period to which the rate relates. (It will be seen later that this kind of death rate is not the same concept as the age specific rate of mortality used in life table calculations—though except where mortality is changing rapidly with age it is not numerically very different). As a first approximation the midyear (or mid-interval) population is accepted as the mean unless irregular or rapid changes in the population (as, for example, during a war) render it necessary to make more precise calculations of the average number actually at risk. Death rates when calculated for a shorter period than a year are often expressed as an equivalent *annual* rate, viz. as the annual rate that would result from the persistence of the same mortality conditions for a full year.

Example

Deaths for 13 weeks to April 3, 1954	154,817
Mean population (thousands)	44,274
Death rate (for the 13-week period) per 1,000	3·50

Equivalent annual death rate $= 3 \cdot 50 \times \dfrac{365}{91}$

$$= 14 \cdot 0$$

5.6 This conversion is merely for convenience since it is often confusing to pass from annual to quarterly rates and therefore desirable to work with rates of the same order of size throughout. The conversion though convenient may often be unrealistic. To assume that the mortality of a particular quarter which includes a widespread epidemic of influenza, could persist for a whole year would not be justifiable but it is usually accepted that conversion is made without such implication. The shorter the interval the more likely it is that the rate will be influenced by some epidemic occurrence or a spell of particularly inclement weather so that while the rate for a very short period is a fact and a true statement of mortality for that period, extreme care should be exercised not to draw inferences about mortality at other times or over longer intervals.

5.7 It should also be borne in mind that where small numbers of deaths are involved, chance fluctuations are likely to be relatively large. For example, suppose we have a population of only 1,000 with over a long period of years an average death rate of 13 per 1,000 per year. This means an average annual number of deaths of 13; but any elementary statistical textbook will tell us that the frequency distribution of the annual deaths will be such that fluctuations to fewer than 6 or to more than 20 will occur in each case as often as once in forty years and that although the long run average will be 13, in any one year it is as likely as not that the number of deaths will be *outside* the range 11–15. Looking at the problem the other way round we can see that a particular year when there was a chance occurrence of say 18 deaths would be a very misleading basis for calculating the underlying mortality. Where populations or rates are small it is advisable to base calculations upon a group of years rather than upon a single year in order to increase the number of deaths involved and thus to reduce the size of the possible error.

Variation of mortality with age and sex

5.8 The diagram 5.1 shows for England and Wales the rates of mortality in England and Wales in 1952 in successive age periods and for each sex. The

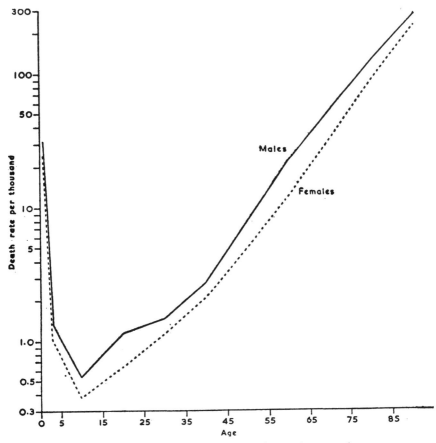

Fig. 5.1 England and Wales 1952, death rates by age and sex

actual rates are shown in Table 5.1. Mortality is highest at the extremes of age. Once the newborn infant has survived the hazards of the first few days of life (see p. 209) mortality falls rapidly and during childhood the risk is very small being very largely confined to that of the occasional lethal infection, which modern treatment with antibiotics and sulpha drugs has made extremely

TABLE 5.1 *England and Wales, 1952—Rates of Mortality per* 1,000

Age Group	Males	Females
0—	31·73	24·74
1—	1·32	1·02
5—	0·54	0·38
15—	1·13	0·64
25—	1·44	1·10
35—	2·74	2·09
45—	7·88	4·91
55—	22·0	11·9
65—	53·3	32·4
75—	122·1	90·1
85+	273·5	227·6

rare, and severe accidental injuries which childish recklessness or lack of adult care sometimes invite. In adolescence the impact and strain of industrial life brings a rise in mortality and these and other factors inherent in the social and economic environment and individual ways of life reacting upon constitutional weakness where that exists, lead to a continuing increase in the risk of death as age advances. At later ages the sheer wearing out of the human frame rather than inimical qualities of the environment becomes the dominant cause of mortality. Ideally if this natural wearing out (true senility) were practically the only cause of death the curves of mortality rates shown in diagram 5.1 would take the form of a J with rates maintained at insignificant levels until advanced ages when there would be a sudden upward rise. Diagram 5.2 shows to what extent successive generations have progressed toward this ideal. This diagram has been drawn by plotting rates which relate to those born in the same year, viz. for those born in 1841 (with births centred on the mid-year) we have the rate at 0–4 in the period mid 1841–mid 1846 because that is the age group through which they pass in this period; the rate at 5–9 in the period mid 1846–mid 1851, the rate at 10–14 in the period mid 1851–mid 1866, and so on.

5.9 Diagram 5.1 also shows the difference between the patterns of mortality for the two sexes. The death rates for females are lower than those for males at all ages. Prior to 1890 there used to be an excess in the death rate of females at adolescence and early adult ages mainly associated with the heavier mortality from tuberculosis in girls; since that time the general level of tuberculosis mortality has fallen so much that this differential has no effect upon the comparison of rates from all causes. Briefly, the higher mortality of males may be explained in medical terms as follows:

(i) In infancy and early childhood, boys are generally more vulnerable to some birth hazards (prematurity, malformation, birth injury), to infection, possibly as a result of some biological factor, and to injuries, possibly as a result of more vigorous venturesome activity; these being the principal causes of death at these ages.

(ii) In early and middle adult life the principal causes of death are accidents and violence, tuberculosis, heart disease and cancer and except for the latter cause the death rates are higher in men. The excessive mortality from tuberculosis in men (except in very early adult life) is of a piece with the generally greater vulnerability of men to respiratory disease of all kinds, not only tuberculosis but also bronchitis, influenza, pneumonia, cancer of the lung (and this greater vulnerability extends to advanced ages). The type of heart disease which is most responsible for deaths in this age group is arterial and described as coronary thrombosis—there is still considerable controversy as to the factors operating to increase susceptibility to this disease—diet, smoking, insufficient physical activity and nervous tension, seem to play their part, and sedentary occupations appear to incur, for these or other reasons, a higher risk. The higher risk of accidents must be regarded as occupational in the broader sense of including, as compared with females, more outdoor movement in traffic, etc., as well as greater industrial hazards.

75

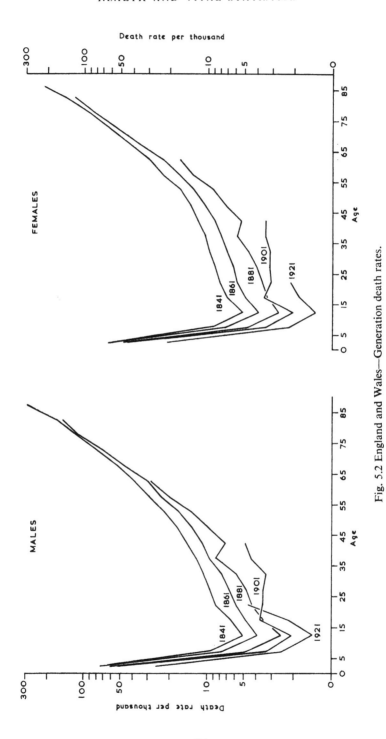

Fig. 5.2 England and Wales—Generation death rates.

(iii) At more advanced ages the process of physical deterioration and lessening resistance to disease associated with general wear and tear appear to proceed faster in men. Age for age cerebral haemorrhages, arterial disease, cancer (especially of the lung) and bronchitis take a heavier toll of males than females.

Marital condition

5.10 The effect of marriage upon mortality is twofold. In the first place those with physical impairments or poor health tend to be less successful, or less willing, to seek partners; and secondly, in women, seclusion from the hurly burly of office and factory of those who are not gainfully occupied has environmental advantages and there appear to be differential effects in certain diseases of reproductive organs—for example mortality from cancer of the uterus is higher in married than in single women while mortality from breast cancer though higher in married than in single women during the childbearing years, is higher in single or in childless married women at older ages—and there are of course still risks associated with childbearing itself. Married men have the advantage of home comforts and someone to look after them when they are sick. The result is that the mortality of married persons is lighter than that of single and widowed persons at all ages in the case of men and at younger ages in the case of women; the mortality of older women is on balance much the same in all marital condition classes.

Cause

5.11 In 1872 William Farr wrote 'The great source of misery of mankind is not their numbers, but their imperfections and the want of control over the conditions in which they live. Without embarrassing ourselves with the difficulties the vast theories of life present, there is a definite task before us— to determine from observation, the sources of health, and the direct causes of death in the two sexes at different ages and under different conditions. The exact determination of evils is the first step towards their remedies.'

5.12 What Farr said about numbers is not so true in many under-developed parts of the world where population pressure is depressing the standard of living but the remainder of the statement has become a fundamental tenet of faith in preventive medicine. Enough is already known of the natural history of diseases and the social and environmental factors in their aetiology to render profitable the study of death rates specific, not only for age and sex, but also for cause—as certified by the medical practitioner in attendance prior to death, or by the coroner in cases necessitating inquest. The study of such rates over periods of time and in different areas may help to indicate the relative weight of various occupational and environmental factors in the different areas and the relative progress made in those areas toward reducing mortality. The contemporary increase both in England and Wales and in USA, of mortality from cancer of the lung and coronary arterial disease (especially in men) is exercising considerable influence on the shape of the curve of death rates with age and provides an example of the need for cause analysis.

77

5.13 Finally there are ethnic factors to be taken into account. For example in Table 5.2 are shown death rates by age, sex, and colour in the USA in 1951 (rates per 1,000 population).

TABLE 5.2 *Death rates in United States* 1951

Age	White		Non-white	
	Male	*Female*	*Male*	*Female*
Under 1 year	33·2	25·1	62·3	48·4
1—4	1·3	1·1	2·7	2·3
5—14	0·7	0·4	1·0	0·7
15—24	1·6	0·7	2·8	2·0
25—34	1·9	1·1	4·8	3·6
35—44	3·8	2·3	8·5	7·2
45—54	9·8	5·4	18·5	15·2
55—64	23·0	12·7	36·4	29·5
65—74	48·4	31·6	53·1	39·9
75—84	105·1	84·5	88·0	72·8
85 and over	211·0	190·1	139·4	116·1

5.14 The mortality of the white population is considerably lighter than among the non-white at all except the extremely advanced ages (when everyone must eventually die and death rates must catch up). To what extent this difference is of truly racial origin or merely reflects different social and economic conditions is not clear but certainly the statistical separation is important. In England and Wales there is as yet insufficient coloured people to render necessary the preparation of separate statistics but there is growing interest in the health problem created by the recent influx of Commonwealth natives with higher susceptibility to tuberculosis.

Certification of cause of death

5.15 Reference has already been made in Chapter 3 to the procedure for death registration and it is relevant here to discuss the certification of cause. Current practice has been summarized by Logan (1953) and the following notes represent a condensed version.

5.16 A medical practitioner who attends a person in his last illness is required by law to give a certificate stating the cause of death and to send it in the prescribed form, to the local registrar of births and deaths.

5.17 Any person who knows or suspects that a death was due to other than natural causes has the common-law duty of informing the coroner or police, and this duty rests also upon doctors. The fact that a death may have been reported to the coroner does not absolve a doctor from the requirement to issue a death certificate.

5.18 The local registrar has a special duty to report to the coroner any death which he thinks may have been unnatural; but he must also refer to the coroner

(1) When there is no medical certificate either because no registered practitioner was in attendance or because for any other reason the registrar is unable to obtain a certificate.

78

(2) When the death followed an operation necessitated by an injury; or the death occurred during any operation or before recovery from an anaesthetic.

(3) When the death was due to poisoning of any kind, or to abortion, or to an industrial disease.

(4) When the certifying practitioner had not seen the deceased either after death or within fourteen days before death. However, it is not necessary that he should have done both.

(5) When the death was directly or indirectly caused by any sort of accident, violence, or neglect, or when the cause of death is unknown.

Form of Death Certificate

5.19 The part of the death certificate that requires the greatest care in its completion is the section for the statement of the cause of death, the form of which has been established by international agreement. This section, in the certificate used in England and Wales and in Northern Ireland, but not in Scotland, is arranged as follows:

CAUSE OF DEATH	
I	I
Disease or condition directly leading to death.*	(a) .... due to (or as a consequence of)
Antecedent causes.	(b) ....
Morbid conditions, if any, giving rise to the above cause stating the underlying condition last.	(c) .... due to (or as a consequence of)
II	II
Other significant conditions, contributing to the death, but not related to the disease or condition causing it.	....

* This does not mean the mode of dying, such as, for example, heart failure, asphyxia, asthenia, etc., it means the disease, injury, or complication which caused death.

5.20 Part I of this section is used for stating the direct cause of death together with, in the reverse order downwards, the medical conditions, if any, that led up to the final illness. The last of these antecedent conditions to be recorded, which will be the one that arose first, is called the 'underlying cause of death', and it is this condition that is selected by the Registrar General for statistical tabulation when more than one cause of death is mentioned on the certificate.

5.21 Part II of the cause of death section is for the mention of any other conditions that had something to do with the death but did not by themselves play the major part or enter into the sequence of events directly leading to death and reported in Part I.

5.22 A typical certificate might read

  I (a) Peritonitis
      due to
    (b) Perforation of duodenum
      due to
    (c) Duodenal ulcer
  II Epithelioma of skin of cheek

5.23 In such a case the underlying cause of death would be 'duodenal ulcer' and the epithelioma would not be regarded as entering into the chain of events leading up to death though it contributed in some minor degree to the failure of the deceased to survive.

5.24 Medical practitioners are expected to provide sufficient detail to enable the underlying cause of death to be assigned to its proper category in the International Statistical Classification of Diseases, Injuries and Causes of Death.* In describing a new growth they are expected to state the variety—for example, carcinoma; the primary site, if known; and for some organs, such as the stomach, intestine and uterus, also the part of the organ where the growth originated—for instance, lesser curvature of stomach, sigmoid colon, uterine cervix. Pneumonia should be described as, for example, lobar or bronchopneumonia; and if it occurred as a complication of another disease, such as influenza or measles, this should be stated. If the death is attributed to haemorrhage its source and cause should also be stated. Childbirth should not be mentioned alone—the complication should be stated, and where there may be doubt it should be made clear whether the complication arose before, during, or after delivery. (For further examples see 'Medical Certification of Cause of Death', WHO, Geneva, 1952.)

Additional Information: Medical Inquiries

5.25 Sometimes when a certificate is being issued the certifier knows that later on, possibly when a necropsy or laboratory report has been received, he may be able to supply additional information, or may indeed wish to revise his original statement. The death certificate therefore is designed so that the certifier may indicate that he 'may be in a position later to give, on application by the Registrar-General, additional information as to the cause of death for the purpose of more precise statistical classification'. The Registrar, immediately he registers the death, sends a 'medical inquiry' to the doctor, asking whether he is now able to give any additional information.

Old Age

5.26 Certification of the cause of death of very old people is often difficult, the attending physician being in doubt whether to specify the various pathological conditions present or whether to certify 'senility'. Some old people die from quite definite and important diseases that can affect persons of any age, as, for example, pulmonary tuberculosis or cancer, and in these cases no question arises but that the death should be ascribed to the fatal disease. Other people die in old age with a number of pathological conditions present

* *Manual of the International Statistical Classification of Diseases, Injuries and Causes of Death*, Vol. 1, 1967; Vol. 2 (Alphabetical Index), 1967, WHO, Geneva.

that have originated mainly from the process of ageing, as, for example, arteriosclerosis or myocardial degeneration. If among these senile conditions there is one that has mainly contributed towards causing the death to occur when it did, this condition should be given preference upon the death certificate, with old age or senility (these terms are synonymous) either unmentioned or shown entirely as a contributory condition. The third and last group of elderly people are those fortunate few who die without any particular disease or degenerative condition playing a recognizably major part, and in such cases it is reasonable and correct to certify that death was due only to old age.

5.27 It must be borne in mind that though medical students are given training in the practice and purposes of death certification, and though the majority of medical practitioners take considerable interest in maintaining a high standard of reporting, there are sources of inaccuracy in the certification of causes of death and therefore in the statistics based upon these certificates; and it implies no criticism of medical practice to say that statisticians should sustain a healthy reluctance to regard the recorded causes as precise statements. Essentially they are statements of medical opinion however well informed and even when based on post-mortem investigation.

5.28 In the first place, there are the difficulties referred to in relation to old age—the true succession of events leading to death may be so overlaid by other concurrent conditions as make it difficult to discern a single underlying cause. It would be easier if multiple causation were analysed but this would involve complicated multidimensional tabulations. Secondly, there is a tendency for medical practitioners to use terminology in different senses—in most professions there is such a tendency for terms to vary in meaning by personal usage—and a slight change of phraseology may make considerable difference to the cause assignment. As stated below, much has been done to secure uniform terminology but variability still remains. Thirdly there are differences in the diagnostic resources available to doctors, in the length of their training and in the era of their training (ideas change in medicine as in other disciplines). Finally there is ordinary human fallibility from which doctors cannot be expected to escape. All diagnostic procedures (and even medical documentation), are subject to 'observer error' just as other physical measurements are, in the sense that two different observers may arrive at different determinations. In the physical sciences the error is reduced by replicated measurements; in medical diagnosis replication is not often possible for sheer lack of resources.

5.29 The use of uniform and precise language in the description of morbid conditions which will often be complex is essential to statistical classification. In addition, uniformity is necessary in the method of selecting and stating which of several contributory conditions is the underlying cause of death or the primary morbid condition. Both the language and the codes themselves have developed with experience in statistical classification and the advance of medical science.

5.30 The first attempts in modern times to prepare a scientific classification were made during the eighteenth century. Most eminent among these pioneers were Sauvages (1706–77), Linnaeus (1707–78), and William Cullen (1710–90). No system, however, secured universal acceptance. In his letter to the Registrar General published in the *Registrar General's First Annual Report for 1837*, Dr Farr wrote: 'The advantages of a uniform statistical nomenclature, however imperfect, are so obvious, that it is surprising no attention has been paid to its enforcement in Bills of Mortality. Each disease has in many instances been denoted by three or four terms, and each term has been applied to as many different diseases: vague, inconvenient names have been employed, or complications have been registered instead of primary diseases. The nomenclature is of as much importance in this department of inquiry, as weights and measures in the physical sciences, and should be settled without delay.'

5.31 When civil registration was established in 1837, Cullen's nosology was in general use in the public services. This had been published in 1785, and by 1837 it was considerably out of date because of the progress of pathological anatomy, and was found to be an unsatisfactory instrument for the type of statistical classification which Dr Farr wished to introduce. Dr Farr, therefore, framed a classification of his own, and with slight modifications to meet advances in medical science, this list was used in the *Registrar General's Annual Reports* until 1880.

5.32 The revised list introduced in the Report for 1881 formed the basis of the classification used in the General Register Office of England and Wales until 1900. A new list was published in 1901 and used during the ensuing decennium. Since 1911 the *International List of Causes of Death*, revised at approximately decennial intervals, has been used for the analysis of causes of death.

5.33 The same considerations as had led Dr Farr to draw up his own statistical nosology, and the growing desire to secure comparable statistics from different countries, led to an attempt to introduce a classification which would be internationally acceptable. At the 'First Statistical Congress' held in Brussels in 1853, Dr Farr and Dr Marc d'Espine of Geneva were asked to prepare lists of diseases suitable for the classification of causes of death in statistical offices. Their lists, based on different principles, were presented to the Second Statistical Congress in 1855, but neither was accepted. At a later date the Congress adopted a classification in use in Paris. This list, though revised at intervals, did not find general favour, and as late as 1893 no two countries in the world used precisely the same forms and methods for the statistical classification of mortality.

5.34 At the session of the International Statistical Institute (the successor of the old 'Statistical Congress') held in Chicago in 1893, Dr Jacques Bertillon, Chef des Travaux Statistiques de la ville de Paris, presented, on behalf of a special committee appointed by the Institute, a draft list of causes of death for international use. This list was adopted by the Institute and became known as the 'International List of Causes of Death'. It followed the principle adopted by Dr Farr in arranging the diseases as far as possible by their anatomical sites.

5.35 In October, 1897, the American Public Health Association recommended the use of the List in the United States, Canada and Mexico, and suggested its decennial revision to keep abreast of the advance of medical science. The proposal was adopted and taken up by the French Government which, on six successive occasions (in 1900, 1909, 1920, 1929, 1938 and 1948) invited other Governments and interested organizations to send representatives to Paris to participate in what became known as the International Commission for the Decennial Revision of the International List of Causes of Death.

5.36 The Conference held in 1948 was the last to be convened by the French Government, responsibility for the revision of the List now being vested in the World Health Organization. This last Conference unanimously adopted a new and extended list of diseases, injuries and causes of death, designed to provide a basis for compiling both mortality and morbidity statistics, which had been drafted by a group of experts from the United Kingdom, Canada and the United States and revised by an International Committee of experts appointed by the World Health Organization Interim Commission. This new list, known as the International Statistical Classification of Diseases, Injuries and Causes of Death, was approved in July, 1948, by the First World Health Assembly. This classification has since been revised periodically by international agreement.

Principles of the International Statistical Classification

5.37 In general the broad groups have followed the principles of the previous International Lists of Causes of Death. The classification deals first with diseases caused by well-defined infective agents: these are followed by categories for neoplasms, allergic, endocrine, metabolic and nutritional diseases. Most of the remaining diseases are arranged according to their principal anatomical site, with special sections for mental diseases, complications of pregnancy and childbirth, certain diseases of early infancy, and senility and ill-defined conditions including categories for symptomatic conditions to which a specific diagnosis has not been attributed. There are categories of diseases and morbid conditions, categories for external causes of injury, categories for the nature of injuries. A decimal system of numbering has been adopted in which the detailed categories are designated by three digit numbers. The first two digits generally denote significant groups within which the third digit separates specific disease entities or a classification of disease by site. There is a dual system of classification of injuries—by nature (prefixed N) and by external cause (prefix E). The code as published by the World Health Organization is prefaced by detailed rules of application which themselves form the subject of international agreement.

5.38 For the actual scheme of arrangement reference should be made to the latest issue of the Classification.

5.39 The First World Health Assembly also adopted the 'Nomenclature Regulations, 1948'. The purpose of these Regulations, which replaced the International Agreement relating to Statistics of Causes of Death signed in London in 1934, was to ensure as far as possible that mortality and morbidity statistics were compiled and published on a comparable basis in accordance with the Classification. The regulations were amended in 1956 to relax the obligations of certain articles which were regarded as too demanding.

5.40 The first classification devised by Dr Farr for the analysis of causes of death was published, together with a statement of the principles on which it was based, in the *First Report of the Registrar General* (pp. 92–100) and modifications were published in subsequent Reports. When the International List was adopted in 1911 after its second revision, the Registrar General published the first *Manual of the International List of Causes of Death* adopted for use in this country. Revised editions of the manual were published after each decennial revision; the manual in use until the end of 1949 being based on the fifth revision, made in 1938 and brought into use by the General Register Office from the beginning of 1940. From the beginning of 1950 the standard *Manual of the International Statistical Classification of Diseases, Injuries and Causes of Death* (which also contains the text of the Nomenclature Regulations), was used.

5.41 The object of such a manual is two-fold. In the first place it ensures uniformity of practice in tabulation by providing an assignment to one or other of the titles of the International List of any cause stated on a certificate, and by giving the rules to be followed in selecting a single cause of tabulation out of two or more recorded on the same death certificate. In the second place it defines the scope of each title in the List by indicating what kinds of entries on certificates of cause of death are assigned to it.

5.42 Prior to 1940 a system of rules had become established in the General Register Office for selecting the cause for statistical tabulation when more than one cause appeared in the death certificate. The rules were incorporated in successive editions of the *Registrar General's Manual of the International List of Causes of Death* (2nd, 3rd and 4th Revisions). When the 1927 form (forerunner of the International Certificate) was introduced in England and Wales it was thought advisable to adhere to these rules until the new certificate became familiar to the medical profession. The method of selection was not varied in 1927 except that the time sequence on the certificate was used occasionally to determine the choice between two diseases of equally high preference or between two local diseases.

5.43 In 1935 a random sample of 10,000 death certificates showed that obvious misunderstanding of the method of using the form had become comparatively rare, and that there was no longer any need to delay the adoption of a method of selection based upon the certifier's opinion on the order of the causes expressed by their arrangement on the certificate. The sample also showed, however, that such a change of method would cause important alterations in the assignment of deaths, which would be reflected in the death rates. It was decided, therefore, that from 1936 to 1939 deaths would be assigned by both the old and the new methods. From these data, corrective factors or conversion ratios, could be calculated to ensure statistical continuity of death rates. A description of the changes and a full list of conversion ratios were published in the *Registrar General's Statistical Review* (Part I) for 1940, Appendix B (i). During the years 1936–38 assignment was made in accordance with the 1929 List and each method of selection; for the year 1939, assignment was made by the 1929 List and the old system of selection by rules on the one hand, and by the 1938 List and new system of selection on the other, the latter forming the basis for the published tabulations for the year 1940.

5.44 The introduction of the International Statistical Classification of Diseases, Injuries and Causes of Death presented similar problems of bridging the change-over from the 1938 List in such a way as to ensure statistical continuity and comparability. Causes of death in 1949 were reclassified in accordance with 6th Revision procedure and detailed figures for 1949 based on the new classification were published in the *Registrar General's Statistical Review of England and Wales* for the two years 1948–49, Text, Medical. This volume also included a table showing some of the principal effects and changes resulting from the 1948 revision and a table showing factors for conversion from the old (1938) classification to the new. With the taking of the classification into general use by Member States of the World Health Organization and adherence to the related rules, the major part of the scheme to secure international comparability foreshadowed at the 1938 Conference has been completed.

Tabulation Lists

5.45 An Intermediate List of 150 causes and an Abbreviated List of 50 causes were agreed upon at the same time as the International Statistical Classification of Diseases, Injuries and Causes of Death. They were designed for use in certain tabulations which do not relate to the territory of a Member State taken as a whole, and the Abbreviated List is being used for appropriate tables in the *Registrar General's Statistical Review*. Until 1949 an 'Abridged List' was used by the General Register Office for similar purposes. This list comprised thirty-six groups of causes, and there was a supplementary list of thirty-six sub-divisions of the Abridged List. A similar list, broken into two parts with thirty-six causes in each, and based on the International List, was introduced in 1950.

The American Standard Nomenclature

5.46 Another important classification has been developed in the United States of America. Developments in this field in North America during the nineteenth century were similar to those in Europe and culminated in the 1928 Conference of the New York Academy of Medicine, the primary object of which was to produce a nomenclature that would be accepted as standard throughout the country. Under the editorship of Dr Logie the first draft was approved in 1931. In 1940 the American Medical Association took over formal responsibility for regular revision. The fourth edition was published in 1952. This is more of a refined nomenclature for the clinician who wishes to attain standard specificity in the description of the causative agent of a disease and the site of the body affected than a statistical classification, though the fact that it has numbered rubrics to facilitate diagnostic indexing has led to some confusion about its objective and it has sometimes been wastefully applied to statistical use in the mistaken belief that greater refinement must always be better than less.

5.47 A dual system of listing is employed: (1) by topography following eleven main anatomic divisions with progressive decimal subdivision to specific sites, e.g. $244 \cdot 7 =$ synovial membrane of wrist, the first digit, 2 — —, indicating 'muscoloskeletal system'; the second digit, — 4 —, indicating 'joints'; third digit, — — 4, indicating 'joints of *wrist*'; and the fourth digit, $\cdot 7$ indicating 'synovial membrane'; (2) by aetiology following thirteen main categories with decimal subdivision, e.g. $448 =$ frostbite, the first digit, 4 — —, indicating 'trauma or physical agent'; the second digit, — 4 —, indicating 'heat or cold'; and the third digit, — — 8, specifying 'freezing: frostbite'.

5.48 In specifying a disease the topographical code is written first separated by a dash from the aetiological code, viz. Adenoma of liver = 680—8091.

6			Digestive system	8		New growths
	8		Liver	0		New growths of epithelium
		0	Liver, generally		9	Tumours of glandular epithelium origin
					1	Adenocarcinoma

5.49 There is no real competition between the Standard Nomenclature and the International Statistical Classification, the former being used for clinical indexing where standards of diagnosis ensure that a high degree of specificity can be regarded as reproducible in the sense that the same condition will always be assigned and, sought by, the same number, and the latter for broader grouping in indices and for official vital statistics of international comparability. The current edition of the Standard Nomenclature gives for each entity not only the Standard code number but also the code number of the International Statistical Classification.

Grouping of causes for tabulation

5.50 Comparisons of the course of mortality over periods of several years in different local areas and especially in different countries, are complicated by the changes in classification that have been made at successive revisions of the International Lists and by differences in diagnostic or certification practice. For example in 1940 in England and Wales a revised International List of Causes was introduced simultaneously with the abandonment of the rules of selection which had hitherto operated in the selection of joint causes of death. This change produced sharp discontinuity in the rates of mortality for certain of the principal causes of death, notably heart disease, bronchitis, pneumonia and other respiratory diseases, cancer and nephritis. The following statement shows the combined effect of these two changes upon the death statistics:

Changes of assignment of deaths to causes—England and Wales 1940

Cause	Approximate change in numbers of deaths as a percentage of those formerly assigned to this cause
Influenza	—11
Cancer	—3
Diabetes	—30
Heart disease	—10
Other circulatory	—6
Bronchitis	+100
Pneumonia	+5
Other respiratory	+50
Nephritis	+12
Diseases of pregnancy, etc.	+10

5.51 The Registrar General tabulated statistics on both bases in advance of the change and thus was able to publish in the *Statistical Review* for 1940 approximate factors by which pre-1940 figures for every disease could be converted to the new basis to overcome the discontinuity.

5.52 With regard to differences in diagnostic practice it is, for example, impossible to compare the mortality from respiratory diseases in England and Wales, where many deaths are assigned to bronchitis, with mortality in the United States of America where few deaths are assigned to this cause.

5.53 A more common trouble is that if an attempt is made to trace through a number of years the mortality from a particular cause, it may be found that the disease is sometimes shown separately and sometimes grouped with other diseases, and even then it may change its class from period to period.

5.54 In the light of these difficulties Pedoe (1946) has emphasized Bradford Hill's caution (1948) that 'in making comparisons between death rates from different causes of death at different times or between one country and another it must be realized that one is dealing with a material which is in Raymond Pearl's words "fundamentally of a dubious character"'; and has formed the opinion 'that mortality by causes (when dealing with statistics of a whole country) is only of significance when grouped together to give a few main classes. Even then trends must be watched closely for possible transfers among these main classes.'

5.55 It therefore seems advisable for the purpose of comparing mortality trends to analyse deaths in broad groups. For example, by grouping together deaths from heart disease, other diseases of the circulatory system, intra-cranial lesions of vascular origin, nephritis, and bronchitis (owing to its frequent concurrence with heart disease and the fact that most deaths from bronchitis are among older persons) a general picture is obtained of the trend of degenerative disease. This group in 1954 covered 57 per cent of all deaths in England and Wales, and it may seem a very large group to put together; it is doubtful whether separation would achieve any real increase in definition.

5.56 Next in importance come deaths from cancer and malignant tumours —a simpler and more homogeneous group but one requiring careful statistical treatment. It is difficult, especially in dealing with particular sites, to separate the effect of improved diagnosis from absolute changes in mortality. Thus the registered death rate from cancer of the lung, bronchus, and pleura in males aged 55–64 in England and Wales rose from an average of 128 per million in the decade 1921–30 to 2,145 in 1952. There is no doubt that a part of this increase is due to a progressive increase in the efficiency of radiological detection. The effect of improved case finding is often cumulative. As more cases are found, so there is an increased tendency to look for them.

5.57 Nevertheless despite the need for caution on this account it is clear that in contrast with the relative stability of rates of mortality for cancer of other sites, there has been a real and substantial rise in mortality from lung cancer, especially in men. Recent investigations, as indicated in Chapter 16, point to environmental factors and therefore to the possibility of preventive action.

5.58 The death rate of tuberculosis was at one time an important index of the average level of living and especially of the extent of balance between nutrition and energy expenditure, but the dramatic fall in mortality since about 1947 when streptomycin was introduced as an effective chemotherapeutic agent, and when antibiotics generally rendered lung surgery a safer operation, has destroyed the indicator value of this rate. Nevertheless as a chronic in-fectious disease which strikes and disables younger persons, tuberculosis is still worthy of separate attention (especially in less developed countries which have not yet fully shared the benefit of improved case-finding and treatment).

5.59 Deaths from pneumonia and influenza form an important group since these are not only affected by periodical epidemics of influenza or other respiratory infection but also by external factors such as cold weather and atmospheric pollution. Here again the introduction of antibiotics and sulpha drugs has invalidated comparison with years prior to World War II.

5.60 The death rate from the common fevers of childhood such as diphtheria, measles, scarlet fever and whooping cough is now very low and these might be treated as a single group; but the increasing epidemic character of poliomyelitis demands for this disease separate statistical treatment.

5.61 The incidence of peptic ulcer is considered to be related to environmental factors; ulceration arises from trauma of gastric mucosa through dietary disturbance or duodenal irritations as a result of psycho-physiological disturbances and in both cases mental distress and over-intense living play an important part in aetiology. Here again modern surgery has effected a considerable reduction in the lethal quality of these lesions but it may still be worth while to separate the deaths into a separate gorup. Other digestive diseases might then be combined in one broad category.

5.62 Diabetes is another disease of especial interest since it has been said that it affects chiefly those people who are financially able, and inclined, to indulge in over-eating and under-exercising; and it is therefore a disease, the mortality from which may be correlated with the level of living, even though it has been reduced to small proportions by insulin therapy.

5.63 If disease is a penalty which society pays for the mode of living it adopts, there is one other penalty which is worth recording, namely, the death risk from accident and injury.

5.64 Infant mortality must be given special attention for reasons which have been set out in that part of Chapter 11 which has been devoted to it (p. 209).

5.65 Maternal mortality is an extremely small part of the total death risk but it is still an important subject of study because pregnancy is not, or should not be, an illness, and the birth of a child should not be in the least associated with death if this risk can be eliminated; and the approach to its elimination indeed forms an indication of the relative efficiency of the maternal care and obstetric services. Maternal mortality was falling only very slowly until the introduction of the sulphonamides, in the middle 'thirties, resulted in a substantial decline in the mortality from puerperal infection. Since that time puerperal sespis has lost its position as the most serious mortality risk of pregnancy, and has been replaced by toxaemia, haemorrhage, and other accidents (trauma of pelvic organs, etc.), but even for these causes mortality has been declining. The Ministry of Health in England and Wales collects confidential reports on all maternal deaths; these reports are initiated by local health authorities but they are finally completed by regional obstetric specialists who sift information from all those concerned in the care of the mother in order to be in a position to express an opinion as to whether or not the death could have been prevented by better medical care.

5.66 The following Table 5.3 provides an example of this grouping for comparisons (a) between two different points of time in England and Wales; (b) countries in the same year, viz. 1950. The information required for this

TABLE 5.3 Rates of mortality per 1,000 for groups of causes for different countries

Cause Group (International List Nos. in brackets)	England and Wales 1940		England and Wales 1950		1950 only Scotland		Northern[2] Ireland		Union[1] of South Africa		Canada		New[2] Zealand		France		Netherlands		U.S.A.[3]	
	M	F	M	F	M	F	M	F	M	F	M	F	M	F	M	F	M	F	M	F
Tuberculosis (all forms) (001–019)	0·88	0·55	0·47	0·27	0·59	0·48	0·53	0·43	0·29	0·17	0·29	0·23	0·26	0·17	0·76	0·41	0·21	0·17	0·30	0·15
Other infective and parasitic diseases (020–138)	0·39	0·24	0·14	0·09	0·14	0·08	0·14	0·11	0·28	0·21	0·13	0·09	0·14	0·09	0·19	0·15	0·13	0·10	0·15	0·09
Cancer and malignant tumours (140–205)	1·87	1·68	2·06	1·84	2·02	1·83	1·62	1·53	1·22	1·15	1·31	1·22	1·45	1·31	1·76	1·70	1·50	1·44	1·35	1·31
Diabetes (260)	0·11	0·15	0·06	0·11	0·06	0·15	0·05	0·09	0·07	0·15	0·09	0·14	0·08	0·16	0·07	0·11	0·06	0·11	0·12	0·20
Vascular lesions affecting central nervous system (330–334); Diseases of the heart and circulatory system (400–468); Bronchitis (500–502); Nephritis (590–594)	7·09	6·23	6·65	6·42	6·31	6·20	5·70	5·57	3·68	2·86	4·58	3·67	4·83	4·15	3·80	3·88	2·78	2·97	4·55	4·19
Pneumonia and influenza (480–483; 490–493)	1·21	0·82	0·52	0·37	0·51	0·45	0·55	0·55	0·70	0·57	0·44	0·37	0·29	0·27	0·74	0·74	0·29	0·30	0·36	0·27
Ulcer of stomach and duodenum (540–1)	0·24	0·06	0·18	0·05	0·20	0·04	0·10	0·04	0·08	0·02	0·08	0·02	0·12	0·03	0·05	0·04	0·08	0·02	0·09	0·02
Other diseases of the digestive system (550–572; 581)	0·39	0·29	0·21	0·18	0·25	0·21	0·23	0·18	0·40	0·30	0·27	0·19	0·17	0·14	0·44	0·31	0·15	0·12	0·26	0·18

89

table has been mainly derived from the *Demographic Yearbook* of the United Nations. This annual publication is an invaluable source of information of vital statistics in the different countries of the world. The coverage of the mortality statistics varies according to the extent of death registration and the degree of cause classification undertaken within the different countries.

Correction for residence

5.67 It has already been pointed out in an earlier chapter that, in calculating a death rate, there must be correspondence between the numerator and the denominator; only those persons must be included in the denominator as at risk, who, if they had died, would have been included in the numerator.

5.68 It is the normal practice in most countries to estimate populations for local areas on the basis of usual residence, since these are the persons in respect of whom local administration accepts responsibility for the provision of social services of various kinds.

5.69 It follows that correspondence between denominator and numerator in the calculation of death rates is more conveniently achieved by adjusting the deaths in the numerator to the same usual residence basis. It is therefore the practice in England and Wales and in most other countries including the United States of America to code death registrations according to the usual residence of the deceased and thence to tabulate the deaths by area of residence before calculating local area death rates. For the most part this is a straightforward procedure which gives rise to no difficulty other than the tedium of coding and punching additional holes in machine cards, but there are certain groups for whom, at death, it is difficult to determine a usual residence, e.g. inmates of mental institutions, or long stay hospitals, or long term convicts in prisons, most of whom have ceased to retain any claim to a home address and who are to all intents and purposes 'usually resident' in their respective institutions. It is the practice in the General Register Office of England and Wales to transfer to the area of usual residence all deaths in acute general hospitals and, in other hospitals (chronic sick and mental), those of patients who have been in hospital for less than six months but not to transfer deaths of inmates of welfare institutions covered by Parts III and IV of the National Assistance Act, 1948. This is the same criterion as is used to determine 'usual residence' at the census.

5.70 A difficulty immediately arises that a medical officer of health of an area with a small population may find that the accidental presence of a large long stay institution in his area with many 'non-transferable' deaths occurring within it may greatly inflate the local death rate. It has always been possible in reporting the death rate to explain the source of this inflation but owing to fears that such explanation would not be fully understood medical officers of health have not unnaturally striven to reduce the number of 'non-transferable' deaths by pleading that institutions are not of such a long stay character as to prevent transferability. An alternate mode of procedure would be to recognize the fact that every member of population has a risk of terminating life in a long stay institution and that despite the uneven geographical distribution of such institutions the deaths within them should be distributed among local authority areas in proportion to their populations. This method has been adopted in principle by the General Register Office of

England and Wales; the particular mode of its application is that the redistribution is incorporated in the Area Comparability Factor (see p. 94) which also adjusts the crude death rate for the difference between the national and the local population structure by age. Multiplication of the crude death rate by the area comparability factor thus produces a rate appropriate to a population with an age structure similar to that of the country as a whole and with only a proportionate share of the national total of deaths in long stay institutions. See para. 6.14.

REFERENCES

FARR, W. (1872) 35th Annual Report of Registrar General.
HILL, A. B. (1948) Principles of Medical Statistics, *Lancet*, London.
LOGAN, W. P. D. (1953) *Lancet*, ii. 1199.
LOGAN, W. P. D. (1953) *Brit. Med. J.*, i. 1272.
PEDOE, A. (1946) *J. Inst. Act.* 73.213.
United Nations (1953) *Stat. Papers Series*, M.19.
United Nations (1955) *Demographic Year Book* 1954, UN, New York.
WHO (1957) *Manual of International Statistical Classification of Diseases, Injuries and Causes of Death*, Vol. 1, 1957; Vol. 2 (index), 1957, WHO, Geneva.
WHO (1952)—*Medical Certification of Cause of Death*, WHO, Geneva.
HEASMAN, M. A., and LIPWORTH, L. (1966) *Accuracy of Certification of Cause of Death. General Register Office Stud. Pop. and Med. Subj: No. 20 H.M.S.O.*

CHAPTER 6

MORTALITY INDICES: LIFE TABLES

6.1 In 1954 the crude death rate in Bournemouth was 15·4 per 1,000 living and the corresponding rate for Corby was only 6·5. These two figures do not indicate the real difference in the mortality risks besetting the population of the two towns. Bournemouth is a coastal town attractive to older retired persons—in 1951 nineteen per cent of the population was aged sixty-five or more—and this means the population is abnormal by virtue of a shortage of young persons. The effect on the death rate is to reduce the denominator without proportionately reducing the numerator (because young people do not contribute many deaths) and thus to inflate the rate. On the other hand Corby is a new and rapidly developing town growing up round an expanding steel works; many young families have moved there and in consequence the population is short of old persons. This affects the numerator more than the denominator and deflates the crude mortality rate.

6.2 Consider the following example—

Age	Area A			Area B		
	Population (thousands)	Deaths	Death rate per 1,000	Population (thousands)	Deaths	Death rate per 1,000
0—4	280	1,400	5·00	220	2,200	10·00
5—24	900	900	1·00	810	1,215	1·50
25—44	910	2,730	3·00	900	2,970	3·30
45—64	720	14,400	20·00	780	11,700	15·00
65 and over	310	38,750	125·00	350	38,500	110·00
All ages	3,120	58,180	18·65	3,060	56,585	18·49

6.3 The crude death rates are 18·65 and 18·49 but their general similarity conceals the fact that the age specific rates in area B are higher at young ages and lower at older ages than in area A, i.e. the age incidence of mortality is very different. But the age structure of the population of B is so much older than that of A that it produces an elevation of the crude death rate to compensate for the lighter age specific mortality rates.

6.4 It must be borne in mind that the crude death rate is a weighted average of age specific rates in which the weights are the numbers of the population in the respective age groups, i.e. if $m_{x,t}$ is the death rate at ages x to $x + t$ and $P_{x,t}$ is the population in the same age group, the total deaths will be $\Sigma P_{x,t} . m_{x,t}$ where the summation is over all age groups, and the total population $\Sigma P_{x,t}$ so that the crude death rate is

$$\frac{\Sigma P_{x,t} . m_{x,t}}{\Sigma P_{x,t}}.$$

92

6.5 Clearly if the values of $P_{x,t}$ are increased for older ages at the expense of the younger ages then notwithstanding the constancy of the age rates of mortality, the crude death rate will rise. The weights used in such an average are therefore important.

The need for a single figure index

6.6 Before taking this any further we should consider why it is that an average should be used at all. It ought to be evident that since mortality varies with age, and population age structure varies with area, then in comparing mortality in two different areas we ought to look at the age specific rates. However it is difficult mentally to assimilate a large number of rates and for many purposes, (e.g. for brevity in description, ease in manipulation, etc.) it is desirable to have a summary measure to accomplish what the mind finds difficult to do unaided, i.e. to epitomize the whole experience. This is, of course, the fundamental object and justification of any type of average.

6.7 It will be understood that this desire for a single measure or average is increased by virtue of the fact that mortality varies with many other characteristics such as sex, marital condition, ethnic origin and social conditions, etc., so that for really thorough comparisons a very large number of refined specific rates may be involved.

Standardization

6.8 We have seen that the crude death rate is one such average but that it suffers from the defect that the weights used in its calculation are the local age group populations, i.e. they vary from area to area. Nevertheless, this defect is not serious for the very large number of areas whose population have a structure of the same general character, and the crude death rate is indeed widely used in such circumstances. Where there is no precise knowledge of the population structure, i.e. where only the total deaths and the total population are known, there is, of course, no alternative to this procedure. Where the age structure is known however, i.e. where the age specific rates of mortality are known there is no reason why we should not avoid, in calculating the average death rate, using weights which vary from area to area, by deciding to use a fixed set of weights, i.e. a *standard* population structure. Such an average rate then becomes a *standardized mortality rate*. Since populations can vary in their sex proportions at each age it is usual to standardize rates for *persons* for this source of variation also.

Direct standardization

6.9 Employing the same notation as before but using the symbol ^sP to indicate the standard population and remembering that the rates are specific also for *sex* and the summation is over all ages (and, for persons rates, is performed for *the two sexes* separately);

$$\text{Standardized mortality rate} = \frac{\Sigma^s P_{x,t}\ m_{x,t}}{\Sigma^s P_{x,t}}$$

Indirect standardization

6.10 Where, for example, a large number of district rates of mortality require standardization on the basis of the national population, the direct method would entail a very large amount of computation; moreover age specific rates and age analysis of the population may not be available for the districts.

6.11 It would clearly be a simpler process if we could find a factor F such that, when the crude death rate of a district is multiplied by it, the result is equal to the standardized mortality rate, viz

$$\left[\frac{\Sigma P_{x,t}\ m_{x,t}}{\Sigma P_{x,t}}\right] \times F = \left[\frac{\Sigma^s P_{x,t}\ m_{x,t}}{\Sigma^s P_{x,t}}\right]$$

where the values of the bracketed expressions are known but not necessarily the individual elements in the summations.

6.12 To calculate F we use the specific rates for the standard population in this equation instead of the district rates (which may not be known).

$$F = \frac{\Sigma^s P_{x,t}\ {}^s m_{x,t}}{\Sigma^s P_{x,t}} \div \frac{\Sigma P_{x,t}\ {}^s m_{x,t}}{\Sigma P_{x,t}}$$

i.e. if the district population were subject at each age to the same mortality as in the standard population its crude death rate would still be different from that of the standard population to the extent that the age structure of the district population differs from that of the standard population. If the district population is of an older age structure the crude rate will be inflated and F, to correct for this inflation, will be correspondingly less than unity, e.g. if the inflation is $33\frac{1}{3}$ per cent, F will be $100/133\frac{1}{3}$ or $0 \cdot 75$. F will only apply to similar degrees of distortion, i.e. to circumstances where the general pattern of mortality is similar to that of the standard population since we have assumed that the distortion is the same even though ${}^s m_{x,t}$ has been substituted for $m_{x,t}$, but it is usually valid to make this assumption. We still require $P_{x,t}$. These age group populations will be available at times of population census and except when violent population changes are taking place it may be possible to assume that they remain sufficiently stable to permit the use of F, once calculated, throughout the intercensal period and until the next census makes it possible to recalculate F.

6.13 If we write ${}^s c$ for the crude death rate in the standard population and $n_{x,t}$ for the *proportion* of the local population in the particular age group x to $x + t$, i.e. $n_{x,t} = \dfrac{P_{x,t}}{\Sigma P_{x,t}}$ then the equation for F can be transformed to

$$\frac{1}{F} = \Sigma n_{x,t}\ ({}^s m_{x,t} \div {}^s c)$$

and this simplifies the calculation since the factors $({}^s m_{x,t} \div {}^s c)$ can be calculated once and for all and then accumulatively multiplied by the appropriate set of n's (directly into an automatic calculating machine) to give $1/F$, whence the reciprocal yields F.

6.14 In England and Wales factors similar to F are used by the Registrar General to adjust local death rates to the national population structure (i.e. in this case the standard population death rates are the national rates for the current year) and these factors are then called *Area Comparability Factors*. The method of calculation removes altogether the effect of local concentration of long-term institution inmates. Reference should be made to the introductory notes of the Annual Statistical Review Part I.

Choice of a standard population

6.15 Up to 1941 the Registrar General of England and Wales published

(a) Death rates for each sex standardized for age, and a death rate for persons standardized for sex and age, for all causes combined;
(b) for selected causes of death, age-standardized rates for males and females separately.

6.16 The standard population used was that of England and Wales in 1901. The direct method was employed. Specimen figures are given in Table 6.1.

TABLE 6.1 *England and Wales—Death rates 1871–1940*

Period	Crude death rates per 1,000 living			Standardized rates per 1,000 living		
	Persons	*Males*	*Females*	*Persons*	*Males*	*Females*
1871–80	21·4	22·7	20·1	20·3	21·8	20·0
1881–90	19·1	20·3	18·1	18·6	20·0	17·3
1891–1900	18·2	19·3	17·1	18·1	19·5	16·7
1901–10	15·4	16·4	14·4	15·2	16·6	13·9
1911–20	14·4	15·9	13·0	13·5	15·0	12·2
1921–30	12·1	12·9	11·4	10·6	11·8	9·5
1931–40	12·3	13·1	11·5	9·3	10·6	8·2

6.17 It will be seen from these figures that owing to the ageing of the population from 1871 to 1940 the higher death rates at older ages received growing weight in the crude death-rate which became more and more in excess of the average based upon a standard population. According to the crude persons rate mortality decreased over the period by 43 per cent; but the standardized rate was reduced by 54 per cent.

6.18 It will be noticed that the standardized rate for 1931–40 is only 9·3 per 1,000 compared with a crude rate of 12·3. This is because the population of 1901 had a 'young' age structure (32·4 per cent at ages 0–14 and only 4·7 per cent at ages 65 and over) favouring a low aggregate mortality. Such rates (which were in effect abstract figures rather than crude rates actually experienced) could only be compared among themselves and would be too low for comparison with any other countries where rates have not been reduced to the same or at least to a closely similar standard.

6.19 The fact that standardized rates are low or 'young' looking does not destroy their value for depicting the mortality trend freed of distortion due to changes in population. It is possible that the choice of standard population might affect the relative emphasis given to mortality at younger ages (where improvement has been greater) and so might affect to a small extent the degree of decline in aggregate mortality. The Registrar General of England and Wales reported the following figures in an Appendix to the Medical Tables of the *Annual Statistical Review for 1941* as supporting criticism of the use of the 1901 standard:

95

Mortality rate and period	Standard population used as basis	
	1901	1939
Standardized rates of mortality (all causes) per 1,000:		
Persons: 1901	16·9	19·6
1939	8·5	12·1
per cent reduction	50	38

	1901	Mean of 1938–39
Males:		
per cent change 1938 to 1939	−0·6	+1·6

6.20 One answer to this criticism has already been given, viz. that the 50 per cent and the 38 per cent reduction are of the same order of size but differ to the extent that the 1901 population is 'younger' than the 1939 population and so gives proportionally more weight to the mortality at younger ages where most of the 1901–39 improvement occurred; the two series refer to different average ages and are, strictly speaking, non-comparable though in fact they tell very much the same story. Neither is 'right' or 'wrong'; it is a matter of choice of the set of weights which most accords with judgment as to the relative importance of old or young mortality. Where the per cent change in mortality, as between 1938 and 1939 is virtually zero, a change in the standard population can produce a change in sign but since no one would treat −0·6 or +1·6 per cent change in a single figure index as having much significance this is hardly an important criticism.

6.21 Nevertheless, the General Register Office regarded these differences as defects and also regarded the 1901 population as too youthful and inappropriate to current conditions. For these reasons it was decided in 1941 to cease to standardize strictly. A new Comparative Mortality Index was introduced which represented the ratio of aggregate mortality in the year of observation to that of a base year (1938), on the basis of a population structure *intermediate* between the two years.

CMI (year x) $= \Sigma m_x (n_x + n_{38}) \div \Sigma m_{38} (n_x + n_{38})$ where m_x and m_{38} are the sex age death rates for years x and 1938 and n_x and n_{38} are the proportions within corresponding sex age groups of the total populations of the respective years.

6.22 Thus the CMI was a ratio of standardized death rates and did not have the characteristics of death rate itself and it was age adjusted in a manner which varied from year to year, offending to an increasing extent against the very principle of standardization. It has never been adopted by any other country. In 1958 the CMI was abandoned by the General Register Office in favour of the so-called 'standardized mortality ratio'. This is another method of achieving comparability which does not involve a standard population as such. It is a comparison of actual deaths in a particular population with those which would be expected if 'standard' age specific rates applied. (See p. 125.) This in our symbols is

$$\frac{\Sigma P_{x,t}\,{}^s m_{x,t}}{\Sigma P_{xt} \cdot m_{x \cdot t}}$$

which can be written

$$\frac{\Sigma P_{x \cdot t} \cdot m_{x \cdot t} \left({}^{s}m_{x \cdot t}/m_{x \cdot t} \right)}{\Sigma P_{xt} \cdot m_{xt}}$$

i.e. it is a weighted average of age specific mortality differentials ($^{s}m/m$) where the weights are the actual deaths in each age group.

6.23 In the United States of America Mortality Statistics for 1911, the standard population used was that of England and Wales 1901 thus enabling accurate comparison to be made between the mortality experiences of the two nations. In recent times however it has been considered preferable to use a standard more appropriate to American conditions and for age-adjustment in the *Vital Statistics of the United States 1945* (the Annual Report of the United States Public Health Service), for example, the age distribution of the USA population of the 1940 Census was used without regard to sex, colour, or other characteristics.

6.24 The International Statistical Institute recommended that the population of Sweden of 1890 should be used for standardization for international comparison but later abandoned this proposal in favour of a composite European population based on the census populations in or about 1900 of a large group of European populations (ISI, 1917).

The development of standardized measures

6.25 The first reference to a standard rate occurs in Farr's report of 1855 (16th Annual Report of the Registrar General, 1853) and this was to the crude death rate of 17 per 1,000 expressing the level of mortality of certain 'healthy' districts. This concept was later used (20th Annual Report) to calculate a standard 'natural' death rate for London in order to assess the excess mortality of the Metropolis. Essentially this represented 'indirect' standardization. It appears that the direct method was due to Ogle who read a paper on the subject to the International Statistical Institute in 1891 recommending the use of an international standard population (though the direct method had in fact been employed in the Annual Report of the Registrar General for 1885). Brownlee (1922) urged the use of the 'life table death rate', i.e. 'the ratio of the number of deaths of persons above any defined age to the number living above that age in a stationary population' (a population distributed on the basis of the 'living' column of the relevant life table—see p. 101). This, as we shall see later, is the reciprocal of the expectation of life. Brownlee justified the use of the standardized death rate for all causes combined by its direct linear relationship with the life table death rate (to an accuracy of one third per cent) but refused to accept the standardized rate for specific causes, owing to the absence of this relationship. Yule (1934) pointed out that the standardized death rate as calculated by the direct method could be expressed as a weighted mean of ratios of age rates with the deaths in the standard population age groups as the weights, i.e. this rate was not independent of the standard population; thus, for example, standardized death rates for the two sexes were not comparable. Yule also criticized the indirect method since in this case the weights were not constant for all comparisons. He preferred the equivalent average death rate, i.e. a rate standardized by reference to a population with equal numbers in the age groups. This is an

D   97

arithmetic mean of the rates for age groups up to some convenient limit, such as 65 (beyond which it becomes unrealistic). In the discussion on Yule's paper Derrick suggested that the former's criticism arose from an attempt to pursue specific comparison of age rates in a summary measure designed to avoid such specificity.

6.26 This kind of criticism was perhaps a rather theoretical expression of a discontent which was crystallized in more practical terms by Yerushalmy (1950) who recalled that in normal direct standardized comparison, as Yule had stressed, the age rate ratios were weighted by the deaths in the standard population with the result that undue representation was given to mortality at old ages where deaths were heavy and secular improvement slight while little account was taken of mortality at younger ages where deaths were few but improvement considerable. In order to give more representation to this important improvement at young ages he suggested weighting so that equal proportionate changes in age rates affect the mortality index equally (as the standardized rate now becomes) no matter at what ages these changes occur.

6.27 Starting with the normal expression for the standardized death rate we have—

$$\text{Standardized death rate} = \frac{\Sigma m_{x,t} \, {}^s P_{x,t}}{\Sigma {}^s P_{x,t}} \tag{1}$$

$$\text{(which Yule transferred to)} = \frac{1}{{}^s P} \Sigma \left(\frac{m_{x,t}}{{}^s m_{x,t}}\right) {}^s d_{x,t} \tag{2}$$

Where ${}^s d_{x,t}$ is the number of deaths in the standard population corresponding to ${}^s m_{x,t}$ and ${}^s P$ is the total standard population.

6.28 Yerushalmy effectively replaces ${}^s d_{x,t}$ by t giving

$$\frac{\Sigma t \cdot \left(\frac{m_{x,t}}{{}^s m_{x,t}}\right)}{\Sigma t} \text{ i.e. the age specific}$$

mortality differentials are given equal weight in averaging them. Liddell (1960) suggested using ${}^s P_{x,t}$ rather than the arbitrary weight t. This reduces still further the weight given to older ages. The method was proposed as appropriate to occupational mortality where the active age groups are of salient interest. It would be possible also to use $P_{x,t}$ rather than ${}^s P_{x,t}$ if the latter were not available (Doering and Forbes, 1939). Kohn (1951) has proposed that if there is to be prior assessment of the weight to be given to a particular age group in averaging improvement then there would be an advantage in separating the derivation of weights from the deaths or death rate of the age group for the disease involved, and in producing a system of weights which would be capable of universal application, Kohn suggests using the reciprocal of the age of death—in practice the reciprocal of the midpoint of the age interval of each group, viz.

$$\text{mortality index} = \frac{\Sigma m_{x,t} \, ({}^t/_a)}{\Sigma ({}^t/_a)}$$

where t = class interval
a = age at midpoint

98

6.29 This goes even further in according increased weight to the younger ages. As Kohn pointed out his index may be readily varied in its sensitivity to changes at particular ages by adjustment in the weight differential, e.g. one might modify the gradient in representation by using log a or $\sqrt{a}$, etc. Kohn's index does not refer to standard mortality and is a different kind of average from those considered above.

Years of life lost

6.30 The study of mortality changes may be extended by considering the years of life lost by each death rather than by simply counting the number of persons whose lives were terminated; the underlying concept being that a man dying at the age of say thirty might but for the 'accident' of death have lived to the remainder of his normal span and that it might be a greater achievement to prevent his death than to save the life of a man aged ninety who cannot have much longer to live. There is nothing new in this idea. Price (1769) compared the expectation of life in the towns with the more 'natural' expectation in the country—'the further we go from the artificial and irregular modes of living in great towns the fewer of mankind die in the *first* stages of life and the more in its last stages.' In 1843 when Farr published in the 5th Annual Report of the Registrar General the English Life Table No. 1 he commented that even in the most favourable circumstances the mean life attained was then twenty-five years shorter than the 'three score and ten'. Later (1859) he addressed the Royal Society on the use of the most favourable expectation of life (on the 'Healthy District' Life Table) as a yardstick of public health, and returned to the subject again (1875) in a supplement to the 35th Annual Report of the Registrar General, where he measured 'the effect of the extinction of any single disease on the duration of life'.

6.31 In more recent times Karn (1931) also considered the effect of the elimination of certain causes of death upon the expectation of life and Dublin and Lotka (1936) dealt fairly extensively with the years of life forfeited on death from various specific causes. Dempsey (1947) used the same concept to measure the importance of the decline in tuberculosis mortality and was taken to task by Greville (1948) for using expectation of life at birth less age at death instead of expectation at death. Dickinson and Walker (1948) elaborated the study by the consideration of working years lost as distinct from total years lost. Controversy about the correct span of life was crystallized by Haenszel (1950) who re-emphasized that in considering the lives saved by the removal of a cause of death the expectation of life used to measure the saving must take account of the removal of that cause at later as well as earlier ages; this is the 'zero mortality' assumption. Haenszel introduced a system of using, in the construction of standardized rates of mortality, *expectations* rather than the usual weights of *deaths* which give insufficient emphasis to improvement at younger ages. The standardized rate now becomes a standardized rate of lost years of life (per 1,000 population or other appropriate unit).

6.32 Other recent references to the concept of loss of years of life and applications of the measure have been made by Martin (1951) who made calculations of years lost up to age seventy based on successive English Life Tables; Snow (1953) who expressed the mortality statistics of Western Australia in terms of the 'useful years lost' with the result that heart disease and cancer were displaced in importance by automobile accidents, and other accidents and coronary diseases became prominent; and Stocks (1953) who compared the loss of future working life from cancer, respiratory tuberculosis and accidents.

6.33 Accepting the principle of age-sex-standardization in an era of changing population structures there remains the choice of the 'normal span of life' to be used in measuring years lost on death. While this choice offers a stimulating philosophical pursuit it is largely irrelevant. There is no precise or absolute measure since a current life table is necessarily based upon the mortality of the lives now dying and is never exactly reproduced; and any 'projected' life table even constructed with 'zero mortality' considerations judiciously applied might be more realistic but would nevertheless be entirely arbitrary and speculative. Logan and Benjamin (1953) have suggested that it is more practicable to take refuge in the fact that the assessment of mortality improvement requires *relative* indices rather than absolute measures and for an index have proposed to take as the limit of 'normal' life that age in the life table at which the number of lives surviving is less than ten per cent of the original entrants, viz. the maximum span within which ninety per cent of persons die and is survived only by an abnormally longeval ten per cent. For males this was 85 and for females 88 years of age in round numbers and at current levels of mortality. For purposes of further illustration it was proposed to distribute the years of life between the working age period, 15–64, and the remainder. For a man dying at age 20 in 1952 it would therefore be assumed that a total potential loss of years of life (for index purposes only) of 65 years was incurred, and 45 of those years would be in the working age range. On this basis the mortality of 1952 represented a total loss of 238 years, and a loss of 76 working years per thousand population. If the specific mortality rates of 1848–72 were applied to the 1952 population, these losses would be raised to 1,004 and 497 years respectively. Comparable figures are shown below.

TABLE 6.2 *Years of life lost per 1,000 population—England and Wales*

Mortality of period	Persons		Males		Females	
	Years lost per 1,000		*Years lost per 1,000*		*Years lost per 1,000*	
	15–64	Total*	15–64	Total*	15–64	Total*
1848–72†	497	1,004	542	1,047	455	964
1952	76	238	92	266	61	211
1952, per cent of 1848–72	15	24	17	25	13	22

* Total to age 85 (males) and 88 (females).
† Standardized on the 1952 population.

6.34 If the proportionate improvements shown in this table are compared with those shown in Table 6.3 based upon conventional mortality rates it will be recognized that this index does give more weight to the relatively greater reduction of mortality at younger ages, since it now suggests that male mortality (in terms of total years lost) has been reduced to one-quarter and female mortality to almost one-fifth of the earlier level—this is comparable with the reduction in death rates below age forty-five.

100

TABLE 6.3 *England and Wales—Mortality in 1848–72 and* 1952

Period	Mean population (thousands)	Death rate per thousand	Death rates per thousand											
			Males						Females					
			0–	1–14	15–44	45–64	65+	All ages	0–	1–14	15–44	45–64	65+	All ages
1848–72	20,029	25·73*	202·66	16·12	9·81	23·94	95·63	23·45	162·28	15·80	9·64	20·62	86·27	21·42
1952	43,940	11·32	31·74	0·78	1·81	13·70	79·43	12·21	24·74	0·58	1·31	8·06	58·79	10·50
1952 per cent of 1842–72		44	16	5	18	57	83	52	15	4	14	39	68	49

* Standardized on the 1952 population.

6.35 A table showing this index has been introduced on an experimental basis in the Quarterly Return of the Registrar General of England and Wales (Appendix C of issue for quarter ended June 30, 1954). A method of calculation for local areas was given as follows—

(a) to calculate 'all cause' death rates for the local area in the age groups 0–4, 5–9, 15–24, 25–44, 45–64, 65 and over;

(b) to multiply these rates by standard weights; the weight for a particular age being the product of the average years 'lost' by each death and the proportion of the England and Wales population in each age group. [It will be readily seen that the local death rates when multiplied by the proportions of the England and Wales population in each age group and summed would yield a standardized death rate. If the products include for each age group also the years lost per death then clearly this produces an age and sex standardized rate of 'years lost'.]

(c) The years lost are obtained by deducting the mean age at death in each age group for England and Wales from 85; (alternatively for the 'working life' comparison, by deducting the mean age at death or 15 whichever is the greater, from 65).

The life table

6.36 Another way of summarizing a mortality experience is by means of the life table, i.e. a table which shows, on the basis of current mortality rates, the number out of 1,000 births (or some other convenient starting number, termed the 'radix' of the table) who survive to certain specified ages and the numbers dying between these successive points of age. A full life table gives this information for each integral age from nought to an upper limit beyond which it is convenient to regard the number of survivors as negligible. (As it is impractical to have a fraction of a survivor it is necessary to choose a radix large enough to allow for whole numbers to be surviving at these advanced ages.) Shorter tables (abridged life tables) are commonly produced which give the survivors and deaths for five-year intervals. Table 6.4 (p. 102) is an example of an abridged table based on the mortality of England and Wales, 1952.

Notation

6.37 The symbol l_x is conventionally used to denote the number surviving to the exact age x and d_x is used to indicate the number dying between exact age x and the next age shown in the table. The average number alive between

101

TABLE 6.4 *Abridged Life Table, 1952, England and Wales*

Age x	Males		Females	
	Survivors l_x	Deaths d_x	Survivors l_x	Deaths d_x
0	10,000	309	10,000	241
1	9,691	22	9,759	18
2	9,669	13	9,741	10
3	9,656	10	9,731	7
4	9,646	7	9,724	6
5	9,639	28	9,718	20
10	9,611	24	9,698	17
15	9,587	43	9,681	25
20	9,544	64	9,656	37
25	9,480	61	9,619	47
30	9,419	74	9,572	57
35	9,345	102	9,515	78
40	9,243	149	9,437	118
45	9,094	257	9,319	179
50	8,837	447	9,140	272
55	8,390	699	8,868	402
60	7,691	988	8,466	606
65	6,703	1,313	7,860	916
70	5,390	1,533	6,944	1,314
75	3,857	1,605	5,630	1,731
80	2,252	1,278	3,899	1,857
85	974	974	2,042	2,042

age x and $x + 1$ is denoted by L_x. This is the average of l_x for all values of x between exact age x and exact age $x + 1$ i.e. $\int_0^1 l_{x+t} \, . \, dt$. Alternatively we consider a population generated by l_0 births annually, spread uniformly over the year. At any one time the number aged, say, 46 years and 23 days would be $\dfrac{l_{46 \cdot 063}}{365}$ and the number living at age 46 last birthday would be

$\dfrac{1}{365} [l_{46} + l_{46 \cdot 0027} + l_{46 \cdot 0054} + \ldots \ldots + l_{46 \cdot 0630} \ldots \ldots + l_{46 \cdot 9973}]$ and if we made the interval progressively smaller we would reach a limit of $\int_0^1 l_{46+x} \, . \, dx$ or L_x so that in a stationary population generated by l_0 births annually and subject to the life table mortality, L_x is the number aged x last birthday.

6.38 Other symbols are

$m_x =$ the death rate at age x last birthday in the ordinary vital statistics sense of the ratio of annual deaths at age x last birthday to the average population at age x last birthday during the period of measurement. As an average population at risk is involved for which a mid-period population is often used as an approximation, this is sometimes referred to as a *central* death rate.

$q_x =$ the probability of dying within one year of attaining exact age x.

$p_x =$ the probability of surviving at least one year after attaining exact age x. [The word 'probability' here is used merely in the sense of the proportionate mortality or survival and p_x and q_x are expressed as proportions *per unit* so that $p_x + q_x = 1$. If $p_x = 0 \cdot 5$ this means that according to the life table one half of those who attain age x also survive to age $x + 1$.]

$T_x =$ the total population aged x and over in a stationary population generated by constant births and subject to the life table mortality. From what has been said already about L_x it will be seen that T_x is the cumulative sum of L_x for all values of x up to the end of the table.

$\mathring{e}_x =$ the complete expectation of life, i.e. the average period in years (including fractions of a year) lived beyond age x by those who attain exact age x. We shall see later that $\mathring{e}_x = T_x/l_x$.

Rates of mortality and probabilities of death

6.39 The two functions m_x and q_x represent different concepts. The first represents the average risk to which the population is subjected during its passage through the year of age x to $x + 1$; the second represents the total effect of the mortality pressure in terms of those who fail to survive the whole year without reference to its variation over the course of that year. The two measures are related by the fact that $m_x = \dfrac{d_x}{\displaystyle\int_0^1 l_{x+t}.dt}$ and $q_x = \dfrac{dx}{l_x}$.

6.40 If the deaths are uniformly distributed over the year of age (as they are, approximately, except at birth and at extreme old age) then $\displaystyle\int_0^1 l_{x+t}.dt$ (or L_x) is approximately the population of the middle of the year of age, viz. $l_{x+\frac{1}{2}} = l_x - \frac{1}{2}d_x$.

6.41 We may then write

$$m_x = \frac{d_x}{l_x - \frac{1}{2}d_x}$$
$$= (d_x/l_x) \div [1 - \tfrac{1}{2}.(d_x/l_x)]$$
$$= q_x \div (1 - \tfrac{1}{2}.q_x)$$

and $\quad q_x = \dfrac{2m_x}{2 + m_x}, \qquad p_x = \dfrac{2 - m_x}{2 + m_x}$

6.42 Thus when m_x had been derived, the values of q_x and p_x required to produce the life table may be derived from these simple relationships. In the first year of life mortality is varying rapidly and it is necessary to break up the year of age into intervals during which more uniform mortality may be assumed and to calculate q directly for these intervals by having regard to the related births, i.e. those among which the deaths may be assumed to have occurred.

6.43 As an example of this method reference may be made to the Decennial Supplement of the Registrar General for England and Wales 1931 Part I Life Tables, p. 28 where it will be seen that for English Life Table No. 10 (deaths of 1930–32 and census population 1931)

$$q_0 = q_0^{(0-3 \text{ months})} + q_0^{(3-6 \text{ months})} + q_0^{(6-9 \text{ months})} + q_0^{(9-12 \text{ months})}$$

where $q_0^{(0-3 \text{ months})}$ = probability of dying in the first quarter of the first year

$$= \frac{\text{deaths in 1930, 1931 and 1932 (age 0–3 months)}}{\frac{1}{2}b^4_{1929} + b_{1930} + b_{1931} + b_{1932} - \frac{1}{2}b^4_{1932}}$$

where b^4_{1929} = births in fourth quarter of 1929 which would on the average be exposed to risk of death at age 0–3 months for one half of the following quarter

[Note also that reference back to births was also necessary for those ages which correspond to generations at times of sharp fluctuation in the birth rate for here again in the absence of stability it is not possible to assume that the mid population is also the average population.]

6.44 As a further example of this method we may note that in the annual calculation of abridged life tables by the Registrar General for England and Wales, q_0 is obtained by adding together the infant mortality rates per related birth (see p. 210) for ages—under 1 month, 1–3, 3–6, 6–9, 9–12 months. Deaths are assumed to be uniformly spread over these short intervals, so that in the first month the average population is $\frac{1}{2}(l_0 + l_{\frac{1}{12}})$ and so on.

6.45 When the column of p_x has been derived it is a simple matter to start with a convenient radix $l_0 = 100,000$ and to find $l_1 = l_0 \times p_0, l_2 = l_1 \times p_1$ etc.

6.46 It should be noted that since $d_x = l_x - l_{x+1}$ by definition, then $l_x = d_x + d_{x+1} + d_{x+2} \ldots \ldots$ (see reference to Halley's Table and the Northampton Table below).

6.47 At advanced ages the data are always scanty and age statements are unreliable. It is usual therefore to assume an arbitrary trend to run off the table either by fitting a mathematical curve to the later part of the q_x column (or drawing a freehand curve) and extrapolating. It is common to adopt a curve named after Gompertz who used it to express a law of mortality, viz. $m^x = Bc^x$ where B and c are constants. Any degree of approximation adopted is not important since the values of the rates at these advanced ages have little effect on expectations of life over the main body of the table.

Actuarial methods

6.48 Life tables themselves have no greater mystery about them than any other statistical tables showing the frequency of occurrence of specified events or of numbers of persons in specified categories. Any difficulty arises mainly in the calculation of the appropriate population at risk corresponding to the observed deaths from which it is proposed to derive the basic death rates—or probabilities of death if these are to be derived directly. The fundamental techniques for this purpose especially where the data are not in census form require more extended treatment than can be accommodated here and reference should be made to appropriate textbooks. (See for example Actuarial Statistics Vol. II by J. L. Anderson and J. B. Dow, Cambridge University Press, 1948.)

History of life tables

6.49 The first actual life table was constructed by Edmund Halley (1656–1742) for Breslau in 1687–91. Males and females were not distinguished in it and like the Northampton Table below it was virtually based on deaths alone. It is fair to add (as has been pointed out by Greenwood [1948]) that Halley realized that the population was not stationary and made some correction for the excess of births over deaths. The first life table used for the purpose of determining the rate of premium to be used for life assurance was Dr Price's Northampton Table published in 1873. This was based on the death returns for a parish in Northampton in 1735–80, i.e. it was assumed that these could be added up from the lowest age to provide an estimate of the corresponding population at risk just as in the life table $l_x = d_x + d_{x+1} + d_{x+2} \dots$ This assumption would only be justified if in fact the population were stationary i.e. generated like the life table l_x column from constant births with constant mortality and no external migration. Dr Price was under the misapprehension that the population of this parish was stationary, judging by the number of infantile baptisms. However, at the time the data were recorded, there were a large number of Baptists in Northampton, who repudiated infantile baptism. The consequence of this oversight was that the living were understated and Dr Price assumed the mean duration of life to be twenty-four years, when it was really about thirty years. Unfortunately, his table was made the basis for the Government annuity schemes; and the same error which gave the insurance offices unduly high premiums induced the Government to grant annuities too large for the price charged, resulting in a loss to the public funds of about £2 millions sterling before the error was corrected.

6.50 Dr Price also constructed a correct life table from the population and deaths in Sweden, which was the first national life table ever made, and redounds much more to his fame than the Northampton Table.

6.51 The Carlisle Table was constructed in 1815 by Mr Milne, from the observations of Dr Heysham, upon the mortality of two parishes in that town in the years 1779–89, and two enumerations of their population in 1779 and 1787. It represented an advance in life table technique, being based on a proper estimate of the population at risk. At the time it was constructed it showed results too favourable for the whole country; but owing to the decrease of mortality which followed, it became more applicable.

6.52 The Carlisle Table, although based on scanty and uncertain data, was largely employed in insurance work for many years. Later, many individual insurance offices investigated their mortality experience, alone or in combination with other offices. The experience of insured persons is that of persons who have been selected either by medical examination or some kind of enquiry as to their fitness and tables based on such experience are not applicable to the general population.

6.53 In 1843 the Seventeen Offices' Experience was published, and later the Twenty Offices' Experience. The last named was published in 1869, and included the Healthy Males (H^m) table. This table, compiled by the Institute of Actuaries, soon became the standard table, and remained so until the issue of the British Offices' Tables, based on data relating to the period from 1863 to 1893, which were supplied by sixty British offices. The work of compilation was carried out by the Institute of Actuaries and the Faculty of Actuaries jointly. The O^m table of this work, for male lives, took the place of the H^m table. In 1912 the Government Annuitants' tables were published. After the 1914–18 war the Institute of Actuaries and the Faculty of Actuaries in Scotland undertook the joint collection of life office statistics of the mortality of annuitants from 1900–20, and produced the $a(f)$ and $a(m)$ tables in 1924 which were of special interest in that these forecast the mortality considered likely to be appropriate to those purchasing annuities in 1925.

6.54 Under the same auspices the Life Offices again combined to produce statistics and tables (A 1924–29) relating to the mortality of assured lives in 1929—two additional tables, a Light and a Heavy table were used to indicate the range of variation between different offices. About the same time a permanent organization was set up (the Continuous Mortality Investigation C M I) for the continuous collection of data. A further annuitants' table the a(55), projected for purchases in 1955, was issued in 1953 and in 1956 an assured lives table based upon the experience of 1949–52 was reported. It has become the general practice to tabulate data in the census form.

6.55 Similar co-operative ventures have been organized by the Society of Actuaries in America, the most notable of these (from a vital statistics point of view) being the studies of the mortality of insured lives with specified medical impairments. The most recent of these—the Impairment Study 1951 —was based on the records of twenty-seven offices in USA and Canada and covered an average duration of exposure of more than six years for 725,000 impaired lives. Mortality differentials were assessed for a large range of impairments, e.g. heart murmurs of various kinds, epilepsy, asthma, duodenal ulcer, diabetes and goitre to mention only a few. Generally the assessment was made by comparing actual deaths with those expected on the basis of a standard table for different ages and durations of policy.

6.56 The national experience of England and Wales has been made the subject of a series of life tables published by the General Register Office.

6.57 *English Life Table, No. 1.* Dr Farr constructed his No. 1 Table, based on the census returns of 1841 and the deaths of the same year (Registrar General's Fifth Report). Thinking, however, that the records of one year's deaths might be open to challenge owing to the short time embraced in them, he constructed the *English Life Table, No. 2.* This is founded on the census enumerations of 1831 and 1841, and the deaths of seven years, viz. those in 1841 and the three previous and three subsequent years. The difference between these two English life tables is slight.

6.58 *The English Life Table, No. 3,* constructed by Dr Farr, was based on the census enumerations of 1841 and 1851, and upon the 6,470,720 deaths registered in the seventeen years 1838–54.

6.59 The near agreement between the results obtained by these three English life-tables is very remarkable, and shows that, notwithstanding annual fluctuations, there was a fairly stationary mortality during 1838–54 (which, we may add, continued up to the year 1871). The latter fact led Dr Farr to abandon his intention of constructing a fourth English Life Table down to 1872.

6.60 *The Healthy Districts Life Table* was constructed by Dr Farr on the basis of the mortality during the five years 1849–53 in sixty-three selected

English districts, which showed, during the decennium 1841–50, a mean annual death rate not exceeding 17 per 1,000 persons living. As pointed out by Dr Farr, it expressed 'very accurately the actual duration of life among the clergy and other classes of the community living under favourable circumstances'. It represented also a standard of healthiness already attained, and was therefore useful for purposes of comparison. This table is printed in the Thirty-third Annual Report of the Registrar General.

6.61 *The English Life Table, No. 4* by Dr Ogle, published in the Supplement to the Thirty-fifth Annual Report of the Registrar General, dealt with the national experience in the decennium 1871–80, and those (*Nos. 5* and *6*) by Dr Tatham with the corresponding experience of 1881–90 and 1891–1900.

6.62 *The New Healthy Districts Life Table*, by Dr Tatham, gave a valuable index of sanitary and social progress. Thus, whereas in 1849–53, the period dealt with by Dr Farr's Healthy Districts Life Table, 'less than 6 per cent of the total population lived in districts the crude death rates in which were below $17 \cdot 5$ per 1,000; in 1881–90, on the other hand, no less than 25 per cent of the population lived in districts the crude death rates in which fell below $17 \cdot 5$ per 1,000, and $4\frac{1}{2}$ per cent in districts the crude death rates in which did not reach $15 \cdot 0$ per 1,000'. When differences of age and sex constitution were allowed for by obtaining death rates in a standard population, it was found that about one-sixth of the entire population, or 4,606,503 persons, had death rates below 15 per 1,000 in 1881–90. This new healthy districts table was therefore calculated on 46 million years of life, a basis more than nine times as great as that of the older table. In the corresponding Healthy Districts Life Table for 1891–1900 it was found practicable to utilize the experience of an aggregate population of 4,447,485 in 260 districts whose death rates did not exceed 14 per 1,000.

6.63 For the decennium 1901–10 much more abundant information was supplied. The making of national life tables for this period was entrusted to Mr George King, FIA, FFA, whose report should be on the shelf of every student of vital statistics.* In this report he describes the method of construction of full and abridged life tables, and the following life tables are given:

(1) Life tables for England and Wales for males and females, respectively, based on the experience of the ten years 1901–10 (No. 7), and corresponding to the English Life Table No. 6 for the decennium 1891–1900.

(2) Life tables for England and Wales, for males and females, based on the census of 1911 and the deaths of the three years 1910–12 (No. 8).

(3) Life tables for females only, according to marital condition, single, married, or widowed, based on the census of 1911 and the deaths in 1910–12.

(4) Sectional life tables, for males and females respectively, for—
   (*a*) The administrative county of London.
   (*b*) The aggregate of county boroughs.
   (*c*) The aggregate of urban districts.
   (*d*) The aggregate of rural districts.

*Supplement to the *Seventy-fifth Annual Report of the Registrar General*, Part I, Life Tables (Cd. 7512).

These were based on the deaths in 1911 and 1912, and on the estimated population in the middle of each of these years.

6.64 Subsequently Part II of the same supplement, dealing with life tables (Cd. 1010) was issued, containing a series of abbreviated life tables prepared by Dr E. C. Snow.

6.65 *Life Tables No. 9 for 1920–22, No. 10 for 1930–32 and No 11 for 1950–52* were undertaken by the Government Actuary. In tables 9 and 10 the census populations and deaths grouped in five-year age periods were graduated to remove irregularities due to errors of age statement, etc. and rates of mortality were derived at quinary age points; rates for individual ages were obtained by interpolation. In connection with English Life Table No. 9 an extensive analysis was made of variation of mortality between different geographical areas and complete sets of rates were given for County Boroughs in Northumberland and Durham (heavy mortality) and Eastern Counties Rural Districts (light mortality). Full life tables were provided for Greater London. In the 1931 Decennial Supplement regional comparisons were made; rates for individual ages 0–84 for each sex were given for Northumberland and Durham County Boroughs and for the Eastern Region Rural Districts; and life tables for Greater London were given. Mortality rates at quinary age points were compared for single, married and widowed women. In table No. 11 the rates, not the population and deaths separately, were graduated. Mortality was compared for different marital conditions and for different areas (the standard regions, the urban/rural aggregates, Greater London, Wales and Scotland). Tables for Scotland and Northern Ireland were also constructed by the Government Actuary and were published separately.

6.66 *United States Life Tables*, 1890, 1901, 1910 and 1901–10, were published by the Government Printing Office, Washington (1921), giving an explanatory text, mathematical theory, computations, graphs, and original statistics. The text of this report forms a textbook of points relating to life tables. The methods employed in constructing the life tables for persons, males and females, for white persons and negroes, for foreign born and native born, for rural and urban sections, and for selected registration states, were similar to those used in the construction of the English Life Tables for 1901–12. The report embodied also a useful comparison of survivorship, death rates, and expectation of life at each age for twelve countries, in most instances for the period 1901–10.

6.67 In 1936 the Bureau of the Census published a further volume incorporating previous tables but including also tables for 1920–29, and for 1929–31 (around the census of 1930). At the census of the United States in 1940, life tables based on the census population and the deaths in 1939–41 were prepared by T. N. E. Greville and were published in 1946. The tables deal separately with white negroes, and other races as well as the total population, of each sex. The methodological chapters are extensive and of great interest to serious students of actuarial techniques but are beyond the scope of this book. Abridged life tables relating to individual calendar years have been prepared since 1945 by the National Office of Vital Statistics and have been published in the vital statistics of the United States.

Methods of calculating abridged life tables

6.68 For normal vital statistics it is unnecessary to undertake the labour of producing a full life table with all the many refinements that may be necessary to avoid chance irregularities in the progression of probabilities of death from one age to another. The main summary character of the table may be achieved by producing the abridged form especially where it is only desired to make broad comparisons between successive years in the same country or between different countries at the same period of time.

6.69 Various methods of calculating abridged life tables have been suggested.

George King's Abridged Life Table

6.70 This method described by King in 1914 proceeds from an assumption that the data are normally in grouped form, e.g. quinary totals of deaths and mean population.

6.71 Grouped data of numbers at risk and deaths from which pivotal* values are obtained for a particular year of age within the group range. These pivotal values are obtained by formulae such as $u_7 = 0 \cdot 2w_5 - 0 \cdot 008 \, \Delta^2 w_0$
where u_7 = pivotal value of population (or deaths) at age 7
w_5 = quinary sum of observed populations (or deaths) for ages 5 to 9.

The summations involved here have the advantage of smoothing or graduating the data, i.e. removing chance irregularities.

6.72 Division of pivotal deaths by populations gives pivotal values of q_x whence p_x and $\log p_x$ are obtained. From these pivotal values of $\log p_x$ $\log {}_5 p_x \left(\text{i.e. } \log \dfrac{l_{x+5}}{l_x} \right)$ must be derived and thus values of l_x, l_{x+5}, l_{x+10} by successive multiplication from the chosen radix.

6.73 The two formulae used are—

$$w_5 = 5u_0 + 7 \, \Delta u_0 + 1 \cdot 6 \, \Delta^2 u_0 - 0 \cdot 2 \, \Delta^3 u_0$$
$$w_6 = 5u_0 + 8 \, \Delta u_0 + 2.6 \, \Delta^2 u_0 - 0 \cdot 2 \, \Delta^3 u_0$$

where in the first form w_5 relates to $\log {}_5 p_{x+5}$ and u_0 relates to $\log p_x$ at pivotal points.

6.74 Using the second form on l_x gives $\Sigma_6^{10} \, l_{x+t}$ Final summation gives $N'_x = \Sigma l_{x+1}$ and $\mathring{e}_x = \dfrac{N'_x}{l_x} + \tfrac{1}{2}.$

6.75 King himself did not use the abridged method below the age of eleven but later users have extended the range to cover all ages. Disadvantages of this method are that values emerge at central ages rather than terminal ages of quinary groups, also special adjustments are needed at the beginning and end of the tables where third central differences are not available. (At the youngest ages formulae corresponding to those of 6·73 are $w_0 = 5u_0 + 2\Delta u_0 - 0 \cdot 4 \Delta^2 u_0 + 0 \cdot 2 \Delta^3 u_0$ $\quad w_1 = 5u_0 + 3\Delta u_0 - 0 \cdot 4 \Delta^2 u_0 + 0 \cdot 2 \Delta^3 u_0.$)

E. C. Snow's method

6.76 Snow's approach (1914) was to find empirical relations, based on pre-

*'Pivotal' connotes use as estimated values at fixed reference points, ages 7, 12, etc.

109

existing tables, between $m_{x,t}$ and $_tp_x$ and between $\frac{l}{l_x}\Sigma_0^t l_{x+t}$ and $_tp_x$. Thus we have for five-year groups:

Ages over 10

Range of death rate $m_{x,5}$	Equation for $_5p_x$	Range of $_5p_x$	Equation for $\frac{l}{l_x}(\Sigma_0^4 l_{x+t})$
0—0·00300	$_5p_x=0\cdot99995-4\cdot8883\,m_{x,5}$		
0·00300—0·00370	$_5p_x=0\cdot98152+5095\cdot5(0\cdot00383-m_{x,5})^2$	1·0—0·9750	$\frac{l}{l_x}(\Sigma_0^4 l_{x+t})=$
0·00370—0·00550	$_5p_x=0\cdot95419+247\cdot824(0\cdot01423-m_{x,5})^2$		$3\cdot0914+1\cdot9084\,_5p_x$

Ages under 10

5—10	$_5p_5=0\cdot99838-4\cdot68181\,m_{5,5}$		$\frac{l}{l_5}\Sigma_5^9 l_t=2\cdot2504+2\cdot7556\,_5p_5$
2—5	$_3p_2=0\cdot99883-2\cdot78784\,m_{2,3}$		$\frac{l}{l_2}\Sigma_2^4 l_t=1\cdot4959+1\cdot5105\,_3p_2$
1—2	$p_1=0\cdot07434+0\cdot92488\left(\frac{2-m_1}{2+m_1}\right)$		
0—1	$p_0=1-$(infant deaths per birth)		

$m_{x,t}$ is calculated in the normal way from grouped data $_tP_x$ is then obtained from tabulated values and l_x follows directly. Values of $\Sigma_0^t\frac{l_{x+t}}{l_x}$ are computed from the standard equations and $\Sigma_0^t l_{x+t}$ follows by multiplication by l_x. $\mathring{e}_x$ is obtained from the relation $\mathring{e}_x=\frac{l_{x+}l_{x+1+}\cdots}{l_x}-\frac{1}{2}$. This method while very rapid may not apply to different countries or periods of time and experiments would be needed before it could be safely used.

Reed and Merrell Abridged Life Table

6.77 The Reed and Merrell approach (1939) is, like Snow's, to find a functional relationship between $m_{x,t}$ and $_tp_x$.

6.78 It was found that when values of $m_{x,t}$ were plotted against $(1-_tp_x)$ that a curve could be fitted of the form,

$$(1-_tp_x)=1-\exp\left(-t\cdot m_{x,t}-a\cdot t^3 m_{x,t}^2\right)$$

giving $(1-5p_x)=1-\exp\left(-5.m_{x,5}-(0\cdot008)\,(5)^3\,m_{x,5}^2\right)$

6.79 Special formulae were derived for initial ages,

$$q_0=1-\exp\left(-m_0[0\cdot9539-0\cdot5509m_0]\right)$$
$$q_1=1-\exp\left(-m_1[0\cdot9510-1\cdot921\,m_1]\right)$$

6.80 All these values have been tabulated and the conversions merely involve looking up values in relevant tables. Progression to l_x is then a simple computing stage.

6.81 From l_x it is possible to obtain T_x directly (for ages > 5) where quinary groups are used, by means of the relation:

$$T_x = -0\cdot20833\, l_{x-5} + 2\cdot5\, l_x + 0\cdot20833\, l_{x+5} + 5\Sigma_1\, l_{x+5a}$$

6.82 For ages under 5, Reed and Merrell fitted equations of the form $\Sigma_0^t L_{x+t} = al_0 + bl_x + cl_{x+t}$ to twenty-four Uunited States Life Tables varying from 1901 to 1930. Finally $\dfrac{T_x}{l_x} = \mathring{e}_x$.

Greville's Abridged Life Tables (1943)

6.83 Transition from $m_{x,t}$ to $q_{x,t}$ is effected by

$$q_{x,t} = \frac{m_{x,t}}{\dfrac{1}{t} + m_{x,t}\left[\tfrac{1}{2} + \dfrac{t}{12}(m_{x,t} - 0\cdot09)\right]}.$$

(The constant $0\cdot09$ is alternative to $\log_x c$ where c is derived by fitting Gompertz's Law $m_{x,t} = Bc^x$ to $m_{x,t}$.)

6.84 Rates of mortality for initial ages are found from births and deaths to obtain a starting value of l_x and then the abridged method is applied. L_x is obtained from the relationship

$$\Sigma_0^t L_{x+t} = \frac{\Sigma_0^t d_{x+t}}{m_{x,t}}$$

assuming that $m_{x,t}$ applies to the life table population as to the actual population whence T_x is found by summing back from the highest age, and thence $\mathring{e}_x$.

U.S. Abridged Life Tables (1945)

6.85 This method, also attributable to Greville, involves construction of an abridged table by reference to a standard full table—in this case the United States 1939–41 Table. It is assumed that the $m_{x,t}:q_{x,t}$ relationship in the standard table may be applied to the particular calendar year for which an abridged table is required apart from

(i) the terminal age group 75+, where it is assumed that $\mathring{e}_{75} = r/m_{75}$, r being the ratio of the terminal group death rate in the actual data of standard table to that of the standard table population.

(ii) q_0 which is calculated directly from death and birth data.

ΣL_x is derived by assuming that the standard table ratios $\dfrac{t.l_x - \Sigma_0^t L_{x+t}}{\Sigma_0^t d_{x+t}}$ remain unchanged when values l_x and d_x of the abridged table are substituted.

Institute of Actuaries (1914)

6.86 When King's method was published in the *Journal of the Institute of Actuaries* the Editors suggested an alternative procedure which retains the data in a grouped form throughout.

6.87 Let $m_x^{(t)} = $ central death rate per five years for a five-year age group x to $x + 5$.

The approximate formula

$$\log {}_5p_x = -Mm_x^{(\frac{1}{2})}\left\{\frac{1 + m_{x+5}^{(\frac{1}{2})} - m_{x-5}^{(\frac{1}{2})}}{24}\right\}$$

$$= -Mm_x^{(\frac{1}{2})}(1 + a_{0/12})$$

where $a_0 = 1^{st}$ central difference of $m_x^{(\frac{1}{2})}$, is used to derive ${}_5p_x$.
$M = (2 \cdot 30258)^{-1}$

6.88 The expectation in five-year intervals is then obtained by the continued formula

$$\tfrac{1}{5}e_x^{(\frac{1}{2})} = {}_5p_x [1 + \tfrac{1}{5}e_{x+}^{(\frac{1}{2})}]$$

whence e_x follows from the formula

$$e_x = e_x^{(\frac{1}{2})} + 2 - \tfrac{1}{5}\left[\frac{1}{{}_5p_{x-5}} - {}_5p_x\right].$$

Current General Register Office Abridged Life Table

6.89 This is published annually in the September Quarterly Return and is computed from the estimated home population in any period and total deaths registered in that period.

6.90 Values of l_x and $\mathring{e}_x$ are given for individual ages up to five and then at five-yearly intervals up to age eighty-five.

6.91 $m_{x,5}$ is converted to ${}_5p_x$ by the relationship ${}_5p_x = \dfrac{2 - 5m_{x,5}}{2 + 5m_{x,5}}$ except

at ages 1 to 4 where the individual age relationship $p = \dfrac{2 - m}{2 + m}$ is used and at

age 0 where the first year of life is subdivided into 0–, 1–, 3–, 6–, 9–12 months and infant mortality is calculated on the basis of related births to give q_0 by summation.

6.92 ΣL_x is obtained by assuming l_x to be linear over each interval of time used whence T_x and $\mathring{e}_x$. It is assumed that $\mathring{e}_{85} = 0 \cdot 99 (m_{85+})^{-1}$

Comparison of methods

6.93 Table 6.5 shows selected values of $\mathring{e}_x$ for females based on mortality in England and Wales in 1954 as derived by the methods described above.

TABLE 6.5 *Expectation of life computed by different methods*

Age	King	Snow	Reed, Merrell	Greville 1	Greville 2	Actuaries	GRO
0–	73·05	73·08	73·15	73·92	73·04	73·18	73·05
5–	69·92	69·99	69·99	69·81	69·93	70·02	69·93
15–	60·10	60·11	60·00	60·04	60·15	60·24	60·15
25–	50·38	50·39	50·35	50·40	50·44	50·54	50·44
35–	40·82	40·94	40·86	40·93	40·89	40·95	40·89
45–	31·56	31·63	31·65	31·67	31·63	31·63	31·63
55–	22·85	22·89	22·95	22·96	22·91	22·91	22·91
65–	15·00	15·02	15·08	15·07	15·04	15·00	15·04
Time Index	2·2	1·0	1·3	1·5	1·1	1·2	1·0

6.94 It will be seen that there is good agreement between the various methods; especially when one bears in mind that some involve arbitrary treatment at initial and final ages. The bottom line of the table compares the time taken (by the same operator) to complete the table to the $\mathring{e}_x$ column using a standard desk model of automatic calculator, and fixing the time for the GRO method as unity. There is little to choose between Snow, Greville (standard table), and the General Register Office methods. It should be added that the electronic computer can be programmed to produce a complete life table from crude data. Where there is access to a computer there may be little saving in restricting the calculation to an abridged table.

Expectation of life

6.95 The word 'expectation' can only be applied appropriately to measurement of lifetime in the sense that the 'expectation of life' is the average number of years lived by people 'in the long run'. In practice we do not know what might happen 'in the long run' because mortality is constantly changing and we cannot observe the 'long run' under stable conditions. Nothing is more certain than that the mortality of the past will not be reproduced in the future. Yet we find it convenient to consider the average lifetime of those who have recently died as a guide to future expectation and it is useful and fair to do so within limitations.

6.96 We must also take note that expectation of life has no meaning at all, not even an approximate one, except in relation to some starting age, because in this matter of survival 'the race is to the swift', and those who are nearer the winning post and have tested their stamina have a better prospect of finishing than those just setting out who have yet to survive the full rigours of the course. This may not be commonly appreciated. It might be thought perhaps that since the expectation of life at birth (i.e. calculated from birth) was 67 years for men, then all men reaching age 65 have only two further years to live on the average. In fact, however, the expectation at birth is calculated by averaging the lifetimes of all males born, some of whom die *before* 65; whereas the expectation of life at 65 is calculated only in relation to those who die *after* age 65 and this select band of men live, on average, for another twelve years. A simple example will make this clear. Suppose our population under observation consists of four* men who die at ages 55, 59, 66 and 88. These four men at the time of their birth were destined to live on the average for $\frac{1}{4}[55 + 59 + 66 + 88] = 67$ years. So we say the expectation at birth is 67. On the other hand, starting from age 65, we only consider those who are still alive (those who are dead have no expectation) viz. those who die at 66 and 88, and these live 1 and 23 years, i.e. an average of 12 years, beyond age 65. The expectation of life at age 65, $\mathring{e}_{65}$, is thus 12. In quoting expectations of life it is essential to specify the age beyond which the expectation is calculated.

6.97 The expectations are always calculated separately for the sexes whose experiences are so different that the concept of an average sexless *person* has no meaning in this context.

6.98 So far we have over-simplified the calculation by saying that we

---

* We would not actually be so foolish as to calculate an expectation based on a handful of lives—the calculations are normally based on hundreds of thousands of completed lives (deaths).

compute the expectation at birth* in any one mortality experience by adding up the ages at death and dividing by the number of deaths. In practice we base the calculation not on the *actual* deaths but on the deaths that would occur in a hypothetical life table population, i.e. a stable population supported by a constant number of births and experiencing the rates of mortality implied by the *actual* deaths. The reason for this is that a sudden rise in births would introduce into the calculations, based on *actual* deaths, an undue

TABLE 6.6 *Expectations of life according to Abridged Life Table*, 1952
(*Home Population*), *England and Wales*

Age	Males	Females
0	67·06	72·35
1	68·20	73·14
2	67·35	72·27
3	66·44	71·34
4	65·51	70·40
5	64·56	69·44
10	59·74	64·58
15	54·88	59·69
20	50·12	54·83
25	45·44	50·03
30	40·72	45·27
35	36·02	40·52
40	31·39	35·84
45	26·86	31·26
50	22·57	26·82
55	18·64	22·57
60	15·11	18·52
65	11·97	14·76
70	9·27	11·38
75	6·96	8·45
80	5·15	6·09
85	3·62	4·35

number of infant deaths (very short lifetimes) associated proportionally with the extra births, and this would depress the average total lifetimes. Since extra infant deaths would merely be proportional to the extra births, death *rates* would not be disturbed. Therefore a population 'generated' by reference to constant births and the death *rates* would not be affected by such a fluctuation in annual births.

6.99 Table 6.7 shows the changes that have taken place in the expectations of life at different attained ages since 1838–54. One important fact to be specially noted as pertinent to an appreciation of mortality trends as reflected by the expectation of life is that if child mortality is reduced so that, to take a single but exaggerated example, all those who formerly died before age 10 survive an additional 40 years, then the deaths at ages beyond 50 will be unaffected. Thus, though the expectation of life at birth will be increased, the expectation at 65 will be unaltered. Something like this has been happening. The major gains in mortality have indeed been at young ages and much less progress has been made at advanced ages. In consequence the

* The only difference in the calculation of expectation at a later age x, is that we first subtract x from the age at death and ignore deaths prior to age x, before averaging.

expectation at birth for males has risen by 26 years from 40 in 1838–54 to 66 in 1950–52, while at age 65 the expectation has only increased by a mere year or so, from 10·8 to 11·7. Even for females, who have experienced greater improvement in longevity, the increase at age 65 is only about 3 years.

TABLE 6.7 *Expectation of life at different attained ages—England and Wales—1838–1952*

Sex	Age	Expectation (years) based on assumption of continuation of mortality of						
		1838–54	1891–1900	1901–10	1910–12	1920–22	1930–32	1950–52
Males	0	39·9	44·1	48·5	51·5	55·6	58·7	66·4
	15	43·2	45·2	47·3	48·6	50·1	51·2	54·4
	25	36·1	37·0	38·9	40·0	41·6	42·5	45·0
	45	22·8	22·2	23·3	23·9	25·2	25·5	26·5
	65	10·8	10·3	10·8	11·0	11·4	11·3	11·7
Females	0	41·9	47·8	52·4	55·4	59·6	62·9	71·5
	15	43·9	47·6	50·1	51·4	53·1	54·3	59·0
	25	37·0	39·4	41·5	42·8	44·5	45·6	49·4
	45	24·1	24·2	25·5	26·3	27·7	28·3	30·8
	65	11·5	11·3	12·0	12·4	12·9	13·1	14·3

REFERENCES

Actuaries, Institute of (1914) *J.I.A.*, 48, 301.

BROWNLEE, J. (1922) M.R.C. Spec. Rep. Series No. 60.

DEMPSEY, M. (1947) *Am. Rev. Tub.*, 86, 157.

DICKINSON, F. G., and WALKER, E. L. (1948) 'What is the Leading Cause of Death?', Chicago, *A.M.A. Bulletin*, 64.

DOERING, C. R., and FORBES, A. L. (1939) Proc. Nat. Acad. Sci. (Wash.), 25, 461.

DUBLIN, L. I., and LOTKA, A. J. (1936) *Length of Life*, New York, Ronald Press.

FARR, W. (1843), 5th Annual Report of Registrar General.

FARR, W. (1859), Trans. Roy. Soc. 1859, 838.

FARR, W. (1875), 35th Annual Report of Registrar General.

GREENWOOD, M. (1948) Medical Statistics from Graunt to Farr C.U.P.

GREVILLE, T. N. E. (1943) Record of Am. Inst. Act., 32, 29.

GREVILLE, T. N. E. (1947) Vital Statistics—Special Reports 23, 241.

GREVILLE, T. N. E. (1948) *Am. Rev. Tub.*, 87, 417.

HAENSZEL, W. (1950), *Am. J. Pub. H.*, 40, 17.

KARN, M. N. (1931) *Annals of Eugenics*, 4, 279.

KING, G. (1914) *J.I.A.*, 48, 294.

KOHN, R. (1951) *Can. J. Pub. H.*, 42, 375.

LIDDELL, F. D. K. (1960) Brit. J. Ind. Med. 17, 228.

LOGAN, W. P. D. (1950), *Population Studies*, 4, 132.

LOGAN, W. P. D., and BENJAMIN, B. (1953) *Monthly Bull. Min. Health & P.H.L.S.*, December, 244.

MARTIN, W. J. (1951) *Medical Officer*, 86, 151.

PRICE, R. (1769) *Phil. Trans.*, 59.

REED, R. J., and MERRELL, M. (1939) *Am. J. Hyg.*, 30, 33.

Registrar General, England and Wales (1875). Supplement to 35th Annual Report.

Registrar General, England and Wales (1936). Decennial Supplement, 1931. (1957) Decennial Supplement 1951.

SNOW, E. C. (1914) Registrar General, Supplement to 75th Annual Report.

SNOW, D. J. R. (1953) Rep. Commissioner for P. H. West. Australia, 1951.

STOCKS, P. (1953) *Brit. Med. J.*, ii, 847.

YERUSHALMY, J. (1950) *Am. J. Pub. H.*, 41, 907.

YULE, G. V. (1934) *J. Roy. Stat. Soc.*, 97, 1.

CHAPTER 7

ENVIRONMENTAL FACTORS AFFECTING MORTALITY

7.1 It has already been noted that mortality varies with age and sex. It is important to note also that there are important factors affecting mortality concerned not so much with endogenous or constitutional variations as between, for example, males and females but with exogenous factors arising from the varying conditions in which people live, work, play and sleep.

Marriage

7.2 We have earlier drawn attention (p. 77) to the effect of marriage upon the mortality for certain causes—arising partly from the selective force of marriage itself, partly also because the contentment and happiness of married life are favourable to well-being and partly (in specific causes for women) from sexual expression, pregnancy and childbirth. It is hardly possible to isolate the separate effects of marital selection (the less fit being less inclined or finding it more difficult to find partners) and of marriage itself. As proof of the selective force of marriage it should be noted that married women's mortality is generally lighter than that of single women (except at advanced ages) and that an exceptional rise in marriage rates with many 'marginal' marriages of spinsters who would not normally marry tends to increase the mortality of married women as a whole.

Climate

7.3 The influence of climate can only be separated with difficulty from that of other conditions of environment. No useful comparison bearing on this point can be made between the general death rates of communities possessing fairly good vital statistics but living in different climates. Australia, New Zealand, South Africa and Canada all furnish instances of remarkably low death rates associated sometimes with sub-tropical summers and extremely cold winters. Where a country is notoriously unhealthy this is usually in a large measure due to the endemicity of malaria or of other insect-borne diseases often along with parasitic diseases, e.g. ankylostomiasis. These causes can be removed and are being removed.

7.4 Climate has a marked influence on the prevalence of particular diseases, e.g. malaria or yellow fever where a high temperature is needed for effective multiplication of the vectors of infection. Diphtheria and scarlet fever prevail little in tropical countries. The prevalence of tuberculosis in some tropical areas is not a product of the climate but of other social factors coupled with racial susceptibility or lack of immunological protection. The common cold and influenza are found the world over but respiratory disease other than tuberculosis is not prevalent in dry sunny climates.

116

Season

7.5 More is known of the influence of season than of climate on the death rate. In former times the chief groups of diseases responsible for seasonal variation in the death rate in England and Wales were diarrhoeal diseases and respiratory diseases, but improvements in hygiene (especially food hygiene) have much diminished the force of the former while advances in the use of antibiotics and sulpha drugs have reduced the fatality of the latter; the lowering of the mortality levels has naturally reduced the amplitude of seasonal fluctuation except when an influenza epidemic intervenes (as in 1951). Fig. 7.1 shows the weekly deaths in London in four-weekly periods in 1921 and 1951 for the following groups of diseases—

All causes
Enteritis
Influenza, bronchitis and pneumonia
Heart disease.

7.6 As has been indicated (p. 73) the best way of comparing mortality in smaller and possibly unequal intervals of the calendar year is to convert the death rates into equivalent annual rates by multiplying the rate for n days by $\frac{365}{n}$.

7.7 Seasonal variation of infectious disease is discussed in the relevant chapter.

Density of population

7.8 One of the greatest influences militating against health in the past has been the increasing gravitation of the population into crowded cities. By 1851 above half the population of England and Wales had become aggregated in towns. In 1921 only $20 \cdot 7$ per cent of the population remained in rural districts and in 1951 this proportion had fallen to $19 \cdot 2$ per cent. In 1951 two-fifths of the population were concentrated in the six major conurbations* (the term given to certain large agglomerations of urban areas which represent towns that have outgrown their administrative boundaries). In earlier days when the process of town expansion was unregulated, town life was associated with many inimical factors—streets instead of fields; unsatisfactory dwellings instead of country cottages; dust and belching smoke and noise instead of sunshine and clean air and quiet; a preponderance of indoor occupations; crowding together of the population with enhanced opportunities for the transmission of infectious disease; bad drainage and risks of contamination of water supplies; importation of food from areas far distant from sources of supply with consequently increased opportunities for its infection and decay. Many of the worst elements of town life have been removed or mitigated by enlightened local government and by the general rise in standards of hygiene in the day to day life of the community at large. Many town dwellings are superior in space, heating, ventilation and sanitation to the country cottage. The town often has the advantage of more extensive medical services. Indoor

* Tyneside, West Yorkshire, South East Lancashire, Merseyside, West Midlands, Greater London.

117

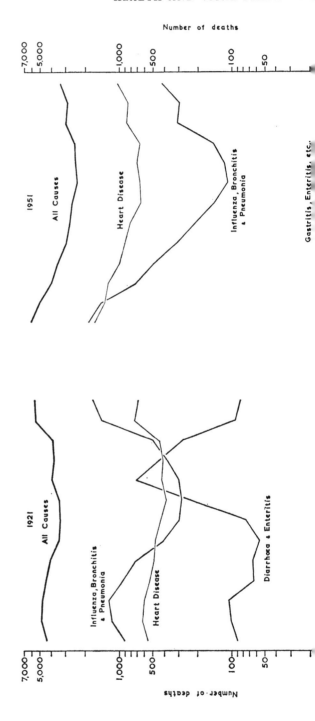

occupations still predominate but factory and office conditions are immeasurably better. The smoke and the noise and the herding together remain however; and if modern medicine and improved nutrition have together greatly lessened the toll of infectious disease, more rapid and more voluminous traffic has not only increased the speed with which epidemics spread within a town and from one town to another, but provided greater opportunities for accidents.

7.9 That the urban differential in mortality still exists may be seen from the following age-standardized death rates per 1,000 in 1961 in England and Wales.

Conurbations	13·0
Urban areas with population of 100,000 and over	13·0
Urban areas with population of 50,000 and under 100,000	12·4
Urban areas with populations under 50,000	12·5
Rural districts	11·5

There has been some controversy as to whether there is any direct relationship between mortality and density of population as such, viz. as measured by the number of persons per square mile of the area in which they are resident. Farr (1843) found an approximate arithmetical equality between the ratio of the death rates of two areas and the sixth root of the density of the population but he himself was doubtful of any implied law. Newsholme (1891) himself showed that the relationship did not provide a basis for predicting the mortality in large tenement blocks. It has since become abundantly clear that ill health springs not simply from the closeness with which people live together but from a whole complex of social and economic factors which may be associated with such crowding.

7.10 Local authorities have done much, especially in areas of new development, to produce high quality housing in pleasant and open surroundings. The schoolroom and the workshop alike are now planned to provide the most comfortable conditions possible. However it still remains true that health is related not only to bricks and mortar and to medical services but is also dependent on mode of occupation and personal habits (in turn determined by intelligence and educational background) and nutrition; the level of living is associated with the level of income however much the strength of this association has been weakened by positive social security measures.

7.11 It is difficult to disentangle the separate influence of particular elements in the general complex of social conditions, since these elements are all interdependent. Those who can afford an expensive house can also afford to be well fed and well clothed, and by the same token are rarely in dirty or unhealthy occupations; they are usually well educated and know how to take care of their health. One condition implies all the others.

7.12 Benjamin (1953) studied the correlation between the death rates in 1931–33 from tuberculosis in twenty-eight London Boroughs and the incidence of certain social factors in those boroughs. These factors were—

(b) Social Index. Percentages of males whose occupations were assigned to social classes IV and V at the 1931 Census.

(c) Percentage of population in private families living at a density of more than one and a half persons per room at 1931 Census.

(*d*) Percentage of males aged fourteen and over unemployed at 1931 Census.

(*f*) Mean weights of school children expressed as a percentage of the London average, 1938.

(*g*) Attendances at tuberculosis dispensaries per case on the registers, 1932.

(*h*) Gross expenditure on the tuberculosis dispensary service in £s per case on the dispensary register in each borough in 1931.

(*m*) Percentage of occupied males aged fourteen and over, engaged at the 1931 Census in the twelve occupations which had the highest mortality from pulmonary tuberculosis during 1930–32.

(*p*) Proportion of persons per 1,000 total population whose birthplace was shown as Ireland at the 1931 Census.

(*o*) Major public open space and private open space, allotments and water-ways per cent of total existing acreage as shown in L C C Draft Development Plan, 1951. (This is the position before development and broadly indicates the open space existing for many years.)

7.13 Factors *b*, *c*, *d* were intended to measure social conditions and in addition it was considered that *c* would also measure the epidemiological influence of overcrowding apart from the economic conditions associated with poor housing conditions. The nutritional status of the boroughs was roughly indicated by *f*. Factors *g* and *h* were intended to measure the strength of the tuberculosis services. The occupational risk was intended to be indicated by *m*. Irish immigration could not be ignored and so factor *p* was introduced. Open spaces were referred to index *o*. Much of the information required for the calculation of the indices was only measured accurately at the Census of 1931, and it was for this reason that the analysis was based on the period 1931–33. Index *f* was based on 1938 because no other data were available, but it is not thought that at 1931 the borough pattern would have been different.

7.14 Essentially and briefly the statistical method of analysis was as follows: If the movement of factor *A* is *not* independent of that of factor *B*, the two factors are said to be correlated. The strength of the correlation or association (without prejudice to the question of whether or not the relationship is causal) is commonly measured by an index known as the coefficient of correlation (*r*). If the dependence is complete (i.e. a change in *A* is always accompanied by a change in *B*), then *r* has its maximum value of unity. If there is complete independence, *r* is zero. Intermediate strengths of association are indicated by values of *r* intermediate between zero and 1. If *A* and *B* tend to increase together, *r* has a positive sign; if *A* increases when *B* decreases and *vice versa r* has a negative sign. The coefficient is itself subject to sampling error and *r* must be significantly different from zero when this error is taken into account, for the association to be accepted.

7.15 Consideration was first given to zero order correlation coefficients— i.e. coefficients obtained by considering only the twenty-eight pairs of values of *z* (mortality from pulmonary tuberculosis) and *b*, etc., without taking into account the possibility that both *z* and *b* might be related to *c* and that the first association might conceal the second. Later, *partial* coefficients were obtained for the association, for example, between *z* and *b* when the indirect effect of other factors was deliberately removed from the calculations—i.e.

effectively c, d, f, etc., were held constant while the variation of z with b was observed.

7.16 The zero order correlations were as follows;

Index z (Mortality from pulmonary tuberculosis) with:

$b + 0\cdot725$	$c + 0\cdot688$	$d + 0\cdot679$
	$f - 0\cdot512$	$g + 0\cdot072$
$h - 0\cdot256$	$m + 0\cdot601$	$p - 0\cdot564$
		$o - 0\cdot296$

7.17 There were thus statistically significant associations between mortality and all the social or economic factors.

7.18 Neither attendances at dispensaries nor the expenditure on these clinic services was significantly associated with mortality in 1931 (when treatment had less effect on mortality than now). This does not mean of course that the dispensary service was futile. It merely indicates that these factors were not sensitive indices of the influence of the service upon mortality.

7.19 The occupational risk gave strong association.

7.20 At first sight the proportion of Irish born in the population was of significance, but the correlation coefficient is unexpectedly negative. One might have expected more tuberculosis where there were more Irish born in view of known nationality (birthplace) factors, but on reflection it seems there is a simple and at least plausible explanation. Many of the Irish who come to work in London are engaged in personal service (often residential), so that relatively more would be found in better circumstanced boroughs (in 1931). On the other hand they are not numerous enough to raise the mortality rate significantly even if they do suffer a high tuberculosis incidence.

7.21 The inverse correlation of tuberculosis mortality with open space was *not* statistically significant.

TABLE 7.1 *Zero order correlation coefficients*

	b	c	d	f	g	h	m	p	o
z	$+0\cdot725$	$+0\cdot688$	$+0\cdot679$	$-0\cdot512$	$+0\cdot072$	$-0\cdot256$	$+0\cdot601$	$-0\cdot564$	$-0\cdot296$
b		$+0\cdot719$	$+0\cdot836$	$-0\cdot591$	$+0\cdot183$	$+0\cdot070$	$+0\cdot626$	$-0\cdot464$	$-0\cdot135$
c			$+0\cdot903$	$-0\cdot636$	$+0\cdot261$	$-0\cdot193$	$+0\cdot915$	$-0\cdot403$	$-0\cdot463$
d				$-0\cdot583$	$+0\cdot349$	$-0\cdot007$	$+0\cdot816$	$-0\cdot469$	$-0\cdot352$
f					$-0\cdot209$	$+0\cdot313$	$-0\cdot470$	$+0\cdot402$	$+0\cdot333$
g						$+0\cdot075$	$+0\cdot210$	$+0\cdot114$	$-0\cdot174$
h							$-0\cdot201$	$+0\cdot133$	$+0\cdot174$
m								$-0\cdot333$	$-0\cdot378$
p									$+0\cdot345$

The position of the coefficient by row and column indicates the two indices between which association is measured.

7.22 None of the factors treated above was independent of the others, as can be seen from the table (7.1) of zero order correlation coefficients. Social class (b), for example, was strongly correlated with housing (c), nutrition (f), occupation (m) and Irish birthplace (p). If therefore there is an association between tuberculosis mortality and Irish birth there will also apparently be an association between tuberculosis and social class.

7.23 Which is the direct and which the indirect of the correlations demonstrated above? This question can be answered only by calculating the partial correlation coefficient between z and b, z and c, etc., while the influence of other factors is removed (the effect is as though, while z and b are considered, the other factors c, d, etc., are not allowed to vary among the boroughs and so cannot influence the direct association between z and b).

7.24 Table 7.2 gives values of the partial correlation coefficients found for the several multiple regression equations which were evolved.

7.25 In the analysis g and h were excluded owing to their lack of significance and d was omitted owing to its obvious overlap with b and c. The order of introduction of the factors was determined after experimentation with many combinations.

TABLE 7.2 *Partial Correlation coefficients between Tuberculosis Mortality* 1931–33 *and Factors Specified*

	b	c	f	m	p	o
Equation Multiple Regression	Social class (proportions in IV.V)	Housing density (per cent living more than 1½ per room)	Nutrition (mean weights per cent London average)	Per cent in high mortality occupations	Irish born proportion	Open space (per cent of total borough area)
1.	+0·73	—	—	—	—	—
2.	+0·45	+0·35	—	—	—	—
3.	+0·44	+0·32	−0·022	—	—	—
4.	+0·44	+0·20	−0·0048	−0·047	—	—
5.	+0·39	+0·20	+0·046	−0·043	−0·36	—
6.	+0·36	+0·18	+0·040	−0·042	−0·34	−0·019

No.	Regression Equation	Source of Variance	Sums of Squares	Degrees of Freedom
1.	$z = 0·0103b$	Variation explained by b	0·2994	1
2.	$z = 0·0067b + 0·0044c$	Increment explained by addition of c	0·0325	1
3.	$z = 0·0067b + 0·0043c − 0·0020f$	f	0·0003	1
4.	$z = 0·0067b + 0·0054c − 0·0045f − 0·0027m$	m	0·0007	1
5.	$z = 0·0055b + 0·0050c + 0·0041f − 0·0023m − 0·0036p$	p	0·0306	1
6.	$z = 0·0056b + 0·0048c + 0·0035f − 0·0022m − 0·0035p − 0·00024[o]$	o	0·0415	1
		Residual	0·1653	21
			0·5703	27

7.26 The second equation of Table 7.2 takes into account the average social status of the borough and the average degree of mild crowding in dwellings—i.e. the combined effects of economic level and facilities for exposure in the home. The small increment in variance explained by c indicates that much of the 'housing' effect has been stolen by 'social class' *simply because it was introduced first* and is highly correlated with housing. Fairly strong association with these two factors *together* is demonstrated with a contribution of 58 per cent of sums of squares. In equation 3 the independent effect of nutrition (bodyweights of children) is introduced—i.e. the effect not already contained within social class and housing and 'stolen' by those two factors—but no significant association exists and there is no further appreciable effect on the variance absorption. Equation 4 is a surprise, for the partial correlation coefficient for m is not significantly different from zero; on the other hand the consequent reduction in the partial coefficient for housing density suggests that the factor of employment in the specified occupations is not a direct tuberculosis risk so much as an association with the social background common to these low-grade occupations (c and m are highly correlated—see Table 7.1).

7.27 Equation 5 shows that the introduction of the proportion Irish born produces a partial correlation coefficient of −0·36, which is only just below the 5 per cent significance level. The negative sign of the correlation coefficient and the fact that the coefficient of correlation with social class is reduced to 0·39 indicates, however, that as suggested above we are measuring here not an influence of place of birth so much as the influence of the social status of the borough. By the inclusion of o (equation 6) the other coefficients for social class and housing, etc. are only slightly reduced, while the partial correlation coefficient for o is almost zero (compared with zero order $-0·296$). This indicates also that o is not independent of b or c. As has been commented elsewhere (Benjamin and Nash, 1951), those who live in areas with little open space are commonly those who cannot afford to live in better residential areas and cannot afford good housing and other amenities.

7.28 The general conclusion to which these calculations led was that there was little gain in introducing the factors other than social class and housing density and that there was very little specific contribution from housing density. It was not possible to find any new factors related to mortality which were independent of economic status. None of the partial correlation coefficients was large enough to be regarded as statistically significant.

Housing

7.29 In so far as housing conditions *do* directly affect health, they normally do so by affecting the incidence of infectious disease. The more a household (of a particular size) is crowded into small or few rooms the greater the opportunity for infection to spread by droplet or direct contact from one to the other. This increase in the facility of transmission of infection is even greater when bedrooms have to be shared by members of the same family or where rooms are used both for living and sleeping; it is also greater, especially for diarrhoeal diseases, where more than one family are compelled to share the same sanitary arrangements (water closets or washing up facilities).

7.30 The important statistics to be measured are, in respect of each household—

> Number of persons—under 15
>   15 and over   } giving persons per room
> Number of rooms — living .   } as an index of crowding
>   sleeping
> Number of rooms used for sleeping by more than one person.
> Use of water closet—sole or shared.
> Use of washing up facilities—sole or shared.

7.31 It is often possible in enquiries into local outbreaks of infectious disease for health visitors or sanitary inspectors to investigate such conditions by house to house enquiry of the dwellings where cases of disease have occurred and, for purposes of estimating differential incidence, of a representative sample of *all* dwellings. For example in a study of the incidence of enteritis in London (Scott, 1953) it was found that the housing density (persons per room) was higher (2·05) in infected houses than in the survey area as a whole (1·38). Infants without any sign of diarrhoea, i.e. with much less evidence of infection, came from less crowded houses than those with diarrhoea. As compared with uninfected households, those with cases of enteritis had a higher incidence of sharing washing up facilities and of sharing water closets.

7.32 Again in an enquiry in a London Borough into the housing conditions of families in which a case of tuberculosis had been notified (Chalke, 1953) it was found that in those households possessing sufficient accommodation for the tuberculous patient to have a *separate bedroom* the incidence of secondary cases was 5·7 per cent compared with 9·9 per cent in households where a separate bedroom could not be provided.

7.33 For general purposes it is necessary to rely on information derived from the population census. It has not yet been possible in a census to distinguish between living and sleeping rooms.

Census statistics

7.34 At recent British censuses the householder has been required to provide information as to the number of persons in the household and the number of usual living rooms occupied by the household: and whether this accommodation constituted the whole of a structurally separate dwelling or was part of a dwelling shared with another household. Information has also been provided about the availability (sole use, shared use, or absence) of piped water supply within the dwelling, cooking stove, kitchen sink, water closet, and fixed bath.

7.35 The tabulations normally show for local areas:

Distribution of dwellings by size (rooms).
Incidence of sharing of dwellings by households
Distribution of households by size (persons).
Density of occupation (persons per room).
Availability of household amenities.

7.36 These factors are cross-balanced to relate housing conditions to household size. Inter-area variations and secular trends are demonstrated.

Occupation

7.37 It is now well recognized that the manner in which a man gains his livelihood and the surroundings in which he spends the greater part of his working hours may have an important influence upon his health. It is equally well recognized that it is difficult to separate the influence of those elements of his environment which are directly associated with occupation as such from those of a more general character associated with his level of income.

7.38 We need to know not only the number of deaths for each cause by age and sex in each occupation (if possible by duration of engagement in the occupation) but also the relative population at risk, i.e. the average numbers engaged in the occupation similarly classified. On a national basis it is not yet possible to obtain information of duration of engagement in the occupation either at census or at death registration. Details of occupation are recorded at the census and, apart from the omission of the durational element, this enables populations at risk to be derived applicable to periods of time close to the census date. Occupation of the deceased is routinely furnished by the 'informant' at death registration and it is customary for the Registrar General of England and Wales to tabulate this information for years surrounding the census, and to prepare a report on occupational mortality for this period as part of the Decennial Supplement. In 1931 the period 1930–32 was chosen but for the most recent investigation (General Register Office 1958) the period 1949–53 was chosen to enable larger numbers to be deployed; finer analysis could thus be made without diminishing the size of the groups to a point at which the rates become liable to relatively large chance errors.

Age standardization

7.39 It is essential in any comparative study of occupational mortality to standardize for age. A crude death rate based on the total population claiming a particular occupation would be liable to mislead in two ways:

(1) The death rate in occupation *A* might be higher than that in occupation *B* although age for age mortality is higher in *B* simply because for example, *B* happened to be a more youthful population either by virtue of reduced longevity or because it comprised a new occupation of fairly recent recruitment. As an example of the first cause the following figures are of interest.

Average Annual Death Rates per 1,000 *Living at each Age Period* 1910–12

	15–	20–	25–	35–	45–	55–	65–74	All ages 15–74
Farmers	0·5	1·5	3·1	4·6	8·6	20·0	51·3	11·6
Coal miners (hewers and getters)	3·2	3·8	4·4	6·7	12·7	30·1	82·3	9·3

The death rates at each age were higher for coal miners but by the same token they were a younger population than farmers and experienced a lower crude death rate.

(2) The total population claiming a particular occupation will include some too young to have incurred any real measure of occupational risk and many too old to have had any contact with the occupational hazard for many years prior to death (though to exclude them does lessen the weight given to postponed effects). In addition statements of occupation are particularly liable to be misleading for older persons (see p.23).

7.40 It is therefore usual in the Registrar General's investigations to restrict consideration to the occupied and retired population of ages 20–65 (with subsidiary examination of the 35–65 group) and to allow for varying age structure within the range by standardization. Separate examination is made of males, single women and married women. The married women are classified by the occupation of their husbands. This is to provide a means of obtaining an indication of real occupational factors. If the wives show the same excess mortality as the husbands for a particular occupation it is implicit that a general environmental or socio-economic factor is involved rather than a true occupational hazard. The methods of standardization are:

(1) For each occupation a standard population is chosen of the same age distribution as that of the whole census population of the particular

125

group considered (all males, single women or married women) but reduced in total size so that it yields 1,000 deaths when the 'all cause' age specific rates for all males (or single women, etc.) are applied to it. Applying the *actual* age specific rates for the occupation gives an index called the 'comparative mortality figure' which is in fact the ratio of 'actual' to 'expected' deaths (where 'expected' means expected on the basis of 'all males' mortality) in a population of *standard* structure. This method was last employed in the 1921 Report.

(2) Age specific rates based on all males (or single women, etc.) are applied to the census population for the occupation to give a figure of 'standard' deaths and the actual deaths are expressed as a ratio (called the 'standardized mortality ratio') to the 'standard' deaths. This index is a ratio of 'actual' to 'expected' in a population not of standard structure but of a structure typical of the occupation and the term 'standardized' is not strictly appropriate. This method was used in the 1931 and 1951 investigations.

These operations are performed separately over the range 20–65 and 35–65.

7.41 The two indices are normally almost equal, but if the excess mortality is concentrated at the ages where the occupation has relatively greater numbers (than in the all males distribution) the SMR gives more emphasis to this excess than the CMF; on the other hand the CMF is affected by random errors in those age rates of mortality for the particular occupation which are based on small numbers—in the SMR they get only the representation of the small numbers actually at risk but in the CMF they get the full representation of the standard population, e.g. in 1930–32 engine drivers at risk at ages 20–35 formed only 7 per cent of the total at 20–65 compared with 42 per cent in the standard population and the CMF was inflated by high apparent mortality at young ages based on small numbers and suspected of error from faulty occupational description at death registration (see p. 131). On balance the SMR is normally adopted since the greater ease with which it can be computed (on a mass scale) outweighs the risk of minor anomalies.

Occupational differences

7.42 The occupations with the twenty highest SMR's (all causes) among 425 occupational groups in the 1949–53 investigation were—

	SMR 20–64 of men	SMR (20–64) of wives (where given)
Royal Navy—other ranks—retired	826	—
Army—other ranks—retired	556	—
Royal Air Force—other ranks—retired	485	—
Slate workers (n.e.s.); slate masons	467	300
Tunnel miners	225	(50)
Getters (mines) (not coal)	222	149
Armed forces—commissioned officers—retired	189	—
Makers of glass and glassware—blowers (not machine hands or bench glass workers)	189	133
Drivers of horse drawn vehicles	189	170
Labourers and other unskilled workers in —All other industrial and commercial undertakings	186	172

	SMR 20–64 of men	SMR (20–64) of wives (where given)
Haulage contractors and managers	175	168
Sand blasters (excluding shot blasters)	173	96
Machine minders—others	160	123
Managers (n.e.s.)	155	—
Workers in chemical and allied trades —Furnacemen, kilnmen	154	164
In coal mines—Hewers and getters (by hand) —below ground	153	146
Land agents, estate agents	150	165
Publicans, owners, etc., of hotels, inns	150	116
Curriers, leather dressers	149	135
Coal mines—coal face coal getters, loaders	148	143

(n.e.s. = not elsewhere specified)

7.43 Occupations with low mortality included, for example, farmers, farm managers (s MR of males 20–64, 70), foremen, overlookers in metal manufacture and engineering (68), civil service higher officers (60), heads or managers of office departments (55), bankers, bank managers, inspectors (76), teachers (not music) (66), costing and accounting clerks (70).

7.44 For many occupations with low mortality the s MR for the wives was also low, e.g. bankers, bank and insurance managers, etc. (husbands 78 wives 82), teachers (husbands 66, wives 77), clergymen of the Church of England (husbands 81, wives 80) indicating that it was not so much the occupation that was healthy as the level of living associated with the occupation. A similar argument (in the opposite direction) could be extended to some of the high mortality occupations in the 1949–53 analysis, e.g. the s MR for the wives of drivers of horsedrawn vehicles (170), furnacemen, kilnmen in chemical trades (164), labourers (172), but in some instances there was a much greater excess mortality in husbands than in wives, e.g.

Husbands SMR		Wives SMR
173	Sandblasters	96
189	Glass blowers	133
160	Machine minders	123
150	Publicans, etc.	116

and this kind of contrast helps to establish prima facie evidence for closer enquiry.

Socio-economic groups

7.45 The inter-correlations between the various social, economic and cultural factors are so strong that it is dangerous and misleading to study any one in isolation. For this reason many workers have regarded it as an economy of effort to concentrate on a single indication of the general level of living with which all other factors are associated in the same general direction. This indication is usually derived from the one objective characteristic which is most easily, most commonly and most accurately recorded: occupation. Sometimes industry, status (employer, manager, foreman, etc.) and whether or not economically active are also incorporated in the one indicating classification.

7.46 The occupational classification used, for example, in England and Wales comprises several hundred unit groups to which one or more individual occupations are assigned depending upon the description on the census schedule (General Register Office 1960).

7.47 Any one unit will embrace a number of different descriptions, viz. 'Glass formers, finishers and decorators' will include 'Achromatic hand, Acider, Artist (glass-decorating), Assembler (bifocal), Embosser, Mirror backer, Colour bander, Glass-tube bender, Lens blocker, Glass blower, Glass calibrator, Nickel carboniser (valves), Glass cutter, Optical engineer, Knobber, Malletter-on, Sticker-on (lens)' and others.

7.48 Each unit, however, will be broadly homogeneous in respect of the job performed (e.g. manual or non-manual, machine or hand, skill involved) and the conditions in which it is performed (indoor or outdoor, clean or dirty, sedentary or ambulant, heat or cold, long or short hours, seasonal pressure, etc.). For presenting differentials associated with general levels of living, however, it is more practical to group units together. The earliest attempts to do this gave rise to the 'social classes' of the General Register Office:

(i)   Professional etc. occupations
(ii) Intermediate between (i) and (iii)
(iii) Skilled Workers *[(a) Mineworkers (b) Transport Workers (c) Clerical Workers (d) Armed Forces (e) Others]
(iv) Intermediate between (iii) and (iv) *[(a) Agricultural Workers (b) Others]
(v)   Unskilled Workers *[(a) Building and Dock Labourers (b) Others]

7.49 The method here is to attribute to each of the occupations distinguished in the classification a ranking based either on social values (for example, that of standing within the community, such as in Great Britain from the 1911 Census onward) or on a score derived from a battery of such values (as in the United States Census of 1960). This has two disadvantages:

(i)   There is a likelihood that the ranking will be influenced by preconceived notions of just those differentials of health or behaviour which the groupings are to be used to discover.
(ii) It is difficult to provide an economic interpretation of the interrelationships of the groups and other social characteristics because of the abstract and subjective character of the ranking.
(iii) The socio-economic homogeneity of the so-called 'social classes' is limited by the fact that whole occupational units only are assigned to a group irrespective of the circumstances of individual workers coded to that unit.

7.50 Nevertheless the social classes do effect a broad division of the occupied population by economic and social circumstances which are more difficult to describe than to recognize.

7.51 To meet the objection raised against the 'social classes' new socio-economic groups were introduced by the General Register Office at the 1961

* Special splits made for mortality investigation purposes 1950–52.

Census as an alternative grouping to social classes. They represent an improvement in environmental homogeneity.

7.52 The method, which was developed in France (Brichler, 1958) and standardized in the European Working Group on Population Censuses of the Economic Commission for Europe, is to derive groups automatically from a cross-tabulation of the four economic classifications normally used in the population census (1) type of activity (active or inactive and in the latter event the type of inactive group, e.g. hospital inmate, housewife, etc.) (2) occupation (3) employment status (employer, manager, etc.) (4) branch of economic activity (industry).

7.53 The individual cells of such a cross-tabulation represent groups with substantial homogeneity of social and economic characteristics and these can be grouped into broader groups to the extent of contraction in numbers of groups that may be desired. An important feature of these groups is the fact that they are not necessarily ranked in any preconceived order; it is claimed only that they are economically *different* not that one group has higher social standing than another. Clearly in material terms the level of living is higher for one group than another so that some degree of economic ordering is inevitable.

7.54 The European Working Group on Population Census of the UN Economic Commission has subjected this system to close study and have recommended a nominal classification based upon it. The General Register Office classification adopted for the 1961 Census conforms to the ECE list though it excludes groups (e.g. workers' co-operatives) which do not apply in Britain. It comprises:

1. Employers and managers—large establishments
2. Employers and managers—small establishments
3. Professional workers—self employed
4. Professional workers—employees
5. Intermediate non-manual workers
6. Junior non-manual workers
7. Personal service workers
8. Foremen and supervisors—manual
9. Skilled manual workers
10. Semi-skilled manual workers
11. Unskilled manual workers
12. Own account workers (other than professional)
13. Farmers—employers and managers
14. Farmers—own account
15. Agricultural workers
16. Members of armed forces

7.55 If deaths can be similarly classified by social class or socio-economic groups the mortality differentials can be examined. If this can be done within the national vital registration system the statistical investigation can be carried out on a large scale. It must be admitted immediately that this is more difficult for socio-economic groups which require for their identification more characteristics than are normally recorded at the registration of deaths; it is, for example, easier to obtain, from the informants, particulars of the deceased's

E   129

occupation than of his branch of economic activity. But if this form of analysis cannot be applied to a combination of census data (populations) and vital registration records (deaths) it can be applied in *ad hoc* studies.

7.56 At the 1949–53 investigation (General Register Office 1958) the following gradients were discernible:

TABLE 7.3 *England and Wales—Standardized Mortality Ratios*, 1949–53

Ages 20–64	Social Class				
	I	II	III	IV	V
Occupied males	98	86	101	94	118
Single women	82	73	89	89	92
Wives of males in specified social class	96	88	101	104	110

7.57 These social class gradients differed both in steepness and in direction for different causes of death. Causes for which mortality rose steeply with social class (i.e. with *less* favourable economic circumstances) included—

	SMR's (*males* 20–64)				
	I	II	III	IV	V
Respiratory tuberculosis	58	63	102	95	143
Bronchitis	34	53	98	101	171
Pneumonia	53	64	92	105	150
Other myocardial degeneration	68	82	94	101	135
Ulcer of stomach	53	71	98	104	144
Malignant neoplasm, stomach	57	70	101	112	130

while the following are examples of causes apparently associated with comparative affluence—

Acute poliomyelitis	295	171	90	63	42
Leukaemia	123	98	104	93	89
Coronary disease, angina	147	110	105	79	89
Cirrhosis of liver	207	152	84	70	96
Diabetes	134	100	99	85	105
Vascular lesions of nervous system	124	104	101	88	101
Suicide	140	113	89	92	117

and some show very little gradient at all, as for example,

Nephritis and nephrosis	102	98	100	94	105

7.58 For a preliminary version of socio-economic groups used in 1951 the SMR's were as shown in Table 7.4.

Difficulties of interpretation

7.59 The interpretation of occupational mortality data is much more difficult than the mere calculation of the indices, complicated though these may appear. There are a number of sources of error and confusion:

(a) *Vagueness of description and coding difficulties*

Occasional vagueness in the entry of occupation in census returns and death registers places a strain upon the capacity of the coding clerk to make

TABLE 7.4 *Standard Mortality Ratios for Socio-economic Groups* 1949–53

Group (Ages 20–64)	Standardized mortality ratios		
	Occupied males	Wives of males in group	Single women
1. Farmers	70	93	72
2. Agricultural workers	75	95	64
3. Higher administrative, professional and managerial	98	96	82
4. Other administrative, professional and managerial	84	81	70
5. Shopkeepers (including proprietors of wholesale businesses)	100	99	97
6. Clerical workers	109	91	75
7. Shop assistants	84	79	82
8. Personal service	113	101	84
9. Foremen	84	91	86
10. Skilled workers	102	105	109
11. Semiskilled workers	97	108	99
12. Unskilled workers	118	111	103

a 'reproducible' assignment to an occupation unit, i.e. an assignment that would be made by any other coder faced with the same description; there is thus no guarantee that in such circumstances the same assignment would be made for the same person at census and at death. Nor is it certain that in cases of death soon after the census date the same description will be used since the informant may refer to the occupation carried out for the greater part of the lifetime of the deceased rather than to the occupation in which the deceased was most recently engaged. For example a police sergeant who retires comparatively early in life may take up a clerical occupation of a relatively minor character to supplement his pension and give him an active interest; at his death it is very likely that the widow or other relative will still consider him to be a 'retired police sergeant'.

There is also a natural tendency for a householder completing a census schedule to elevate the status of his occupation, and for relatives to do the same at the registration of his death. This may take the form of using a description which implies a higher degree of skill or of supervisory capacity than is in fact applicable. If there were the same degree of elevation at both census and death registration there would be errors in the statistics of an absolute character but differentials would not be distorted. However, it has been found that the conditions under which the census is carried out—the prior propaganda, the instructions and examples on the census schedule, the fact that the occupation entry is only part of a more extended discipline (including reference to industry and workplace)—tend to make the census occupation entries more accurate than those made at registration. The absolute degree of error is not however great at working ages and the situation may generally be summarized by saying that status is slightly exaggerated at the census, is rather more exaggerated at death registration, but that the resultant bias in the direction of raising mortality in the higher grade occupations is not, for the ages for which indices are usually calculated, of serious consequence.

(b) Lack of time reference

The studies of occupational mortality are handicapped by the fact that the information both at census and at death is related in most cases to the immediately antecedent occupation. While the census information probably gives a fair approximation to the mean numbers at risk in the different occupations the deaths will be biased in the direction of lighter occupations to the extent to which failing health may lead workers to foresake heavier for lighter employment. The extent of this error is not known; it is probably corrected to some extent by a tendency, noted above, to refer back to the occupation with which the deceased was associated for most of his life. Ideally, deaths and numbers at risk would be classified by duration of employment but the difficulties of obtaining accurate information even at the census, let alone at death registration, are too great to be overcome with present resources.

(c) Separation of specific occupation factors

Reference has already been made to the difficulty of deciding whether excess mortality is due to occupational risk or general social environment and of the use, for example, of the mortality of wives as a control. The mortality index even thus controlled can do no more than establish a prima facie case for closer study within the particular occupation.

Limitations of occupational mortality investigations

7.60 Having regard to these difficulties it must be appreciated that the occupational mortality investigation associated with the census is a very crude diagnostic tool, giving no exact or final answers but throwing into relief differentials worthy of closer study by more precise methods. In this way the investigations have proved of great value in the past. It is probable that in the future longitudinal studies (viz. following up groups of workers throughout their period of employment) in particular industries under the close supervision of medical field workers will be more efficient in revealing true occupational risks. Such studies would not be confined to mortality risks but would embrace also sickness absence, i.e. they would begin at a point nearer the onset of the occupational influence on health.

For a further account of this problem of measuring social and economic factors in mortality and for an extended bibliography see 'Social and Economic Factors affecting Mortality' Benjamin, B. (1965) Confluence Vol. V. Mouton & Co. The Hague and Paris, 88 pp.

Mortality in different parts of the country

7.61 Within England and Wales it has been shown (General Register Office 1955) that 'levels of mortality (standardized for sex and age) tend to arrange themselves into three broad bands that run across the country from south-west to north-east. The highest levels of mortality are found in most of Wales and in the northern counties of England. Counties with intermediate levels of mortality, both in their urban and their rural components, are distributed in a line running from Cornwall north-westwards through the Midlands and on towards the Humber and the Wash. The third area, of low mortality, starts on the south coast at Dorsetshire and likewise runs north-west to include the home counties and continues on towards East Anglia.' This mortality gradient should not be thought of as purely geographical or climatic variation. It is highly probable that other factors are involved particularly the social and environmental influences already referred to in this chapter.

7.62 The following figures are taken from the *Statistical Review for England and Wales for 1950*, Text Volume (medical):

1951 *Census Data*

	Persons per room			Per cent of males 15 and over (occupied and retired) in Social Classes IV and V
Standard Regions	Urban areas of 50,000 or more population	Other urban areas	Rural areas	
Northern	0·85	0·85	0·78	33·9
East and West Ridings	0·74	0·75	0·74	31·6
North Western	0·74	0·72	0·71	31·0
Wales	0·74	0·70	0·72	34·2
North Midland	0·71	0·70	0·70	30·9
Midland	0·79	0·72	0·74	28·9
Eastern	0·70	0·69	0·67	29·1
London and South Eastern	0·68	0·66	0·65	24·6
Southern	0·71	0·67	0·70	26·1
South Western	0·73	0·65	0·68	27·6

7.63 These figures suggest that the higher mortality of the northern areas is associated with greater housing density and less favourable socio-economic conditions. Account must also be taken of the diminished sunlight and greater atmospheric pollution of the industrial north.

7.64 There is scope for research here to identify the important factors. Probably the most profitable course to pursue would be to draw up categories of various factors, e.g. housing, socio-economic groups, urbanization, atmospheric pollution, etc. and then to make a selection of local areas such that there would be a number fitting (roughly homogeneous in respect of) every cross-combination of these classifications. The mortality variance of these areas could then be analysed to show the relative weight and interdependence of the factors.

REFERENCES

*ANTONOSKY, A. (1967) *Millbank Mem. Fd. Quart.*, 45, 31.
CHALKE, H. B. (1953) *Medical Officer*, 89, 183.
BENJAMIN, B. (1953) *Brit. J. Tub.*, 47, 4.
BENJAMIN, B., and NASH, F. A. (1951) *Tubercle*, 32, 67.

*BENJAMIN, B. (1965) Social and Economic Factors in Mortality Confluence, Vol. V. Mouton, Paris.

FARR, W. (1843) 5th Annual Report of Registrar General, p. 20.

General Register Office (1938) Decennial Supplement, 1931, Part IIa.

General Register Office (1960) Classification of Occupations.

General Register Office (1958) Decennial Supplement, 1951, Part II.

General Register Office (1955) Statistical Review, 1952, Text Volume, p. 67.

NEWSHOLME, A. (1891) *J. of Roy. Stat. Soc.*, 54, 70.

SCOTT, J. A. (1953) *Brit. J. of Soc. and Prev. Med.*, 7, 194.

* Both these references contain extensive bibliographies.

CHAPTER 8

THE MEASUREMENT OF MORBIDITY

The meaning of sickness

8.1 Sickness and health are antitheses and are difficult to define except in terms of each other. A morbid condition is a departure from the normal healthy condition and the prevalence of disease can only be assessed given adequate and practical criteria for defining departure from normality. Stocks (1949) has said 'the distinction between living and dead is clear cut, but no such frontier line between sickness and health can be said to exist except in the case of acute illness caused immediately and directly by an external agent. There is a zone between the two states in which the division whether the subject is sick or not depends on definitions or standards of good health, and also on who decides. It is often said that only a physician is competent to decide what a patient is suffering from; but the patient often has to decide whether or not he is ill at all. If he believes himself to be ill, then he is not in normal health; he is consciously suffering from something and therefore sick. On the other hand a person may think he is well, but on examination for some purpose such as life insurance or by mass radiography it is discovered that he has a disease which may at any time cause disability. From that moment he begins usually to suffer inconvenience, if not actual symptoms and then comes into the category of persons who are sick.' In succeeding chapters we shall review some of the problems and techniques that have arisen in the different modes of measurement of sickness applicable to different definitions of ill-health, and to different agencies identifying the ill-health. Apart from the varying standards of health and diagnosis involved there are a number of different unitary concepts involved. Illness is a condition which continues for a period of time. We may, therefore, consider how many sickness periods (illnesses) began in a specified interval or how many terminated during the interval or how many were current at any time during the interval. We have also to distinguish between persons and illnesses, remembering that a person can have more than one illness within an interval and even at the same point of time. An illness may be a new disease or a recurrence of a disease suffered on some previous occasion. An attempt must be made to define the units used on every occasion; in general the term 'incidence' will relate to the emergence of new cases (a 'flow' concept) and 'prevalence' to the numbers existing at a point of time (a 'stock' concept).

Normality

8.2 It is to a large extent the need for standards by which to assess health that has led to the development of social medicine as a distinct discipline. 'If we are to apply the adjective "normal" to the multitudinous structures and

135

functions of which—together with their co-ordinated activity—health is the composite picture, we must understand better what we mean by it and where possible establish standards and measurements of normality. . . . In man, as in other animals, variation is so constantly at work that no rigid pattern— whether anatomical, physiological, psychological or immunological—is possible. . . . There is . . . for each structure or function what may be called a normal range of variability.' (Ryle, 1948.)

8.3 Ryle refers to clinical errors which have arisen from failure to recognize the normal range of variability, and quotes Martin for two examples: (i) the palpability of epitrochlear glands which is present in forty per cent of adult males though once regarded as a symptom of disease, particularly of syphilis (1947), (ii) myotatic irritability of the pectoral muscles commonly present in healthy individuals (a form of the familiar stretch reflex) though often referred to as a suggestive sign of pulmonary tuberculosis or other debilitating disease (1946). There are many other examples. Von Graafe's sign (lid lag) was once thought to be peculiar to thyrotoxicosis but it is now known to be present in other diseases, especially peptic ulcer, and it has no diagnostic value in relation to its hyperthyroid connections (Jackson 1949). A significant proportion of fit young men exhibit a degree of gastric acidity which at one time would have been regarded as pathological and suggestive of duodenal ulceration (Bennett and Ryle, 1921; Campbell and Conybeare, 1924). In 1946 there was published a survey of a group of young students at Harvard 'who had general all-round "normal" reactions'; some of the medical data (Heath, 1946) are shown in Table 8.1.

TABLE 8.1 *Data for 'Normal' Students*

Measurement	No. of individuals	Mean	Range
Pulse: recumbent	259	66·1	40—96
Blood pressure, recumbent mm.Hg.			
systolic	265	114·9	98—146
diastolic	265	71·7	40—92
Red blood cells			
(millions/cu.mm.)	254	5·04	4·25—5·60
Haemoglobin (per cent)	255	97·4	85·4—107·8
Blood sugar (mg. per cent)	147	100·0	84—125
Respiratory ventilation			
(litres/min.)	209	7·0	3·5—14·4

8.4 Though blood pressure tends to rise with advancing age it is difficult to say when this is pathological even though safety margins may be reduced. Hobson and Pemberton (1955) found that in a random sample of old people living at home forty-three per cent had a resting diastolic blood pressure of 100 millimetres of mercury or over and most of these were 'in good health'. Blood pressures fitted a normal curve and the dispersion as indicated by the mean $\pm$ twice the standard deviation was (mm. of Hg):

	Males	Females
Systolic	107·3—236·9	117·4—250·6
Diastolic	55·4—127·4	66·2—131·8

'There was no significant correlation between height of the systolic or diastolic blood pressure and vertigo, tinnitus, angina of effort, clinically detectable arteriosclerosis, radiological size of heart, the subject's well being and activity or albuminuria.' The normal ranges of biochemical values found in elderly males are shown in Table 8.2 (similar variation was found in females):

TABLE 8.2 *Data for Elderly Males*

	No. of subjects	Mean	Dispersion (± 2 s.d.)*
Haemoglobin (g/100 ml)	177	14·4	10·8—17·9
Serum calcium (mg/100 ml)	35	10·1	9·0—11·2
Serum cholesterol (mg/100 ml)	98	268	176—409
Serum Alkaline Phosphatese (K.A. units)	64	8·3	2·7—25·5
Blood urea (mg/100 ml)	50	39·1	26·4—57·8

* Dispersion calculated on lognormal scale and converted into ordinary values.

8.5 The human eye provides an interesting example of successful correlation between elements which vary freely over quite a wide range; though the various components of the optic system (axial length, depth of anterior chamber, refractive power of lens, refractive power of cornea) are each distributed Normally in the population, the distribution of total optical refraction is not normal but is very sharply peaked—the long eye tends to get a flat cornea and lens (Sorsby, Davey, Sheridan, Tanner and Benjamin, 1957).

Abnormality

8.6 It is the successful adaptation of the complex human organism as a whole to the particular variates of composition and function with which it is endowed and to the external environment in which it has to survive that constitutes good health. Account must also be taken of the need to adapt to physical and emotional stresses, and to environmental changes. This adaptation is essential to stability and survival, but it is not satisfactory to measure sickness simply by failure to survive, though in the last resort, e.g. in underdeveloped countries where morbidity statistics are deficient, mortality may be used as an index of general health. Departure from the well-being that constitutes good adaptation is usually identified as 'the point at which either (*a*) the subject began to be conscious of symptoms or some disability or (*b*) someone else decided that disease was present of a nature which could not continue to be ignored without danger to the patient' (Stocks, 1949).

8.7 In the chapters which follow we shall describe the various sources of information about the incidence and prevalence of disease and the measures appropriate to these different sources. It will become clear that the measurement of sickness involves not only the definition of a standard of good health but also differences in concept according to the person making the observations. The *kind* of sickness certified by the general practitioner is different from the kind of sickness complained of by the person interviewed in a sickness survey carried out by lay interviewers; the kinds of sickness pleaded as a

E*

reason for absence from work or recorded in hospital inpatient studies are also different from other kinds of sickness. No measure of sickness should be separated from the conditions of observation.

8.8 It should be borne in mind that a gap still exists between the concept of disease as a wide dispersion of conditions, ranging from some unknown limit of 'health' to a very definite limit of death, and the available indicators of disease incidence and prevalence. Where in the corresponding time scale between incipience of abnormality and death, do the indicators have their reference point? What is the relative sensitivity of the indicators to changes in the well-being of the population? What correlation is there between them? There is still a wide field for research and experimentation, in which a primary part will be played by the 'longitudinal' study, i.e. the carefully controlled follow up of a group of 'healthy' persons of well defined social characteristics in whom the emergence of disease may be closely observed and recorded in its detailed presentation and in proper relation to biological and external environmental factors which may be involved in causation, in the rate of development, or in the possibility of reversion.

8.9 There is a field for research in the development of concepts and definitions for disease measurement. The Statistics Sub-Committee of the Registrar General's Advisory Committee on Medical Nomenclature and Statistics has examined the problem of defining morbidity measures (1954) in two stages: (i) the choice of descriptive words, e.g. the substitution, for the general term 'sickness', of words more specifically describing the character of the condition measured, such as 'sickness absence', 'inpatient care', 'general practitioner consultation'; the substitution of 'inception' (to indicate 'beginning') for 'incidence' which is too broad in current usage; (ii) classification and definition of rates, i.e. distinction between rates relating to inception, prevalence, duration, and fatality respectively. In each case the rate is given a full definition and a short title. In the succeeding chapters reference is made to new cases of disease occurring in a period (inception), to cases of disease existing at a point of time (prevalence), to sickness absence (duration), to frequency rates of consultation. It is important that all such measures should be subjected to close scrutiny in order to ascertain whether their meaning is sufficiently explicit and is capable of precise definition, whether they are the most convenient to calculate, and whether they are most adapted to the purposes for which they were devised. The language of disease measurement is constantly evolving and there is considerable scope for improvement in precision.

8.10 It is essential also that any advance in morbidity measurement should be related to utility. The development of soundly based theoretical concepts is vital to the production of meaningful indices of morbidity. But these indices, and the means whereby the data for their production is derived, must be adapted to such administrative and clinical needs as they are ultimately required to satisfy. These needs include the administration and planning of medical services of all kinds including the assessment of the efficacy of such services and preventive as well as curative medicine. They include the administration of social security services and welfare services in industry. There must be a proper balance between the content of the morbidity measure, the labour in its construction, its use value and not least, the time factor in its release.

Medical records and form design

8.11 It should be borne in mind that all vital and health statistics emanate, at the earliest stages, from symbols written or marks made on paper. If the forms provided are badly designed then the reaction of those responsible for completing them (and nobody *likes* form-filling) will be one of antipathy, with the result that the quality of the recording will suffer. If the questions are illogically arranged in order or ambiguous in meaning then answers may be either incapable of interpretation or frankly inaccurate; and no amount of refinement in later statistical analysis can remedy such defects in the original data.

8.12 In hospital this matter is treated so seriously that there is usually an officer (often designated a medical records officer) specially trained to be responsible for clinical documentation and the custody of medical records. It is his job to see that form design, filing equipment, and coding and classification procedures are maintained at a high standard. A considerable body of technical experience has been built up [Huffman, 1955]. Local health authorities, in the main, have not yet placed sufficient specialized emphasis on the physical conditions necessary to the production of good basic data.

8.13 A few principles of documentation form design may be set down.

(1) *There must be someone to write.*

It is a mistake to think that statistics can be extracted from any aspect of a health service without the expenditure of clerical labour. If the statistics are essential (and they should not be collected otherwise) then this labour must be provided. As there is a limit to the amount of clerical work a clinician or nurse can undertake without detriment to their primary function—medical care—the necessity for clerical assistance should be carefully examined.

(2) *There must be room to write.*

It is useless to expect information to be provided if the space available cannot accommodate even the strict essentials, or if it is tucked away in a corner where it is overlooked.

(3) *The arrangement must be logical.*

Co-operation by respondents will be at the highest level if the dynamic items on the form (i.e. those with a time sequence) follow the natural order in which the events or examinations described took place, and if the static items (invariant with time) are grouped by the proper association of ideas, e.g. items relating to social conditions (occupation, housing, education, etc.) should all be close together. This is especially essential if more than one page is involved since nothing is more irritating than to have to turn pages backward and forward during the taking of a history.

(4) *The content should be minimal and the form should not outlive its usefulness.*

If it can be made apparent that only the essential minimum of information is being sought over the shortest possible time then a bond of confidence will be established between the statistical office and field workers that will be reflected in the quality of the data collected.

(5) *The amount of actual writing should be minimal.*

Where progress notes are required guidance should be given to

139

discourage unnecessary verbosity. Sometimes respondents feel they must write a long story and in doing so omit salient facts. For other types of information the fullest use should be made of self-coding questions which involve only the ticking or ringing of numbers. This principle has assumed much greater importance now that medical records with the aid of computers are being subjected to more extensive statistical analysis. The problem here is one of achieving selective and easy input to the computer. A good deal of the narrative part of a medical record is often irrelevant to statistical analysis however important to actual management of the patient and the selection of information *relevant* to measurement must be made easy. Processing the input to the computer —the sheer conversion of figures written on the record to their magnetic counterparts on tape (including coding operations) is the slowest and costliest part of data-processing and efforts devoted to facilitating this stage (especially mark sensing devices to render manual card punching unnecessary) will pay dividends. It is advisable to seek expert help from the systems analyst associated with the computer installation.

(6) *Paper of the right size and quality should be used.*

Undue compression and excessive size are equally to be avoided, the former for reasons given under (2), the latter on grounds not only of economy but of convenience. If forms have to be folded to be put into a health visitor's bag or into filing cabinets they will suffer. If the form has to last several years it must be of paper strong enough to withstand hard wear.

(7)   Where records are fed into a system involving records of similar medical institutions (e.g. the hospital service) it is essential, if the word 'system' is to have any meaning, for there to be a high degree of standardization. Otherwise comparability between institutions will be impaired if not impossible and costs of data-processing will be raised by inability to apply standard procedures.

REFERENCES

ACHESON, E. D. (1967) Medical Record Linkage, Oxford University Press.

BENNETT, T. I., and RYLE, J. A. (1921) Guy's Hospital Rep., 71.286.

CAMPBELL, J. M. H., and CONYBEARE, J. J. (1924) Guy's Hosp. Rep., 74.354.

Central Health Services Council (1965) The standardization of Hospital Medical Records. Report of Standing Med. Advis. Comm. H.M.S.O.

General Register Office (1954) *Studies on Med. and Pop. Subjects*, No. 8. Measurement of Morbidity, H.M.S.O.

HEATH, C. W. (1946) *What People are: A Study of Normal Young Men*, Harvard University Press, 1946.

HOBSON, W., and PEMBERTON, J. (1955) *The Health of the Elderly at Home*. Butterworths, London.

HUFFMAN, E. K. (1955) *Manual for Medical Record Librarians*, 4th Ed. Physicians' Record Company, Chicago.

JACKSON, W. P. U. (1949) *Brit. Med. J.*, ii, 847.

MARTIN, L. (1946) *Brit. J. Tub.*, 40.49.

MARTIN, L. (1947) *Lancet*, i. 363.

RYLE, J. A., *Changing Disciplines*, Oxford University Press, 1948.

SORSBY, A., DAVEY, J. B., SHERIDAN, M., TANNER, J. M., and BENJAMIN, B., (1957) Med. Res. Co. Spec. Rep. Ser. 293.

STOCKS, P. (1949) 'Sickness in the Population of England and Wales 1944–47'. General Register Office, *Studies on Med. and Pop. Subjects*, No. 2. H.M.S.O.

CHAPTER 9

STATISTICS OF INFECTIOUS DISEASES

History

9.1 Compulsory notification of infectious diseases was first introduced in England and Wales at Huddersfield in 1876. A year later Bolton followed this example. Many other towns soon obtained powers to compel notification by local act and in 1889 a general act, the Infectious Diseases (Notification) Act was passed giving powers to all local authorities to compel notification if they so desired. Ten years later these powers ceased to be merely permissive but became obligatory throughout the country.

9.2 This legislative achievement can be regarded as the culmination of a very long struggle which appears to have begun at least as early as the beginning of the eighteenth century if not before (Newsholme, 1896) when a series of attempts to establish registration of sickness began. Dr Clifton in 1732 urged the registration of illness with special reference to hospitals asking that factual reports should be made, at periodical intervals, of the cases treated. Dr Rumsey, in 1844, in his evidence before the Medical Poor Relief Committee of the House of Commons [1875] suggested a comprehensive plan for the uniform registration of the sickness which affected the poorer classes. In 1848 a Dr Liddle proposed amended forms for the weekly medical returns made by medical officers of Poor Law Institutions to local Boards of Guardians who governed them and the utilization of these returns in general sanitary enquiries. This suggestion was taken up and discussion took place in the medical press of the time of the possibility that the returns might, with suitable modifications, be employed as a basis for the national registration of disease, especially in the recording of epidemics.

9.3 Dr Richardson (later Sir Benjamin W. Richardson) actually operated a scheme for notification and registration of sickness; he collected reports from forty or more doctors, widely distributed over England and Wales and Scotland. These reports were recorded on forms which were posted to them each quarter. Unfortunately Dr Richardson found the work involved more than he could sustain and in the absence of official support and assistance, the scheme of notification was discontinued. This personal pioneer effort was followed by a short-lived co-operative scheme organized by the Metropolitan Association of Health Officers, in 1857, to record sickness attended by Poor Law medical officers, whether in hospitals and dispensaries and workhouses or outdoor cases. The returns were contributed voluntarily by the medical officers. The then General Board of Health undertook to print and circulate the weekly and quarterly tables, and meteorological tables were appended to each publication. Less than half of the medical officers, however, submitted these returns and official publication ceased in the following year. A similar but more complete and longer sustained effort was made in 1860 by the Sanitary Association of Manchester and Salford.

9.4 In 1860 a committee of the Social Service Association passed a resolution recommending the substitution, as vacancies occurred, for the existing non-scientific superintendent registrars of births and deaths of highly qualified medical superintendents, whose duties should include not only registration of births and deaths but also registration of sickness attended at the public expense and, as far as possible, that of sickness attended at public institutions.

9.5 From 1862 the British Medical Association took an active interest. In 1868 a number of local experiments were made in the registration of sickness occurring in public practice, and in 1869 they sent a deputation to the President of the Poor Law Board to emphasize the value of the returns, and of the advantages of this general adoption. In 1874 an appeal was made to the Government for the establishment of a 'National System of Registration of Disease', in the form of a memorial to the Local Government Board. But as Newsholme (1896) commented 'the inertia of officialdom appears to have prevented any practical steps being taken'. Sickness registration was not a measure which it was profitable to pursue in the stress of political party strife, and it was pushed aside for more urgent and politically more attractive schemes. One by one the local voluntary returns died out.

9.6 Then came a reorientation, perhaps a narrowing, in outlook. For about this time Medical Officers of Health in various parts of the country were complaining that their preventive measures were too late; that epidemic diseases had obtained a firm foothold before deaths brought their prevalence to public notice; the desirability of compulsory notification of infectious diseases to meet this difficulty was urged and eventually permitted, at first by Local Acts.

9.7 One of the chief engineers of compulsory notification, Dr Tatham, recorded (1888) as principal advantages arising from notification in his own borough of Salford, the increased proportion of cases admitted to hospital, the subsequent disinfection of places and things, control of school attendance of infectious children, increased detection of sources of infection. Considerable further pressure had to be organized by Dr Tatham before the General Act of 1889 was finally passed.

9.8 Dr Tatham (1888) regarded as complementary to compulsory notification, 'the establishment of a national system of disease registration, limited in the first instance to that of dangerous infectious disease'. He regretted that 'no machinery at present exists by which the information locally collected may be published and rendered generally available'. Dr Tatham had in fact collected information from thirty-two towns and had not only prepared the tables but had printed them on his own copy press. The principal object appeared to be that 'sanitary authorities of one "notification" town may be warned in time of the approach of any infectious disease from other towns of the country'. On the whole Dr Tatham appears to have worked only toward this narrow objective; total morbidity measurement, the complete assessment of ill health in the community, as it now enters into discussions of vital statistics was hardly then envisaged. This is not evidence of narrowness of vision but of the preoccupation with the practical politics and difficulties of medical administration at that time.

9.9 The avowed purpose of notification of infectious disease was to enable a community to 'protect itself against incursions of infectious disease' and to control local outbreaks when they occurred. The object was directly and immediately administrative—to enable the Medical Officer of Health to take some action calculated effectively to restrict the spread of infection, for example to disinfect buildings and clothing, to detect and isolate infectious persons, and to detect and destroy non-human sources of infection.

9.10 The notification of infectious disease is at present governed by the Public Health Act 1936 as amended by the National Health Service Act 1946. The normal method of making a disease notifiable within this legislation is for the Minister of Health to issue a regulation (after consultation). The following diseases are at present notifiable in England and Wales:

Tuberculosis	Whooping cough	Smallpox
Typhoid fever	Meningococcal infection	Measles
Cholera	Plague	Typhus
Dysentery	Leprosy	Malaria
Food poisoning	Anthrax	Scabies
Erysipelas	Poliomyelitis	Puerperal pyrexia
Diphtheria	Encephalitis	Pneumonia

9.11 The form of notification is a matter for local design but a model recommended by the Ministry of Health is usually followed.

Methods of dissemination and recording

9.12 When a disease is made reportable it is necessary to consider a number of related problems, viz. (i) to whom should the disease be reported? (ii) what should be done by way of publication or other means to bring the information to the notice of those who are interested in the facts available? (iii) what statistical organization is necessary?

9.13 In order to take local measures in relation to cases of disease occurring within his own area the Medical Officer of Health is empowered to require that such cases should be reported directly to him in sufficient detail of type of disease, age, sex and place of residence. Though his officers can then take appropriate action upon receipt of this information the Medical Officer of Health will, for better appraisal of the epidemic spread and of the success or failure of his methods, require that cases in the same family be brought together in one record and that some means be contrived to enable him to visualize the chronological and geographical distribution of cases of the particular disease observed. It is then usually desirable that notifications should be recorded in a loose-leaf register or vertical card index with all cases in the same household on the same sheet or card in order of occurrence in time and the sheets and cards arranged by date of first case and street of residence. It would be necessary to make a periodical census of cases and this would be facilitated by the keeping of a running daily record of new cases which could be totalled at weekly intervals. So far as geographical distribution of cases is concerned it might be considered desirable to supplement the register by means of an epidemiological spot map to illustrate visually the paths of spread of the disease. Where food-borne disease is involved it might be

143

advisable to keep a card index of all food establishments in the area and to record on the one card the series of outbreaks in which such an establishment has been involved. Similarly it might be advisable to keep a register of factories or offices to record the results of periodical mass radiography surveys for tuberculosis. In this way establishments requiring special supervision are quickly revealed.

9.14 Medical Officers of Health of other areas will require to be made aware that the outbreak has occurred, and whether (a) it is an outbreak which has not yet reached his area but is likely to do so—this can be estimated by the magnitude of the outbreak and rapidity of development; or whether (b) it is part of a general outbreak in which his area is already involved; or whether (c) it indicates an independent spread from a fresh focus. This does not only apply to medical officers of contiguous areas but in these days of extended communication also to medical officers of remote areas.

9.15 The most economical method of disseminating the information over the widest possible field (including the *international* field) is the publication of a regular epidemiological bulletin summarizing the incidence of disease in all the individual areas. The minimum essential information comprises the number of new cases of a particular disease in a particular district in a given interval of time. The district should be the smallest practicable area and there will necessarily be a compromise between specificity and digestibility of the published bulletin. The interval of time should be the shortest practical unit in order to reduce to a minimum the average length of time between the earliest case included in the bulletin and the publication of the bulletin, i.e. the average staleness of the information. In practice a week is the minimum interval. Advantage has to be taken of the most efficient kind of organization to reduce to an absolute minimum the lapse of time between the end of the interval and the appearance of the bulletin.

9.16 At present the nearest approach to this ideal is provided by the statistics of notification of infectious disease at present published in the body of the weekly return of the Registrar General of England and Wales (a similar publication is issued by the Registrar General of Scotland). It would be an advantage also if less frequently, say, monthly, a bulletin were issued conveying comments and notes by the local Medical Officers of Health upon the important outbreaks during the preceding month including an account of any special action taken and the results of that action. This would eventually add meaning to the weekly figures allowing those reviewing the figures to distinguish true epidemic outbreaks from sporadic and unconnected cases which happen to occur close together in time.

9.17 For epidemiological study and research as distinct from day to day control more detailed information must be brought together and analysed in a refined manner. The various kinds of analyses will be illustrated later.

Responsibility for notification

9.18 Traditionally notification has been made the responsibility of the clinician who either in private practice or in hospital first makes the diagnosis of a notifiable disease. With the extension of pathological facilities there has been a tendency in the observation of many diseases for example in streptococcal infection, meningitis, food poisoning, typhoid, dysentery and tuberculosis to await laboratory confirmation or specification of organism before notification is made.

Present purposes

9.19 The purposes of infectious disease notification under present conditions are—

- (*a*) Access to treatment; the use of notifications to plan allocation of beds or to make a case for the provision of buildings or treatment facilities not hitherto provided.
- (*b*) Local administrative action
  - (i) isolation of infectious cases or sources of infection
  - (ii) prophylaxis
  - (iii) disinfection
  - (iv) after-care
- (*c*) Medical intelligence
  - (i) epidemic control
  - (ii) morbidity indices
- (*d*) Epidemiological research
- (*e*) Diagnostic study

9.20 Objects (*b*) (i), (ii), (iii) and (*c*) (i) are directly administrative and preventive while (*d*) though primarily statistical in character holds the key to local preventive action in the future. Object (*b*) (iv) is not preventive in relation to infectious disease but may reduce the morbidity from sequelae; (*c*) (ii) also is not specific to infectious disease but represents the exploitation of notification statistics by health authorities in the wider purposes of preventive medicine.

(a) Treatment

9.21 If it be part of the public health policy to regard a disease as requiring active medical treatment (apart from isolation) either owing to the danger of the disease itself or of secondary infections then certain problems immediately arise. In the first place recognition of the disease must be encouraged— recognition of dangerous symptoms by the sufferers themselves in order that they may seek medical treatment (this touches upon the field of health education in which notification may play part) and recognition by medical practitioners. We will return to this again in considering object (*e*). Here we consider one particular aspect namely the need for some statistical measure of the extent to which this recognition is successful in different areas at different times. It is evident, for example, from the capricious behaviour of the ratio of notifications to deaths of dysentery in England and Wales that recognition of the disease has been, in recent years, enhanced by improved pathological facilities (Glover 1947). Table 9.1 demonstrates the increased notification that, in the light of the mortality trend must have arisen from earlier examination of stools (with improved pathological facilities) and more efficient detection of Shigella. In this particular example and in others where laboratory tests are of prime importance it must be asked whether nominal records of cases or even numerical measures of incidence are necessary; it could be argued that laboratory activity itself might measure the successful prosecution of the drive for better diagnosis and further, that the fact of there being some positive findings (without exact or complete numerical expression) in an area would be sufficient indication of the presence of disease.

9.22 The problem goes beyond this stage however, for it may be assumed that where the possible sequelae are sufficiently dangerous to make early recognition and treatment a matter of vital importance, then hospital treatment, at least initially, is implied. This being so, there are two aspects. The positive aspect is that of measuring the total incidence and the proportion

TABLE 9.1 *Notified cases, deaths and the ratio of notifications of deaths of Dysentery; and deaths from Enteritis and Diarrhoea—England and Wales 1931–60*

Year	Notified Cases	Dysentery deaths	Ratio of Notifications to deaths	Diarrhoea and Enteritis deaths
1931	836	95	8·8	5,439
1932	924	109	8·5	5,912
1933	783	75	10·4	5,850
1934	763	85	9·0	4,912
1935	1,177	95	12·4	4,998
1936	1,333	72	18·5	5,183
1937	4,167	111	37·5	5,156
1938	4,170	112	37·2	4,968
1939	1,941	96	20·2	4,341
1940	2,860	185	15·5	4,433
1941	6,670	329	20·3	4,654
1942	7,296	198	36·8	4,926
1943	7,905	124	63·8	4,927
1944	13,000(a)	157	82·8	5,018
1945	16,247	165	98·5	5,337
1946	7,870	121	65·0	4,923
1947	3,761	81	46·4	5,859
1948	5,804	61	83·3	3,505
1949	4,519	40	113·0	3,122
1950	17,271	60	287·8	1,765
1960	5,161	1	(b)	189

(a) Corrected notifications are shown from 1944—prior to 1944 the notifications shown are original notifications uncorrected for changes in diagnosis.

(b) Deaths (4) insufficient for ratio to have any meaning.

successfully admitted to hospital; and of the concomitant estimation of the hospital facilities required to sustain this programme. The negative aspect, when the disease has been practically eliminated as in the case of smallpox or diphtheria in some areas, is that of being vigilant and sure of the situation; and certain that no more than minimal reserve clinical facilities *are* in fact necessary. Table 9.2 shows for the County of London from 1931 to 1947 the notified cases of scarlet fever and the proportion hospitalized; and the incidence of and reserve bed accommodation for smallpox. In spite of the introduction of sulphonamide treatment the proportion of cases of scarlet fever admitted to hospital was not materially reduced prior to 1941 but after the commencement of bombardment the shortage of beds compelled a review of policy and severe restriction of admission. The proportion fell in 1941 but rose again as the quieter conditions of 1942 permitted relaxation of restrictions. At the end of the war however the former policy of encouraging admission was finally abandoned and the proportion of cases fell sharply. It is difficult to follow the statistics after 1947 because the National Health Service Act took the fever hospitals out of the control of the Medical Officer of Health and transferred them to Regional Boards covering areas not coincident with county boundaries.

TABLE 9.2 *County of London—Incidence and hospitalization of Scarlet Fever and Smallpox*

		Scarlet Fever		Smallpox	
Year	*Notified cases*	*Admissions to LCC* fever hospitals*	*Ratio of admissions to cases per cent*	*Notified cases*	*Reserve bed accommodation*
1931	12,025	10,752	89	1,452	1,898
1932	14,119	12,771	90	1,131	1,898
1933	21,911	19,909	91	531	1,898
1934	18,238	15,434	85	144	1,898
1935	10,954	9,667	88	—	1,898
1936	10,705	9,394	87	—	1,850
1937	8,455	7,225	85	—	1,850†
1938	8,093	6,932	86	—	200
1939	5,677	4,835	85	—	200
1940	2,498	2,117	85	—	200
1941	2,372	1,798	76	—	200
1942	4,416	3,773	85	2	200
1943	9,477	7,447	79	—	200
1944	4,153	3,061	74	2	200
1945	4,252	2,385	56	3	200‡
1946	4,595	2,180	48	2	200
1947	4,560	1,534	34	3	200

* Direct admissions excluding cases admitted by transfer for convalescence.

† During the year one of the larger hospitals held in reserve for smallpox was in process of conversion to general hospital accommodation.

‡ After the 1939–45 war the LCC made a contractual arrangement with Surrey County Council for London smallpox cases to be admitted to East Clandon, Surrey, Isolation Hospital and the reserve must be regarded as nominal.

9.23 Which diseases fall within the class which we are discussing? There are infectious diseases with chronic phases, such as tuberculosis, requiring long term clinical supervision with possibly prolonged intervening periods of hospital treatment; and diseases like poliomyelitis in which treatment in the acute stage is less specific than palliative but where institutional care is considered desirable in the rehabilitation of paralytic cases; while for diseases like smallpox or diphtheria which require urgent hospital treatment when they occur but which do not occur often, statistical measurement is a necessary prerequisite of the fixing of the minimum bed reserve for the contingency of outbreaks. The figures in Table 9.2 show how it was possible in 1937 to safely reduce the reserve for smallpox in the LCC area.

9.24 Finally there are a group of common fevers which were at one time treated in hospital to a considerable extent but which are now very largely treated in the home; these are diseases like whooping cough, measles and scarlet fever where the risk of secondary infection was formidable but is now reduced to minimal proportions by the specific action of antibiotics on the one hand and by the general improvement in the innate resources of children on the other. Advances in nutritional standards no less than the protective qualities of chemotherapy have played their part in the dramatic fall in the secondary morbidity of the common fevers.

9.25 Another aspect to be considered apart from the provision of beds is the provision of facilities for confirmation of diagnoses where the disease is uncommon and individual clinicians necessarily have restricted experience; as for example with smallpox or rickettsial diseases.

(b) (i) *Isolation*

9.26 It is a fundamental teaching of epidemiology and an inescapable responsibility of those charged with the *control* of communicable disease that sources of infection should be identified and further passage of the infecting organism to susceptible hosts should be prevented. The kind of action indicated may vary. Where sewers are polluting water supplies as perhaps in a typhoid outbreak the chain of infection is broken by purely mechanical repair of the drainage system and purification of the water supply. In the case of a healthy carrier of say amoebic dysentery an attack upon the organism— disturbance of the symbiosis—is made by chemotherapy. Where clinical disease is present the reduction of infectivity is an inseparable concomitant of treatment, as for example in venereal disease. In this instance as in others reduction of infectiousness may be so rapid as to render physical isolation of the infected person unnecessary. In tuberculosis however the bacilli cannot be so easily destroyed and it is necessary to either keep the patient from conveying bacilli to other people by isolating him or at least teaching him to place a barrier of hygiene between himself and his contacts. Grenville-Mathers and Trenchard (1953) have shown a marked decline in the tuberculin conversion rate of children in tuberculosis households when hygiene measures have been instituted in respect of the index (original) infectious case. Though the effects of chemotherapy have been outstanding the segregation of infectious cases has been a major factor in the reduction of morbidity from tuberculosis in this century. In most of these various forms of action there is a common difficulty that the diagnosing practitioner cannot take adequate action upon his own resources; either the resources are insufficient or there is not enough time. Other resources and help from other authorities have to be enlisted, either in the detection of the focus or dealing with it. Thus some system of reporting becomes essential.

9.27 There are some diseases, e.g. poliomyelitis, or measles, or the common cold where the organism is so widespread and the vectors so numerous that control over an epidemic in the community is difficult to achieve. There are too many routes of infection on the one hand and on the other, the primary case cannot be diagnosed in time sufficiently to restrict transmission.

(b) (ii) *Prophylaxis*

9.28 There are some diseases where it has been found practicable and economic to attempt to prevent the spread of infection by reducing the number of susceptibles, i.e. by active immunization. Within this class fall smallpox, tetanus, typhoid, diphtheria, tuberculosis, and whooping cough. [Prophylactic control over typhus, and plague for emigrants or the Armed Forces, must not be overlooked but this hardly affects notification in England and Wales.] In the case of diphtheria it is at present necessary to regard the risk of infection as ever present and to pursue a total compaign which has as its object the immunization of every baby in the first year of life, and re-immunization at school entry. Local registers of personal immunization histories with records of attacks of disease are an essential part of the measures taken to ensure the efficacy of this campaign.

9.29 In England and Wales the Ministry of Health requires every local health authority to prepare a six-monthly return of diphtheria immunizations carried out at different ages in order that the total volume of immunization may be correlated with the number of children estimated to be reaching these ages. Thus, over the whole year 1965 in England and Wales 767,718 primary immunizations were carried out. It was estimated that 56 per cent of children under the age of 16 remained protected.

9.30 In order to estimate the current immunity state in each local area the Ministry also calls for an annual return (Fig. 9.1). From these returns it is

Fig. 9.1 Immunization return.

FORM D.I.1.

DIPHTHERIA IMMUNIZATION
ANNUAL RETURN FOR YEAR ENDED
DECEMBER 31, 1963

LOCAL HEALTH AUTHORITY

C.C.

C.B.C.

This Return should be made by the Medical Officer of Health after he has ascertained the corrected notifications for the calendar year and the number of death registrations transferred to and from the Authority's area by the General Register Office

I. IMMUNIZATION IN RELATION TO CHILD POPULATION

Number of children at December 31, 1963, who had completed a course of Immunization at any time before that date (i.e. at any time since January 1, 1949)

Age at 31.12.63, i.e., Born in Year	Under 1 1963	1—4 1962–1959	5—9 1958–1954	10—14 1953–1949	Under 15 Total
Last complete course of injections (whether primary or booster) A. 1959–1963	22,500	150,000	100,000	80,000	352,500
B. 1958 or earlier	—	—	60,000	100,000	160,000
C. Estimated mid-year child population	50,000	200,000	500,000		750,000
Immunity Index 100A/C	45	75	68		47

149

possible to see not only what proportion of the children in each age group have at some time completed a course of immunization but also to what extent these immunizations are either recent and therefore of high protective value or were made so long ago that the antibody production may have become seriously diminished. In the example shown (the figures are hypothetical) we may see that although 512,500 of the children under age fifteen or 68 per cent have received courses of immunization, only 352,500 or 47 per cent have had these injections in the last five years. The duration of the protective effect of injections of antigen and the manner in which it diminishes with time is not precisely known and probably varies with the individual child; immunity may fall off gradually immediately after injection or it may remain sustained for a number of years and then diminish rapidly, but a conservative approach would suggest that injections carried out more than five years previously should be ignored in assessing the total immunity state of the local child population. This arbitrary convention has been followed in calculating the indices shown at the foot of the return.

9.31 In an immunization scheme which is entirely voluntary there will always be pockets of resistance, and, in a mobile population, there are likely to be localities where groups of children have missed supervision and re-immunization; in such circumstances it is vital that local outbreaks should be reported (particularly in relation to school attendance rather than residence) so that rapid investigation of the local immunization level can be made and, if necessary, emergency measures taken.

9.32 The Report of the Chief Medical Officer of the Ministry of Health for 1951 (1953) gives an account of three outbreaks of diphtheria. In two of these the districts had been free of clinical evidence of infection for at least a year. 'The investigation revealed close links between almost all cases and the carriers detected had all been in close contact with patients. The epidemics were fairly quickly controlled once the carriers had been detected and treated and other contacts immunized or given boosting doses.' The report says 'The need for early examination and swabbing of all close contacts is especially emphasized by the history of the second outbreak. If the carriers . . . had been detected immediately after the occurrence of the first case, and the possibility of skin infection considered, this outbreak might have been curtailed.' The third outbreak was in an area where the disease has never been eradicated and was also combated by the 'vigorous cleaning up of carriers and immunization of children'. Such control by the health authority cannot take place without the reporting of individual cases to form the basis of carrier detection and contact tracing.

9.33 Notification is also necessary to provide statistical appraisal of the success of an immunization campaign; proof of efficacy will not only be demanded by the administering authority and the public who pay for the campaign but will also be necessary to induce successive generations of mothers to participate. Table 9.5 is taken from the text of the *Annual Statistical Review of the Registrar General for England and Wales for 1948–49* (1953) and illustrates the kind of demonstration required.

9.34 For smallpox it has been customary, despite a much reduced risk of importation of the disease into the country, to encourage the routine vaccination of babies partly because the associated reaction is then milder than if the process is postponed to adult ages but mainly because it provides a basic immunity which will last for many years and can readily be boosted when required. If, however, a ring of insusceptible population is to be placed round an outbreak sufficiently promptly then there must be widespread notification of the appearance of infection so that neighbouring authorities may be warned in time.

TABLE 9.3 *Comparative Rates of Diphtheria Notifications and Deaths in* 1949, *per* 100,000 *children who were returned as having been Immunized and as not having been Immunized before the end of* 1949—*England and Wales*

Immunized	1—4	5—14	Total under 15
Number of children	1,843,964	4,315,015	6,229,318
Number of notifications	119	296	417
Number of deaths	4	1	5
Rates:			
Notified cases per 100,000	6	7	7
Deaths per 100 cases	3	0	1
Not immunized			
Number of children	1,148,036	1,545,985	3,332,682
Number of notifications	324	556	909
Number of deaths	37	23	62
Rates:			
Notified cases per 100,000	28	36	27
Deaths per 100 cases	11	4	7

9.35 So far as the statistical appraisal of vaccination is concerned it is useful to relate the new vaccinations carried out in each year at, say, ages under two years to the corresponding population of the same ages. For 1965 in England and Wales the annual returns made to the Ministry of Health by local health authorities showed that the total number of children vaccinated in the first two years of life was 33 per cent of this age group.

(b) (iii) Disinfection

9.36 This purpose is a natural corollary of *b* (i) since we are dealing here with the destruction of sources of infection and this is only another aspect of isolation. This particular aspect however is a specialized service and involves the deployment of disinfectors as distinct from therapeutic agencies. Sections 85 (i), 166–7 of the Public Health Act, 1936 give powers to local sanitary authorities to ensure the disinfection of clothing and premises where these are considered to be a source of infection. The powers apply to occasions when the Medical Officer of Health certifies that such action 'would tend to prevent the spread of *any* infectious disease'. The disinfection is carried out by the local authority only if the occupier fails to take satisfactory action, on notice from the authority. Generally speaking these powers are only applied to instances where apart from the patient, the clothes and premises are the main residual sources of infection and their disinfection is likely to be of practical value. The local authority also has powers under the 1936 Act to impose penalties on any person who 'knowing that he is suffering from a notifiable disease exposes other persons to the risk of infection by his presence or conduct in any street, public place, place of entertainment or assembly, club, hotel, or in a shop'; to exclude infectious children from school; to prevent infectious articles being sent to laundries, or infected books being returned to libraries; to prohibit the owner or driver or conductor of a public vehicle from conveying an infectious person; and where a 'serious risk of infection is caused to other persons' to secure the removal to hospital of a person suffering from a notifiable disease.

9.37 These powers are less employed than formerly but are still regarded as important in the control of infectious disease.

(b) (iv) After-care

9.38 There are some infectious diseases such as meningococcal meningitis or poliomyelitis or encephalitis which if not fatal may yet leave serious disability requiring rehabilitative treatment, institutional and domiciliary, extending over long periods. There are, certain other milder diseases where the risks of sequelae are still important—bronchiectasis as a possible sequela of whooping cough, deafness caused by middle ear infection after measles, are two examples; and indeed none of the common fevers which are regarded as the inevitable social risk of children can really be looked upon as harmless though few untoward effects emerge. Benjamin, Cawthorne and Whetnall (1954) have found that among children with acquired deafness 73·5 per cent have a history of an attack of measles, while in normal children of a similar age group the percentage was only 58·6, indicating the importance played by measles in the aetiology of acquired as distinct from congenital deafness. Bentley, Grzybowski and Benjamin (NAPT 1954) have found suggestive evidence that the additional strain on the respiratory system inflicted by whooping cough may increase the risk that a primary tuberculosis infection will proceed to infiltrate. It is, therefore, an essential part of preventive medicine to encourage adequate after care in all cases of infectious disease, and it is important that the risks should be statistically assessed as in the examples quoted.

(c) (i) Epidemic control

9.39 Control of an epidemic means action taken either to suppress its development, e.g. by cutting all possible channels of spread, or to reduce its dimensions, e.g. by measures of vaccination, or at lowest level to prepare for its effects in order to mitigate them, e.g. mobilization of hospital beds and respirators in an outbreak of poliomyelitis. The necessity for any such action must be predicated upon knowledge.

(a) of the actual or probable inception of an epidemic
(b) of the speed of development of the outbreak
(c) of the probable limit of its development
(d) of the section of the population most likely to be affected
(e) of the seriousness of the outbreak in terms of disability (the more serious the disease the more ruthless may be the preventive action).

9.40 This knowledge is derived very largely from the application of the often empirical laws of past experience to current statistics.

Incidence

9.41 The size of the problem presented by a particular disease is usually measured by the frequency with which new cases arise during a unit interval of time and the severity of those cases as indicated by the need for treatment or by fatality.

9.42 Table 9.4 based on figures taken from *The Annual Statistical Review of the Registrar General for 1960* relates to England and Wales and is illustrative—

TABLE 9.4 *Notified cases in England and Wales*

	1951	1952	1953	1954	1955	1956	1957	1958	1959	1960
Smallpox	27	135	30	—	—	—	4	6	1	1
Diphtheria	664	376	266	173	155	53	37	80	102	49
Scarlet fever	48,744	67,261	61,180	43,026	32,619	33,103	29,547	38,853	47,919	32,170
Measles	616,192	389,502	545,050	146,995	693,803	160,556	633,678	259,308	539,524	159,364
Whooping cough	169,441	114,869	157,842	105,912	79,133	92,410	85,018	33,404	33,253	58,030
Meningococcal Infection	1,390	1,327	1,354	1,246	1,126	1,168	1,016	836	746	632
Poliomyelitis— paralytic	1,529	2,747	2,976	1,391	3,712	1,717	3,177	1,419	739	257
non-para.	1,085	1,163	1,571	641	2,619	1,483	1,667	575	289	121

9.43 In this simple example of incidence we have taken an interval of time —a year—which for infectious disease is often too long. For infections commonly occur in epidemic waves sometimes spreading throughout the community with great rapidity; the number attacked in a unit interval increases until the number of persons not previously attacked (or immunized) —referred to as the susceptibles—has diminished to a point at which this spread is retarded and the epidemic wanes. In order to observe this spread and to design appropriate measures of control we need a short time interval. How short depends upon the rapidity of spread and the steepness of rise in incidence. In a severe influenza epidemic when industrial sickness absence is high and hospital resources strained it may be important to review the situation daily.

9.44 It is of special interest to refer to influenza because it is not a notifiable disease and other indices of incidence must be devised. The following is an extract from records maintained in the London County Council Public Health Department during a period when influenza was prevalent in Europe and was expected here. To save space these figures have been summarized in weekly intervals but it must be emphasized that the original records were compiled on a *daily* basis.

1949 Week ended	Deaths registered from			Patients removed to hospital by Emergency Ambulance Service for Influenza, Bronchitis, Pneumonia
	Influenza	Bronchitis	Pneumonia	
January 15	8	108	53	138
22	3	93	51	167
29	6	89	52	127
February 5	13	150	70	184
12	11	215	98	224
19	33	212	104	292
26	40	155	105	260
March 5	48	137	75	208
12	39	139	83	182
19	31	101	71	146
26	26	79	62	135

9.45 What is important in local health administration is the immediate observation of a real epidemic rise. The actual weekly figures of notifications in London (admin. Co.) shown on p.155 illustrate the beginning of epidemic outbreaks, or seasonal rises in prevalence.

9.46 The significant rise in numbers which usually fluctuate considerably can normally be seen by regarding the weekly numbers in interepidemic times as subject to random variation on the basis of a Poisson distribution (or if the numbers are fairly large, a binomial distribution), i.e. possessing a standard error equal or approximately equal to its square root. Table 9.5 compares the distribution of weekly cases of poliomyelitis in London during the period between the epidemic outbreaks of 1947 and 1949 and immediately preceding the latter outbreak, with that expected on the basis of a Poisson distribution. The mean and variance *are* reasonably close and the week ended June 18th stands out as that in which a significant rise occurred. In the statement below a line has been drawn between two successive weeks when the difference is greater than twice the square root of the earlier week (or average of irregular weeks covering a stable prevalence), i.e. approximately there is less than a 20 : 1 chance that the fluctuation is within the bounds of random fluctuations at the interepidemic level. In this way the development of epidemic conditions can be fixed. If this appears arbitrary it must be stressed that the purpose of

TABLE 9.5 *Weekly notifications of poliomyelitis in London*
(*Administrative County*) 1949

Week ended	Notifications of poliomyelitis	
January 8	4	
15	4	
22	3	
29	4	
February 5	—	
12	2	Number of Weeks = 23
19	1	Mean cases = 1·96
26	1	Variance = 1·77
March 5	—	
12	2	
19	5	
26	2	
April 2	2	
9	3	
16	2	
23	1	
30	1	
May 7	2	
14	1	
21	1	
28	1	
June 4	1	
11	2	
18	6	$6 - 1·96 = 4·04$
25	6	$t = \dfrac{4·04}{\sqrt{1·77}} = 3·0$
July 2	6	
9	6	significant rise
16	13	
23	7	
30	20	

154

this serial record is to initiate control measures in time; it is more important not to miss a significant rise in new cases than to avoid acting prematurely— the criterion of significance must not be too strict.

Disease	Measles		Poliomyelitis		Dysentery		Scarlet Fever	
Year	1952		1953		1953		1953	
	week	cases	week	cases	week	cases	week	cases
Week No.	36	280	21	7	2	19	32	25
shown on left,	37	240	22	1	3	32	33	27
notified cases	38	272	23	5	4	32	34	23
shown on the	39	354	24	4	5	29	35	26
right, of each	40	554	25	4	6	36	36	28
column	41	682	26	6	7	29	37	29
	42	964	27	19	8	50	38	42
	43	1,094	28	27	9	39	39	61
	44	1,252	29	36	10	28	40	58
	45	989	30	34	11	41	41	55
	46	1,208	31	34	12	79	42	81
	47	1,129	32	17	13	60	43	87
	48	1,560	33	14	14	45	44	58

Epidemic curves

9.47 When an epidemic rise in new cases has occurred how long is it likely to continue? What is likely to be the total dimensions of the outbreak? Very often in an epidemic the cases occurring in successive weeks when plotted as a graph (see fig. 9.2) follow a characteristic pattern.

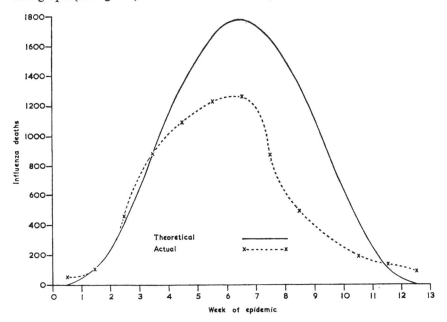

Fig. 9.2 Influenza deaths in great towns, weekly, 1951.
['Great Towns = London, All County Boroughs, and Municipal Boroughs and Urban Districts with populations exceeding 50,000].

155

9.48 Clearly if there were an underlying mathematical law to this 'epidemic curve' and if it were known then at the outset of the epidemic it would be a simple matter to forecast the course of the outbreak, its duration and its total toll of new cases.

9.49 It can be shown that if point infection (instantaneous infection) can be assumed and if the so-called law of mass action applies, i.e. that the number of cases infected by one case is proportional to the number of susceptibles in the community at the time, then a simple relationship arises such that if f_0, f_1 are the numbers of cases in successive intervals of time (equal to the incubation period), x_0 is the instantaneous number of susceptibles and x is the 'steady state' number of susceptibles when 'one infects one'

$$f_1/f_0 = \frac{x}{x_0} \text{ and } x_0 = s.a.$$

where a is the number of accessions of susceptibles to the community in one interval of time, s being the number of intervals required to accumulate x_0 the steady state level. From this relationship it is possible to generate the characteristic type of epidemic curves provided the requisite data are available. This, however, implies prior knowledge of the 'steady state' and is therefore of little value for purposes of forecasting (though of great value in the measurement of periodicity of past epidemics). Apart from this difficulty it is also an unfortunate fact that normal experience rarely conforms to a simple pattern. While most outbreaks reproduce the ascending and descending phases (as exemplified in fig. 9.2) and conform to the bell-shaped pattern, with a varying degree of distortion from symmetry, and while it is often possible to fit a mathematical curve to an epidemic when it is over, it is not possible to be sure what form this curve will take when the epidemic has just commenced. For, to a very large extent, every outbreak is unique.

9.50 To take an example, suppose that in the outbreak of influenza in the 'great towns' in 1951 we had attempted to fit to the weekly deaths a mathematical curve, of the type suitable at the preceding epidemic of 1949, after the third week of the 1951 epidemic. This would produce the continuous line in fig. 9.2. The actual course of the outbreak is indicated by the broken line. So mathematics do not help very much in current epidemic control, though much epidemiological knowledge has been gleaned from retrospective analysis of this type—knowledge for example of the degree of infectiousness of the disease and the extent to which epidemics are brought to a close by the exhaustion of the available susceptible (unattacked or non-immune) population or by other factors known to have been operating. This clearly enables inferences to be drawn about the probable manner of development of subsequent epidemics even though prediction of actual numbers of cases cannot be attempted. An example of this kind of inference can be given in relation to influenza.

9.51 Table 9.6 shows the result of an experimental analysis of pneumonia notifications and influenza deaths in all the major epidemics of influenza in the 'great towns' of England and Wales since 1921. The table demonstrates that in recent outbreaks the rise in deaths has been steeper and the peak has been reached more rapidly than in earlier outbreaks. Attention was drawn to this fact by Logan and Mackay (1951). Therefore only recent outbreaks are

TABLE 9.6 Influenza deaths in the Great Towns of England and Wales from 1921, and pneumonia notifications from 1949

			Influenza								Pneumonia							
Type of Outbreak	Winter of	week ended	Deaths in successive weeks commencing with week preceding epidemic rise				Ratios		Peak number of deaths in t'th week of outbreak		Notifications in same weeks							No. of towns
			0	1	2	3	1/0	2/1	t	Number	0	1	2	3	1/0	2/1	t'th week	
LARGE (Peak week, over 1,000)	1921–22	19 Nov. 21	59	80	128	149	1·36	1·60	10	1,450								96
	26–27	25 Dec. 26	69	86	172	326	1·25	2·00	9	1,023								105
	28–29	5 Jan. 29	99	122	179	321	1·23	1·47	7	2,183								107
	32–33	17 Dec. 32	85	120	303	681	1·41	2·53	6	1,934								118
	36–37	26 Dec. 36	97	325	768	1,100	3·35	2·36	6	1,155								122
	43–44	20 Nov. 43	106	375	709	1,148	3·54	1·89	3	1,148								126
	50–51	23 Dec. 50	54	102	458	890	1·89	4·49	6	1,269	364	502	956	1,300	1·38	1·90	1,664	126
MEDIUM (Peak week, over 300)	1923–24	12 Jan. 24	93	153	236	367	1·65	1·54	8	730								105
	24–25	3 Jan. 25	100	124	142	195	1·24	1·15	9	361								105
	25–26	13 Mar. 26	88	136	136	223	1·55	1·00	5	302								105
	30–31	10 Jan. 31	101	146	242	309	1·45	1·66	7	546								107
	31–32	26 Dec. 31	140	240	412	412	1·71	1·72	2	412								117
	39–40	6 Jan. 40	94	158	291	417	1·68	1·84	7	629								126
	40–41	18 Jan. 41	99	120	176	261	1·21	1·47	4	324								126
	45–46	5 Jan. 46	123	165	174	273	1·34	1·05	5	304								126
	48–49	12 Feb. 49	94	158	251	259	1·68	1·59	5	360	607	879	914	884	1·45	1·04	864	126
	52–53	10 Jan. 53	51	72	132	313	1·41	1·83	5	530	685	686	776	1,174	1·00	1·13	1,443	160
SMALL	1920–21	5 Feb. 21	61	93	103	138	1·52	1·11	4	167								96

157

comparable. In this last three 'large' outbreaks the rise was more than sixfold in the first two weeks; in the last three 'medium' outbreaks the rise over the same period was only to between two and three times the deaths of the pre-epidemic week; while in the last two small outbreaks the rise was less and the second week was in each case the peak. It seems possible from the steepness of the rise in deaths to forecast in the *second week* of the outbreak the ultimate dimensions of the epidemic in terms of mortality. For example it can be seen from the table that in the week ended January 10, 1953, 51 influenza deaths were registered. The standard error of 51 assuming a binomial distribution is about 7 and twice that value 14 so that at a 5 per cent significance level more than 65 deaths would have to be recorded in the following week to indicate a significant rise. In fact 72 were registered and in the next week deaths rose to 132. This rate of increase could have been seen from previous experience, viz. from the ratios of current or previous week's deaths shown in the table, to suggest eventual development of a 'medium' outbreak. The comparable sets of ratios are for 1939–40 when 629 deaths was the peak after 7 weeks and 1930–31 when the weekly deaths peaked at 546 after 7 weeks; so that 600 could be forecast as the peak. In fact deaths in 1953 reached a peak of 530 in the fifth week of the epidemic. Pneumonia notifications are not quite so sensitive for this purpose, but appear to rise more steeply in severe epidemics of influenza.

9.52 Where the disease is such that it attacks a very high proportion of susceptibles, e.g. measles, and does not become epidemic until sufficient susceptibles have accumulated by new births or migrants since the last epidemic, each epidemic tends to follow the same pattern in time and total dimensions. In England and Wales as a whole measles epidemics occur biennially with almost unbroken regularity (in some local areas there is an annual rhythm); notifications which are always minimal in September (whether epidemic year or not) rise rapidly in the ensuing months of the autumn (preceding the epidemic year), reach a peak in January or February and then gradually decline until by the end of April or May the epidemic may be regarded as virtually at an end. Variation from this average timing occurs from epidemic to epidemic. The pattern may develop sooner or later and may cover a varying duration of time, but the general picture remains constant in outline. Under such conditions an epidemic must clearly come to an end because the remaining susceptibles become fewer and farther apart. Late winter increases in incidence occur in interepidemic years but these are minor waves and are not regarded as approaching the order of major epidemics. The statistics on page 159 are illustrative.

In these circumstances, prediction is merely a matter of looking at past records. Whether the rhythm in a particular locality is annual or biennial seems to depend upon whether or not the population is sufficiently far spread to be incompletely covered before the epidemic is arrested by the autumn refractory period.

9.53 There are not many diseases which reproduce the same pattern of prevalence so regularly as measles. Whooping cough, for example, varies irregularly both in timing and extent of epidemic prevalence and such seasonal swing as is exhibited differs considerably from year to year and is not capable of simple description.

Measles

			In peak week		Total in epidemic (approximate)	
	Epidemic rise week ended	*Peak week ended*	*No.*	*% of average weekly births*	*No.*	*% of average annual births*
Town						
	Epidemic year 1952–53					
Birmingham C.B.	4.10.52	14.2.53	1,482	417	20,700	112
Bootle C.B.	10.1.52	16.5.53	76	484	873	107
	Epidemic year 1951–52					
New York City	16.11.51	14.3.52	2,233	71	36,000	22

9.54 Poliomyelitis emerged after World War II as one of the most threatening epidemic diseases, partly by virtue of the high incidence of disablement, often permanent, and the relatively high fatality, and partly by virtue of its capricious periodicity. Vigilance is necessary at all times but particularly in the late spring and early summer months when prevalence tends to rise, even in non-epidemic conditions, and rises rapidly in epidemic outbreaks, Prevalence does not usually decline again until the cooler weather of the late autumn. Regular returns of notifications are essential and during May and June these notifications must be scrutinized daily for signs of the development of epidemic prevalence, partly so that there shall be time to mobilize hospital facilities and partly so that certain essential precautions may be taken, e.g. restriction of tonsillectomy and non-urgent inoculation procedures. More recently the preparation of an effective vaccine and its use on a mass scale has considerably reduced the incidence of the disease.

Geographical spread

9.55 If a disease is known to be travelling along well defined lines of communication it may be possible to prevent spread by interposing in its path a barrier represented by the isolation or restricted movement of the potential infectors and the remainder of the community. Reference has already been made to the need for attempting to record by the use of spot maps the direction of spread of infectious disease. This presupposes the provision of statistics tabulated by intervals of time and subsections of territory to facilitate such examination of the existence of foci and directions of travel. Clearly, even though a disease is conveyed from person to person there would be little point in this statistical operation if the disease were so infectious, either by the multiplicity, ubiquity or invasiveness of organisms involved or by the enhanced susceptibility of those at risk of infection, that spread were rapid and practically uncontrollable. Many abortive attempts were once made to control the spread of measles by the closing of schools; it is still true that a high proportion of susceptible children may be attacked within a few weeks of the commencement of an epidemic. Poliomyelitis falls within the same category though the proportion suffering frank attacks is very small; infectivity is high and transmission rapid so that it is possible to portray channels of spread only in small closed communities where the problem of control is correspondingly much less serious. Where large communities are involved and the challenge is greater the method has so far proved to be futile.

9.56 Difficulties of tracing the spread of disease are naturally greater in large urban areas. In looking at measles prevalence in London* for example it is not often that it is possible to discern any clear passage of epidemic wave from one metropolitan borough to an adjacent borough. Each borough has its own reservoir of infection and its unique fund of susceptibles and an outbreak occurs in a locality when the conditions are favourable; sometimes independently of what is happening in the next locality, sometimes because an outbreak in a neighbouring locality helps to produce favourable conditions. In each of the years 1945, 1946, 1947 the measles cases were grouped into thirteen four-week periods and the number of the period (1–4 weeks = 1, 5–8 weeks = 2 etc.) in which the peak incidence occurred was plotted on the County maps. Contours were drawn where possible around boroughs coming into epidemic peak at approximately the same time. In 1945 it was not possible to put in any contours because the rise was almost simultaneous throughout the County. In 1947 there was a north-east flow from the western border but all else was conjecture and confusing. Only in one year, 1946, was there a clear pattern of spread. In both 1946 and 1947 there was a suggestion that the river might have acted as a partial barrier in slowing up spread, e.g. Stepney and Bermondsey, Battersea and Chelsea. There was a suggestion of a slowing up in spread as between Hammersmith and Kensington, perhaps as a result of large railway sidings and open spaces. There was in all years a rapid spread in the south-east parts of London where the populations were compact and where there were few barriers. (Four weeks is too long a period to distinguish adequately the position of peaks, but any lesser period would only increase irregularities due to the small numbers involved and make the true peaks even more difficult to determine.)

9.57 The dispersion of the peaks was sometimes wide as can be seen from the following figures:

Number of 4-week period	Boroughs with peaks in period 1945	1946	1947
1	—	1	2
2	3	1	3
3	5	4	3
4	15	5	3
5	2	1	1
6	3	6	8
7	—	6	5
8	—	1	3
9	—	—	—
10	—	—	—
11	—	—	—
12	—	1	—
13	—	2	—
Number of Boroughs	28	28	28
Number of period of peak in London A.C. as whole	4th	5th	2nd and 6th

9.58 In estimating the peak period for a particular borough by reference to the County as a whole, there would be a high frequency of error even in

* Reference in these sections is to London A.C. and the metropolitan boroughs as they existed prior to the London Government Act 1963.

1945 when the dispersion was narrow. It is important to bear in mind that the epidemic curve of a larger area is made up by a number of curves of small areas and that the timing and shape of these component curves may differ from each other and from the compositite curve.

9.59 The following figures are of interest:

		Difference in months between times of epidemic peak in the three years 1945–47			
Boroughs		1945	1946	1947	Average
Bermondsey	Southwark	1	2	1	1·3
Lambeth	Battersea	0	1	0	0·3
Deptford	Lewisham	0	0	1	0·3
Hackney	Stoke Newington	0	1	2	1·0
		1945	1946	1947	Average
Chelsea	Battersea	1	5	7	4·3
Stepney	Bermondsey	1	3	3	2·3
Poplar	Greenwich	1	1	0	0·7
Kensington	Hammersmith	1	2	5	2·3
Willesden	Hammersmith	0	5	6	3·7

(The four Average values 1·3, 0·3, 0·3, 1·0 are bracketed together with 0·7)

9.60 Between boroughs where there were few barriers the average difference was small and rarely more than one month. Where the river appeared to exert a resistance to spread the difference was much larger, e.g. Chelsea—Battersea; Stepney—Bermondsey. The apparent exception was Poplar—Greenwich but there was considerable communication through Blackwall Tunnel. Between Hammersmith and either Kensington or Willesden, the lag was comparatively long, perhaps as a result of the railways and open spaces which occupied the north and western boundaries of Hammersmith.

9.61 At the other extreme where the territory surveyed is wide and the population comparatively sparse, it is relatively easy to follow the development of epidemics in space as well as time.

(c) (ii) *Morbidity indices*

9.62 Infectious disease notifications play a part in the measurement of public health, or rather, or public ill-health. Diseases in the infective and parasitic group (1.S.C.001—138) and influenza but excluding the common cold accounted for 12 per cent of days of incapacity in adults aged 16–64 in 1946–47 (Stocks, 1949) and for 34 per cent of school sickness absences in 1947–48 in children under 7 years and 18 per cent of sickness absence in children aged 8–11 (Bransby, 1951). In particular the incidence of tuberculosis is a significant index of the health and well-being of a community. Tuberculosis is still an important cause of death in this country even though, happily, fatality has been declining rapidly in an era of chemotherapy and bold surgery. The prevalence of tuberculosis is highly correlated with the prevalence of other respiratory diseases and is also highly correlated with environmental and socio-economic factors (Benjamin, 1953). The prevalence of infectious disease must be included in the general scheme of morbidity measurements which form the basis of planned public health administration.

9.63 There are deficiencies in the measurement of infectious disease prevalence; variability in the degree of completeness of notification, variability in the criteria of distinction between frank and sub-clinical cases of disease, between notifiable and non-notifiable infection. These deficiencies

F
161

are perhaps less formidable than those which are inherent in any other morbidity measurement; they are capable either of correction or of being discounted in the delineation of secular trends within one locality where conditions may be regarded as homogeneous and constant.

Differentials in age and sex

9.64 Where infectious diseases are endemic, it is merely a matter of time before the infection is encountered and since the period of time involved is short the common fevers are characteristically diseases of childhood. The following table is illustrative (Benjamin and Gore, 1952). The estimated proportions (per cent) of children at the ages of five and fifteen years who will have previously experienced an attack of each disease studied are as follows:

Disease	Percentage of children attacked	
	By the age of 5 years	By the age of 15 years
Chickenpox	20	45
Rubella	7	15
Measles	35	65
Mumps	10	15–30
Whooping cough	25	35
Scarlet fever	4–5	10–12

9.65 Several important age and sex differentials are generally observed and these have been excellently reviewed by Stocks (1949), the following being a summary, though not exhaustive.

Disease	Main differentials
Scarlet fever	Male excess at ages under 3; female excess at school ages, disappearing at 15–24; reappearing at 25 and over.
Measles	Slight female excess in first year of life, no appreciable sex difference between 1 and 10 years and a female excess thereafter.
Whooping cough	Increasing female excess with advancing age.
Poliomyelitis	Male excess at all ages.
Meningococcal infection	Male excess especially in childhood.
Dysentery	Male excess in childhood; female excess at adult ages.

9.66 The statistical examination of such differentials is illustrated by reference to measles in England and Wales in 1944–47.

TABLE 9.7 England and Wales—Measles notification rates per 100,000, 1944–47

Age	Males	Females	Rate for females per cent of rate for males
0—	1,621	1,697	105
1—	4,770	4,739	99
3—	6,537	6,572	101
5—	3,987	4,062	102
10—	452	504	112
15—	105	109	104
25 and over	8·3	14·5	175

9.67 The cumulative proportion of children who at this level of incidence would have been notified before reaching age 15 is approximately estimated as the summation of products r.n. where r is the rate (assumed to apply uniformly over the age group) and n the number of years in successive age groups up to 15, i.e. it is assumed that as a boy passes through, for example, the 5–10 age group the rate of 3·987 per cent applies in each of the five individual years passed through.

Males	Females
$1·621 \times 1 = 1·621$	$1·697 \times 1 = 1·697$
$4·770 \times 2 = 9·540$	$4·735 \times 2 = 9·478$
$6·537 \times 2 = 13·074$	$6·572 \times 2 = 13·144$
$3·987 \times 5 = 19·935$	$4·062 \times 5 = 20·310$
$0·452 \times 5 = 2·260$	$0·504 \times 5 = 2·520$
46·430	**47·149**

9.68 Thus, 46 per cent of boys and 47 per cent of girls would be notified before age 15.

Fatality

9.69 The infectious diseases vary greatly in their lethal effects. Some like chickenpox or rubella rarely have fatal consequences. Others such as meningococcal meningitis carry a serious risk of death. It is usual and useful to measure the risk of death, or the fatality, by expressing the deaths as a percentage of the cases from which they have arisen. The accuracy of the calculation depends upon completeness of notification; for measles, scarlet fever and diphtheria the notified cases represent most of those with recognizable symptoms, but it is generally accepted that only about one half of whooping cough attacks are notified and expressing the whooping cough deaths as a percentage of notified cases overstates the fatality. Where the disease is not notifiable, e.g. influenza, no measurement of fatality can be made except where local surveys may sometimes replace notification.

9.70 The following figures are typical:

England and Wales—1965

Disease	Notified cases	Deaths	Deaths per 100 cases
Measles	502,209	115	0·02
Meningococcal Infection	406	112	27·6
Poliomyelitis	91	19	3·3 (See § 9.71)
Scarlet fever	26,723	1	(a)
Whooping cough	12,945	21	0·16

(a) With only one death, the rate could not be a reliable index.

9.71 One point to be noted is that owing to the time elapsing between onset and death, the deaths of 1965 do not relate exactly to cases notified in 1965 since (a) some of those dying were notified before 1965 and (b) some fatal cases notified late in 1965 will be included in the deaths of 1966 or later. The error is of significance when very sharp and unequal irregularities in incidence occur at the beginning and end of the year so that (a) and (b) do not balance. There is also possible error when the lag between onset and death is long. For example, of the 19 deaths from poliomyelitis in 1965 in the table, 16 were from late affects. The true fatality ratio was $3 \cdot 3$ a record low figure. The correction is likely to be more important when in addition the number of deaths have been declining and also for local areas where the total numbers involved are small.

9.72 Changes in the fatality rate may give an indication of variation in the virulence of the disease, or improvement in either resistance or therapy. Alternatively, where there is other evidence of constancy in true fatality the *recorded* fatality rate may be used as an indication of completeness of notification. Scarlet fever for example has always been fairly completely notified and the reduction in fatality from $0 \cdot 57$ per cent in 1931 to $0 \cdot 08$ per cent in 1950 has been a reflection of a combination of all the factors of improvement mentioned above, reduced virulence, increased resistance, improved treatment. As an example of the other kind of use, the following is an extract from the *Annual Statistical Review of the Registrar General* (Medical Text) for 1950 and relates to whooping cough. 'The notification rate in Wales was much lower than the average for the country as a whole but the high ratio of deaths to notifications taken together with the fact that the death rate per million living was little different from that of the country as a whole, suggests a considerable degree of under-notification.'

Death rates

9.73 Relating the deaths to the population as distinct from cases of disease is also often important. Where the completeness of notification is increasing rapidly (e.g. dysentery) or where the disease is not notifiable at all (e.g. influenza) the death rate may provide the only reliable measure of the severity of outbreak. Apart from this the death rate is a measure of the death toll in relation to size of population and indicates the relative importance of the disease as a cause of death in the community. Among the relatively small number of cases of diphtheria which occurred in England and Wales in 1951 the fatality was if anything higher than ever. Even after excluding cases of long duration the fatality was $4 \cdot 5$ per cent. The death rate was, however, insignificant (1 per million compared with an average of 48 in 1940–44).

(d) Epidemiological research

9.74 Epidemics defy complete explanation. Knowledge of the nature of the pathogens, of their invasiveness, incubation, immunological reactions, mode of spread and of whether they are endogenous or exogenous, is limited and many gaps are still left to be filled by conjecture and hypothesis. It is certain, however, that many steps in the elucidation of the natural history of infectious diseases have been made not at the bedside, vitally important though such clinical observation has been, but rather in the community at large, by the patient (and largely statistical) observation of the dynamics of epidemics as they have occurred. The classical law of mass action from the development of which has emerged the mathematical description of the epidemic curve was developed from observation of the distribution of reported cases in space and time by pioneers such as Farr, Brownlee, Ross and later Soper and Kermack and McKendrick. Where clear laws of periodicity can be substantiated this is a vital gain in preparedness. If the weekly notifications of measles are plotted graphically as for example in Birmingham during 1950–53 (fig. 9.3) a clear picture of the rhythm of measles epidemics is obtained. When the same process is repeated for whooping cough however the picture is not nearly so clear. (Fig. 9.4).

9.75 The discovery of the methods by which infection was transmitted, often made only by the successive elimination of many false suspects, has depended on the reporting of cases and the accurate tracing of paths of spread. In individual outbreaks the careful charting of paths of spread gives much useful information assisting control. The following example has been quoted by Pickles (1939).

Epidemic catarrhal jaundice

A (the first victim)

Not attended personally but said to have had jaundice in July, 1929. It is impossible to trace the infection in his case, but it is significant that he visited Askrigg, a hotbed of infection in June

B (A's sister)

Commenced with the disease on August 23rd and while still obviously jaundiced attended a village fete on August 28th. All those on the line below were present also and developed the disease on the given dates, all 1929.

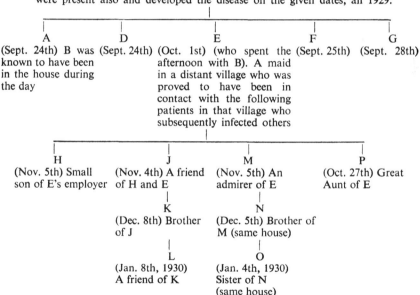

A	D	E	F	G
(Sept. 24th) B was known to have been in the house during the day	(Sept. 24th)	(Oct. 1st) (who spent the afternoon with B). A maid in a distant village who was proved to have been in contact with the following patients in that village who subsequently infected others	(Sept. 25th)	(Sept. 28th)

H	J	M	P
(Nov. 5th) Small son of E's employer	(Nov. 4th) A friend of H and E	(Nov. 5th) An admirer of E	(Oct. 27th) Great Aunt of E
	K	N	
	(Dec. 8th) Brother of J	(Dec. 5th) Brother of M (same house)	
	L	O	
	(Jan. 8th, 1930) A friend of K	(Jan. 4th, 1930) Sister of N (same house)	

9.76 So far as the study of incubation periods is concerned, a careful system of reporting of individual cases is essential to the identification of contacts of the primary or 'index' cases and of the distribution in time of the secondary cases. There is often no unique period for a particular disease but a wide range of observed values—extremes of from 6 to 22 days are accepted for rubella, and 3–20 for diphtheria though the modal values are 16 and 5 respectively. As all quarantine procedures and many prophylactic measures depend upon a knowledge of these ranges, the observation of incubation periods and of possible secular variations is important. If, for example,

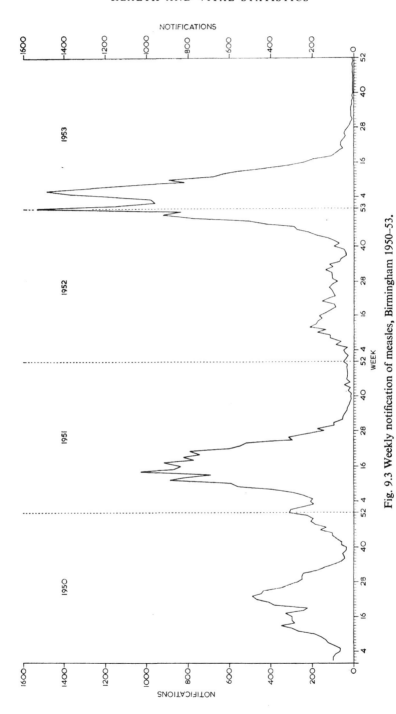

Fig. 9.3 Weekly notification of measles, Birmingham 1950–53.

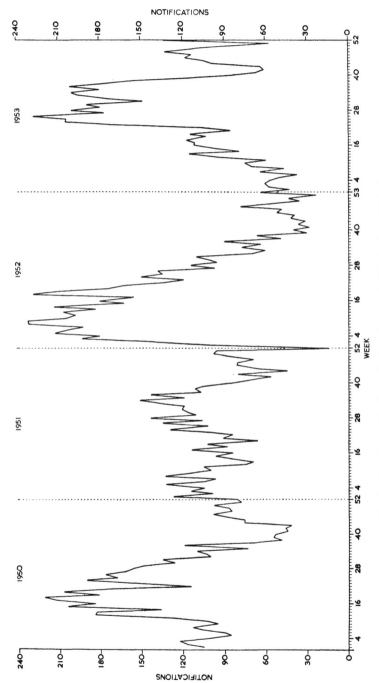

Fig. 9.4 Weekly notifications of whooping cough, Birmingham 1950–53.

records are kept of notifications by *household* so that second cases in the same household can be related to the onset of disease in the first cases, then a distribution of the following kind may be constructed—

Poliomyelitis—Interval between initial and secondary case in the same family

Interval in days	0	1	2	3	4	5	6	7	8	9	10	11	12	13	14+
Cases	61	45	47	41	46	45	26	17	22	9	8	7	3	3	11

Many of these cases have not been infected from the first; of those that were it looks as though the incubation period might well be as long as eight days and occasionally longer.

9.77 Equally the study of immunity involves the differentiating of the susceptible from the insusceptible members of the population in relation to their histories of previous attack. These histories must be reliably known. Human memory is fallible and it is better that there should be permanent personal written records of attacks of infectious disease at least while such studies are being conducted. Widely differing estimates have been made, for example, of the proportion of children who suffer an attack of whooping cough before the age of ten, viz.—

	per cent
Schools Epidemics Committee 1938 (*a*)	60–70
L.C.C. hospitals 1938 (*b*)	30–40

(*a*) Histories of public school entrants: Medical Research Council Spec. Rep. Series 227.

(*b*) Histories of non-whooping cough patients: Benjamin, B. and Gore, A. T.—*Brit. J. Soc. Med.*, vol. vi, p. 197.

These differences are not wholly due to the variations in environmental background but are partly due to differences in the extent to which attacks have been recognized and recorded.

9.78 For mumps the differences are even wider—

	Per cent attacked by age 15
Benjamin and Gore, 1952	15–30
Logan, 1951	25–30
Bransby, 1952	50

Infectiousness

9.79 The infectiousness of a disease has normally been measured by the secondary attack rate, i.e. the proportion of susceptibles who are infected in households into which the disease has been introduced. This measure implies knowledge of the number of susceptibles, defined as those without past history of the disease, since these form the denominator of the rate, and it also implies identification of secondary as distinct from primary cases. Thus, reported cases must be locally classified by household and date of onset and susceptibility must have been recorded by household enquiry. Inasmuch as some members of the household may escape the first chain of infection but may be attacked by infection from one of the secondary cases, and so on, it is possible for susceptibles to be exposed more than once and if, as is often necessary for simplicity, secondary and subsequent cases are aggregated, the susceptibles who are exposed more than once should have all their exposures included in the denominator. This again implies some knowledge of details of spread in the household.

9.80 Hope Simpson (1952) has stressed the difficulty of distinguishing different generations of cases, e.g. of separating true secondaries from coincident primaries (infected from outside the household). The time of onset must be fixed by some conventionally accepted stage in the usual chain of symptoms (e.g. first appearance of rash) and then a graphical plotting of the frequency distribution of onset of cases in time will usually be effective in distinguishing the generations of cases.

9.81 Infectiousness for the same disease may vary with many factors—season, age distribution or density of aggregation of susceptibles, geographical situation, to mention a few. The following illustrative figures are taken from Hope Simpson (1952)—

Secondary attack rate (per cent) in measles in different areas, times and ages

Age Group (years)	Providence, U.S.A. 1929–34	Cirencester, England 1947–51
Less than 1	40·6	40·0
Less than 15	81·1	80·1
15 or more	16·7	16·3

9.82 The correspondence is remarkable and shows that measles behaves in a similar manner in USA and England.

9.83 Where prophylactics are being tested a comparison of secondary attack rates in comparable groups treated with different antigens may indicate the relative degrees of protection conferred by these antigens. A classic example is the whooping cough vaccine trial carried out by the Medical Research Council (1951) from the report of which the following figures have been extracted.

Percentage Attack rate in children exposed to infection in their own homes

Vaccine*	Vaccinated	Unvaccinated
A	22·2	85·0
B	7·3	79·5
C	8·9	90·0
D	30·4	90·5
E	29·8	90·7

* Letters have been substituted for the names of the original table.

9.84 Much can be learned of the aetiology of infectious disease by having regard to social or occupational variations in incidence. This has been especially true of tuberculosis (Collis and Greenwood, 1921; Hart and Payling Wright, 1939) with its indisputable association with poverty, but it has also been the subject of study in other diseases, for example, measles (Breen and Benjamin, 1949) or poliomyelitis (Martin and Hill, 1949; Benjamin and Logan, 1953) and the negative results were just as important in relation to the management of the diseases as were the positive findings for tuberculosis.

9.85 Epidemiological research has been much stimulated by the application of modern probability theory. The classical mathematical models have been deterministic (see, for example, Soper, 1929) in the sense that given rates of infection and accession and removal of susceptibles, the number of new cases arising in a particular interval of time is definite and determined by the proportion of the population which is still susceptible at that time. This leads to an epidemic curve of the type

$$x = m + \int_0^t (a-z)dt \text{ or } \frac{dx}{dt} = a-z,$$

where z = cases per unit time, x = number of susceptibles, a = accessions of susceptibles per unit time, m = steady state, or level, number of susceptibles, when one infects one.

9.86 Bartlett (1949) and Bailey (1950) have stressed that a more complete stochastic model should be used to take account of the fact that the single point on the deterministic curve ought to be regarded as the mean of a probability distribution. The smoothness of observed epidemics which has seemed to support deterministic theory arises from the fact that the statistics observed represent combinations of several restricted epidemics occurring at the same time with attack rates further smoothed by being averaged over finite intervals. Nevertheless, while the deterministic curves indicate the growth of an epidemic when numbers are large, they are not adequate when numbers are small or in the important early stages of an epidemic. The mathematics of the stochastic approach are formidable and lead to equations which are far from simple, but they appear to offer a sounder basis for prediction. One practical advantage may be mentioned. The deterministic theory involved a degree of damping in successive epidemic waves which is not observed in large communities. The stochastic theory does not result in damping terms in the equations and permits recapitulation of epidemic waves more in accord with experience.

(e) Diagnostic studies

9.87 Standards of diagnosis are known to be influenced by environment and attitude. If a disease is known to be prevalent, vigilance is generally raised in intensity—it is well known that during epidemics of, for example, poliomyelitis or whooping cough, a larger proportion of subclinical attacks which would otherwise pass unnoticed are detected and notified; if the disease is known to be common in certain places or certain strata of the population, it is more quickly suspected in those places and strata and there are undoubtedly regional and social variations in diagnostic practices and standards in relation to such diseases as for example tuberculosis or enteritis; if the disease is very dangerous, there is a tendency to err on the side of safety and not to leave anything to chance—this was, until the tendency was obscured by the minimal incidence of the disease, evident in the case of diphtheria where in 1950 in England and Wales confirmed cases amounted to only thirty-four per cent of originally notified cases (Registrar General of England and Wales, 1954). What practitioners are asked to notify may determine to some extent what they look for and there was evidence of this when in 1950 the notification regulations were amended in respect of poliomyelitis specifically to seek a separation of non-paralytic from paralytic cases—the proportion of non-paralytic cases which in hospital admissions of 1949 had been 21 per cent was, in the 1950 original notifications (i.e. uncorrected for diagnosis), 28 per cent (Logan, 1950; Bradley, 1950). The corresponding figure in 1965 was 60 per cent.

Completeness

9.88 Completeness of notification is defined as that combination of comprehensiveness and specificity such that reports cover every clinical case of the disease but include no cases not assignable to the entity in question. Four conditions must be satisfied if completeness is to be achieved:

(i)   the patient must be seen by a medical practitioner
(ii) the practitioner must make a correct diagnosis
(iii) the practitioner must be aware that the disease is notifiable and
(iv) he must actually notify the case.

9.89 It is difficult to determine precisely how completely a disease is being notified, but some indication can be obtained by comparing the notification records with the statistics of incidence derived from other sources, such as morbidity surveys, school absenteeism records, hospital records, public health laboratory records, and certified causes of death.

9.90 Stocks (1949) examined the completeness of notification of certain infectious diseases in England and Wales and came to the following conclusions:

'Thinking of the rates of illness in terms of the typical manifestations of the disease and excluding sub-clinical varieties, doubtful cases and evidences of infection without definite clinical symptoms, the general conclusions as to "completeness" in that sense of notification . . . can be summarized as follows:

Acute poliomyelitis Cerebro-spinal fever Diphtheria Scarlet fever	} Notification is fairly complete
Respiratory tuberculosis	Probably nine-tenths notified
Typhoid and paratyphoid	Probably four-fifths notified
Measles	About two-thirds notified
Pneumonia	From a third to a quarter notified
Whooping cough	From a quarter to a fifth notified
Erysipelas Non-respiratory tuberculosis	} Defective to an indeterminate degree
Dysentery	Notification only fractional.'

9.91 These are estimates for England and Wales as a whole. Completeness is more closely approached in some urban areas where better medical facilities are available. For example it has been suggested (Benjamin and Gore, 1952) that in London 50 per cent of whooping cough is notified.

Correction of notifications by revision of diagnosis

9.92 Prior to 1944 a notification could be withdrawn or the diagnosis amended only by the practitioner who originally notified the case, and in practice only a very small proportion of amendments to notifications were made. Since 1944 provision has been made for the Medical Officer of Health to be informed of any change in diagnosis made not only by the notifying practitioner, as before, but also by the hospital to which the patient may have been admitted. This has proved a most valuable arrangement, as the 'final notifications', i.e. notifications after revision by correction of diagnosis, give a much more accurate picture of the incidence of many of the infectious diseases than do the 'original', i.e. uncorrected or provisional, notifications.

Industrial diseases and accidents

9.93 In England and Wales, under the Factories Act 1937, the following diseases are notifiable to the Chief Inspector of Factories, by the medical practitioner attending the patient where he is of opinion that the disease has been contracted in any workshop or factory. The occupier of every factory or workshop is required at intervals of not less than one year, as prescribed, to send particulars of the age, sex and occupation of all persons in his employment. This makes it possible to calculate incidence rates.

Lead ⎫
Phosphorus ⎪
Mercurial ⎪
Arsenical ⎪
Manganese ⎬ poisoning
Carbon bisulphide ⎪
Aniline ⎪
Chronic benzene ⎭
Toxic jaundice
Toxic anaemia
Compressed air illness
Anthrax (specifying wool, horsehair, skins, hides or other industries)
Epitheliomatous ulceration (from pitch, tar, paraffin or oil)
Chrome ulceration (bichromates, dyeing, chrome tanning, chromium plating or other industries)

9.94 Accidents causing loss of life or disablement for more than three days are also reportable by type, e.g. persons falling from transport, cleaning in motion, gassing, sepsis, engines, handling goods, hand tools, explosions, belts, pulleys, etc.

9.95 A full analysis of the trend of accidents and industrial diseases appears in the Annual Report of the Chief Inspector of Factories.

Notification of infectious disease in USA

9.96 The State Board of Health of Massachusetts in 1874 inaugurated a plan for the voluntary weekly notification of prevalent diseases and over a hundred physicians responded. In 1876 a similar system of obtaining postal-card information from physicians in the State of Michigan was organized and in 1883 Michigan made it obligatory on householders, etc., to notify to the health officer infectious diseases dangerous to the public health. In 1884 a similar law was passed in Massachusetts. This required physicians as well as householders to notify.

9.97 Each of the States makes its own laws and there is therefore some divergence in requirements; but as a rule the attending physician is required to notify to the local health officer who transmits the information to the State Health Department.

9.98 In 1951 the States agreed to co-operate in a uniform scheme of national morbidity reporting to the United States Public Health Service, weekly, with annual summaries by month of year and by county of usual residence.

REFERENCES

BENJAMIN, B. (1953) *Brit. J. Tub.*

BENJAMIN, B. CAWTHORNE, T. E., and WHETNALL, E. (1954) Unpublished.

BENJAMIN, B., and GORE, A. T. (1952) *Brit. J. Soc. Med.*, 6, p. 197.

BIDDLE, D. (1888) *B.M.J.*, ii. 160.

BRADLEY, W. H. (1950) *Monthly Bull. of Min. Health*, 9, 203.

BRANSBY, E. R. (1951) *Medical Officer*, 86, 2231.

BREEN, G. E., and BENJAMIN, B. (1949) *Lancet*, ii. 620.

BREEN, G. E., and BENJAMIN, B. (1950) *Brit. M.J.*, ii. 1473.

COLLIS, E. L., and GREENWOOD, M. (1921) *Health of the Industrial Worker*. Churchill, London.

GREENWOOD, M. (1946) *J. R. Statist. Soc.*, 109, 85.

GRENVILLE-MATHERS, R., and TRENCHARD, H. J. (1953) Proc. R. Soc. Med., 46, 859.

GLOVER, E. A. (1947) *Bull. of Min. Health and P.H.L.S.*, 6, 44.

HART, P. D'ARCY, and PAYLING WRIGHT, G. (1939), *Tuberculosis and Social Conditions*, N.A.P.T.

HOPE, SIMPSON R. E. (1952) *Lancet*, ii. 549.

IRVINE, E. D. (1952) *Lancet*, ii. 724.

LOGAN, W. P. D. (1950) *Monthly Bull. of Min. Health and P.H.L.S.*, 9, 198.

LOGAN, W. P. D., and MACKAY, D. (1951) *Lancet*, i. 284.

London County Council (1933) Report of Medical Officer of Health on the Measles Epidemic (1931–32). No. 2996 P. S. KING.

HILL, A. B., and MARTIN, W. J. (1949) *B.M.J.*, ii. 357.

Medical Research Council (1951) *B.M.J.*, i. 1463.

Ministry of Health (1953) Report of Chief Medical Officer for 1951, H.M.S.O.

NEWSHOLME, A. (1896) *J. Roy. Stat. Soc.*, 59, 1.

PICKLES, W. H., *Epidemiology in Country Practice*, Bristol (John Wright), 1939, p. 114.

Registrar General of England and Wales (1951) *Statistical Review*, 1946–47 Text. Medical H.M.S.O.

RUMSEY, (1875) Essays and Papers on Some Fallacies of Vital Statistics, 1.

STOCKS, P. (1949) 'Sickness and the Population of England and Wales 1944–47', *Studies in Pop. Med. Sub.*, No. 2 G.R.O. H.M.S.O.

TATHAM, J. (1888) *B.M.J.*, ii. 402.

TAYLOR, J., and KNOWELDEN, J. (1964) 'Principles of Epidemiology', J. H. Churchill. 2nd Ed.

CHAPTER 10

TUBERCULOSIS

10.1 Though tuberculosis is an infectious disease there are important differences in aetiology, pathology and in the administration of preventive and curative services which distinguish it from other infectious diseases and give rise to special statistical needs. In the first place we distinguish between *infection*, the invasion of the body by the tubercle bacillus with the concomitant resistant and immunological reactions, and *disease*, the actual colonization of bacilli in tissue or bone and the production of clinical or radiological evidence of successful and threatening invasion. Although this distinction has doubtful pathological validity and is in fact much less clear in practice than as simply expressed here, it is justified statistically since in any population in which tubercle bacillus has been freely circulating a large proportion of the adult population will be found to have been infected before or during adolescence but there will be a relatively small proportion with active disease. In 1949–50 it was estimated that 9–14 per cent of children aged five in urban areas of England and Wales were tuberculin sensitive, and could therefore be assumed to have a history of infection; by age twenty, this proportion had risen to 59–74 per cent. (Medical Research Council 1952.) In contrast the proportion of the population on the registers of tuberculous patients supervised by chest clinics at the end of 1950 was only 0·65 per cent. Thus only a small proportion of those who are infected ever show significant signs of disease, i.e. a spread or infiltration from an original focus of infection. The majority of primary infections heal uneventfully without active treatment and in most cases without the infected person being aware of the infection. These figures are out of date but the contrast remains.

10.2 The disease is notifiable in England and Wales (and most developed countries) but there is some degree of under-reporting mainly because some cases are symptomless and are never detected. Stocks (1949) estimated 10 per cent under-reporting for respiratory tuberculosis. Probably case finding has improved since then. Mass miniature radiography has resulted in the detection of many unsuspected cases of active respiratory disease. Contact surveillance has improved and there has been a generally wider public appreciation of symptomology.

10.3 Notifications are used as a measure of prevalence despite any under-reporting especially since mortality has been falling rapidly and deaths, though completely recorded, bear a changing ratio to the size of the tuberculous population.

The general picture

10.4 The earlier pattern, as indicated by tuberculin surveys in England and Wales, was that the risk of infection (that is the general or average risk in the

174

population as distinct from the risk within a particular tuberculous household) was small in infancy, but rose rapidly after school entry age, at the rate of about four per cent per year of age, until at the age of sixteen about fifty per cent and at age twenty-one about seventy per cent had been infected. At higher adult ages a very high proportion of the population had been infected. In recent years, however, there has been a downward trend in the level of infection and consequently a reduction in positive reactions to tuberculin tests. The tuberculin survey of 1949–50 revealed lower levels of tuberculin sensitivity at all ages than in a survey carried out twenty years earlier (D'Arcy Hart, 1932) and lower than in the comparable subgroups of the Prophit Survey (Daniels, Ridehalgh and Springett, 1948). Between 1954 and 1964 in London the proportion of 13-year old school-children reacting positively to tuberculin tests fell from 14 to 8 per cent.

10.5 To return to the infected persons, we are concerned with the minority in whom the original infection is not confined and healed without physical disturbance but infiltrates into surrounding tissue and causes disease. In many such cases, but not all, this disease is progressive and, if not checked by treatment, lethal. In some cases the natural resistance of the body may eventually prevail and the disease may heal without therapeutic intervention leaving only a scar behind. The proportion of infections which proceed to disease is not exactly known, knowledge being confined to statutory notification.

10.6 Table 10.1 relates notifications to the infected population of England and Wales with the following reservations.

(i) Many cases of disease are never detected or notified—especially those which recover without disability or treatment.

(ii) Some notifications relate not to disease but to primary infection particularly where radiological or other physical changes during the process of healing provoke anxiety and the need for special surveillance.

(iii) The ratios shown in column 4 of the table do not measure the disease potentiality of infections occurring within the age group, since the time interval between infection and diagnosed disease may be long and span the boundaries between age groups.

TABLE 10.1 *Notification of disease among those infected—England and Wales* 1954 (*persons*)

Age	Estimated per cent tuberculin positive	Tuberculosis notifications (all forms) per 1,000 population	Notifications per annum per cent of tuberculin positive
0–1	0·5	0·28	5·6
1—4	5·0	0·53	1·1
5—9	30·0	0·51	0·17
10—14	70·0	1·58	0·23
15—24	90·0	1·05	0·12
25—44	95·0	0·78	0·08
45 and over	95·0	0·47	0·05

10.7 We may estimate from these figures that in England and Wales in 1954 almost all persons had been infected, and that tuberculosis disease would have been notified in about one in fourteen, at some time during their lifetime. Since then the prevalence of infection has fallen considerably but the table serves to illustrate the difference between the risks of infection and of disease.

Notifications of disease

10.8 Tuberculous morbidity has not been conventionally defined and statistically there is no measure other than notifications and the criterion for reporting cases is not specifically related to sickness, disability, or degree of radiologically visible disease but consists either in a belief that the person is a potential infector of others and/or requires medical or social care.

10.9 Notification rates by age and sex in England and Wales in 1964 are shown in Table 10.2. In males the rate for respiratory tuberculosis rises with advancing age; while for females the incidence of notified disease is peaked in the 25–34 age group and thereafter descends rapidly with advancing age. For non-respiratory disease notification is notoriously incomplete though to an indeterminate degree (Stocks, 1949) but taking the figures at their face value it is clear that, as might be expected from association with primary infection, the incidence of non-respiratory forms of the disease is highest in early adult life.

TABLE 10.2 *Primary notifications of tuberculosis—England and Wales, 1964*

Type of Tuberculosis	Sex	Age	Notifications per 100,000 population
Respiratory	Male	0—4	16
		5—14	13
		15—24	34
		25—34	50
		35—44	49
		45—64	63
		65 and over	62
	Female	0—4	15
		5—14	12
		15—24	30
		25—34	34
		35—44	27
		45—64	16
		65 and over	12
Non-respiratory	Male	0—14	2·8
		15—24	6·3
		25—44	8·6
		45 and over	3·7
	Female	0—14	2·9
		15—24	6·3
		25—44	8·9
		45 and over	4·8

176

Mortality

10.10 Death rates by age and sex for each type of disease are shown in Table 10.3. For respiratory tuberculosis the shapes of these curves and the trends of the rates they represent are natural corollaries of the incidence (notification) rates in Table 10.2, for a large proportion of such deaths as occur do so within a few years of notification. Thus in males the rising notification rates with advancing age are reflected by mortality rates rising gradually to a late peak. For females the mortality rates, affected by the peak of the notification rates, rise less steeply.

10.11 With regard to mortality from non-respiratory tuberculosis it has to be borne in mind that disease which terminates fatally may do so in a form which differs from that in which it originated. A number of cases notified as non-respiratory may later develop chronic pulmonary tuberculosis and may ultimately die from that disease. Others notified with local lymphatic or skeletal lesions may suffer miliary extension of disease and may die as a result of lung or meningeal involvement. In general the death risk from non-respiratory tuberculosis is maximal in the early years of childhood (more detailed figures show that the highest death rate is in the second year of life) and rapidly declines to insignificant proportions in adult life. The most fatal of these forms of disease is tuberculosis of the meninges and central nervous system.

10.12 In considering the rates of mortality from tuberculosis at older ages it is important to bear in mind that they represent the experience of earlier generations whose exposure to tuberculosis has generally been at a higher level than more recent generations. Since the disease spread throughout the community each succeeding generation has fared better in combating the ravages of the 'white scourge'. This feature has been extensively analysed

TABLE 10.3 *Death rates for tuberculosis—England and Wales, 1964*

Type of Tuberculosis	Age	Deaths per million	
		Males	Females
Respiratory	0—4	1	3
	5—9	—	—
	10—14	1	1
	15—19	2	1
	20—24	3	1
	25—34	8	9
	35—44	34	25
	45—54	87	25
	55—64	183	33
	65—74	363	48
	75 and over	411	76
Non-respiratory	0—14	1·5	1·3
	15—24	0·9	0·9
	25—44	4·5	2·9
	45 and over	13	11

on a generation or 'cohort' mortality basis by Frost (1939), Springett (1950), Daw (1950) and Spicer (1954), i.e. by following through the mortality experience of successive generations. Generally the results may be summarized by saying that though the secular trend is that the peak of mortality in middle life has moved steadily to later ages and become diminished, this is mainly due to succeeding generations having lower mortality so that the residual (at late ages) of the high mortality of an early generation is greater than the early adult peak of the present generation. The peak is now so late that it does not appear in the published mortality tables which have broad age-groupings at older ages. This has led to the suggestions that more developed communities have been 'breeding out' the disease (i.e. producing, by natural selection, genetic strains of lessened susceptibility) or alternatively that the bacillus itself has become less virulent. There is little evidence to support either suggestion. A much simpler explanation is possible. The problem of tuberculosis is a volumetric problem of a reservoir of infection, i.e. of the quantity of bacilli freely circulating. Reducing the spread of the disease both by isolating diagnosed infectors or reducing their infectiousness by treatment and also by providing fewer opportunities for unknown infectors to infect others in crowded and ill-ventilated workshops, and increasing general resistance to disease by improved social conditions, has resulted in succeeding generations having a reduced risk of meeting heavy doses of bacilli. This process has been tremendously accelerated by the great rapidity with which modern chemo-therapy sterilizes the lesion and renders the patient sputum-negative, and by improved case-finding which has enabled more infectors to be detected and rendered non-infectious. It should be borne in mind that it is indeed a question of how much disease is contracted in early adult life as most of the morbidity of later adult life is due to breakdown of old lesions (Springett [1951]). Indeed this underlies not only the constancy of the cohort pattern but explains some of the deviation from a simple picture to which Spicer (1954) draws attention. The following notification rates for respiratory tuberculosis per 100,000 in England and Wales for (pre-chemotherapy) 1946 and 1964 complete the picture.

Age:		0—	5—	15—	25—	35—	45—	65+
Males	1946	32	46	179	174	125	138	54
	1964	16	13	34	50	49	63	62
Females	1946	28	49	213	141	65	35	16
	1964	15	12	30	34	27	16	12

10.13 The risk of contracting disease in adolescence is clearly diminishing. (There has been some concentration on the detection of the often symptom-free elderly sputum-positive male and this explains the higher rate at 65+.)

Social factors

10.14 Conditions either favouring the transmission of the infecting organism or reducing the host resistance must lead to increased prevalence of disease. On the one hand overcrowded housing conditions or failure to isolate infectious cases from home or industrial contacts and on the other hand malnutrition, fatigue and side effects of poor social conditions foster the disease. The risk of infection from unsuspected or poorly supervised cases of tuberculosis either within their own families or among workmates is high and represents an especially difficult problem owing to the often silent character of primary infection and the effectively long period of 'incubation' before symptoms of disease appear. The precise role of overcrowding in this connection is not clear since it is difficult to separate housing conditions from the whole complex of social conditions (Benjamin, 1953) but there is evidence at least that larger households provide a wider circle through which infection may spread (Benjamin, *ibid.*) and the larger households are usually housed at higher than average density. With regard to poor social conditions, again it is difficult to measure the individual effects of nutrition, occupation, local amenities or medical services and other environmental elements though many attempts have been made [Collis and Greenwood (1921), D'Arcy Hart and Payling Wright (1939), Stein (1951), Benjamin (1953)], but it is clear that the disease thrives more strongly and persistently among the poorer members of the community, and since by incapacitating the wage earner tuberculosis may bring an approach toward poverty, a vicious circle may be created. Tuberculosis is in a very real sense a social disease of great importance.

10.15 Some mention must be made of special occupational risks though again it is difficult to separate these from general environmental influences. The occupational mortality studies surrounding the 1931 Census (General Register Office, 1936) indicated that the ten occupations with the highest mortality from respiratory tuberculosis among males were:

	Standard Mortality Ratio at ages 20–64*
Grinders, metal	275
Potters, waremakers, casters, finishers	233
Glazers, polishers, moppers	230
Barmen	212
Costermongers, newspaper sellers	200
Boot, shoe workers—factory operatives	188
Water Transport—dock labourers	186
Masons, stone cutters, dressers	179
Waiters	178
Hairdressers, etc.	162

* In brief this represents the actual deaths 1930–32 as a percentage of those expected if the average tuberculosis mortality rates for England and Wales, age by age, had been experienced by the occupational group.

In the 1949–53 investigations (General Register Office 1958) the occupations identified as having the highest rates included similar groups—sand blasters, edge-tool grinders, filers, masons, potters and casters, boot and shoe makers, costermongers, dock labourers, hairdressers, barmen and restaurant counter hands—but glazers, polishers, moppers did not have an especially excessive mortality (SMR 106).

10.16 Greenwood and Thompson (Collis and Greenwood, 1921) had many years earlier stressed the powerful influence of the conditions of factory employment in general in facilitating the spread of disease. Later, Collis (1925) in referring to the high mortality from respiratory tuberculosis in printers and shoemakers despite low general mortality stressed that in both occupations the men 'worked indoors under circumstances in which individuals are so congregated together as to facilitate the passage of infection from person to person'.

179

10.17 An investigation of sickness in the cotton, spinning, cotton weaving and printing industries (Bradford Hill, 1927, 1929, 1930), though restricted by lack of data, served to underline the high incidence of tuberculosis in the printing industry.

10.18 Differentiation has to be made between the true occupational risks represented by dust damage to lungs (grinders, potters, glazers, stone cutters) or cross-infection (printers, shoemakers) and the apparent occupational risks which actually arise from the poor level of living of low paid jobs (barmen, costermongers, waiters) where recruitment may also be from persons of poor physique.

10.19 Cairns and Stewart (1951) have discussed the different phasing of the rise and fall of tuberculosis mortality in printers and shoemakers regarding each industry as partially closed communities and have suggested that 'the tuberculosis mortality trends for printers and shoemakers during the fifty years of records represent respectively the declining and ascending phases of two . . . [slow motion] . . . epidemics' such as might occur in the industrialization of trades where the work is light enough to permit the presence of chronic carriers. Evidence of such chronic carriers had been found in a photofluorographic survey of the Northampton boot and shoe industry (Stewart and Hughes, 1949 and 1951) as also had evidence of selective recruitment of workers of poor physique, and of high risks of airborne spread of infection in the factories.

10.20 The classical example of cross-infection risk may be found in the high rate of infection in nurses tending general hospital patients; such patients though not under treatment for tuberculosis form a sick community among whom chronic carriers are likely to be more frequent than in the population at large (Daniels, Ridehalgh, Springett, 1948).

Invalidity

10.21 Stress has already been laid upon the long chronic course of tuberculosis. In the pre-chemotherapy era the average period between notification and death in England and Wales was about 2·2 years (derived from Stocks and Faning, 1944) and these deaths were dispersed over a much longer period. Those who died within a few years of notification may be regarded as a selection of those who were from the outset failing to arrest the progress of the disease and they were probably incapacitated for much of their period of survival. When account is taken of those with more favourable response to treatment much longer periods of survival are involved. In the pre-war period 1937–39 (loc. cit.) 51 per cent of all respiratory cases were alive ten years after notification. In a study of a large body of patients treated by collapse therapy for respiratory tuberculosis between 1937 and 1942 the proportion surviving eight years even among severely cavitated cases was 50 per cent. (Foster Carter et al., 1952). In a study of a normal cross-section of chest clinic cases notified in 1949 and treated by chemotherapy or surgery, the proportion surviving five years was 83·4 per cent (Caplin and Silver 1956). It is probable that prognosis has improved further.

10.22 As to the period of incapacitation, the records of National Insurance (unpublished data) indicate that the median length of spells of sickness claim due to respiratory tuberculosis terminating in 1960–61 was for males 211 days and for females 278 days. Even though results of treatment are infinitely better than a few years ago it is clear that tuberculosis, especially respiratory tuberculosis, prevents the sufferer from carrying on a normal life for a period of many months in most cases, and in some cases for years.

10.23 The total loss to national productivity is thus not inconsiderable. In 1960–61 in Great Britain 6·5 million person-days were lost to industry as a result of tuberculosis in respect of those covered by sickness insurance apart from the loss in respect of non-insured persons. The figure is falling rapidly however. In 1953–54 it was 26 million person-days. It is worth stressing that the majority of new cases in adult life occur at comparatively early ages and that even in recovery (now the rule rather than exception) there may be impairment of function and lack of ability to return to occupations as vigorous as those adopted prior to illness.

Tuberculosis control

10.24 The problem of controlling tuberculosis has been regarded as two-fold:

(1) In the community—identification of infectious cases and prevention of spread by reducing infectivity (treatment and/or isolation).
(2) In the individual—diagnosis and treatment to sterilize disease and to restore function.

10.25 Ideally, these are one and the same problem; in practice in the past it has been too complacently assumed that to treat the known sufferer is to limit automatically the spread of disease. The fallacy is that infectious cases are not always aware that they are suffering, and that a proportion of cases cannot even with the best modern treatment be rendered non-infective. Falling mortality accentuates the problem by prolonging the years during which an infective case can spread disease. In recent years, however, greater emphasis has been placed upon the first part of the dual problem.

10.26 Notification of tuberculosis (to the Medical Officer of Health) is an accepted essential measure of control, as it is of other infectious diseases. In England and Wales, attention was first directed to the spread of infection among the destitute and vagrant population and in 1908 regulations were made compelling poor-law hospital medical officers to notify pulmonary tuberculosis found among cases under their care, to the local sanitary authority (County or County Boroughs, outside London; the Metropolitan Boroughs, within London). In 1911, notification was extended to cases of pulmonary tuberculosis in public hospitals (i.e. not entirely supported by patients' contributions). From January 1, 1912, all cases of tuberculosis coming to the notice of a medical practitioner became compulsorily notifiable.

10.27 The arrangements for notification in England and Wales are governed by the Tuberculosis Regulations of 1952. Briefly they are as follows:

Diagnosis—is sometimes made by the general practitioner, but is more commonly made, finally, by the Chest Physician of the local chest clinic (under the control of the Regional Hospital Board through the local Hospital Group Management Committee) after referral by the general practitioner and after radiological and bacteriological examination.

Notification—Upon diagnosis the Chest Physician (or other medical practitioner making the diagnosis) reports the case to the County or County Borough Medical Officer of Health. The report states name, age, sex, address, occupation and site of the tuberculous lesion. The County Medical Officer of Health has a definite part to play in co-ordinating services since the local health authority pays a fraction of the salary of Chest Physicians and provides the nursing staff for assistance at the clinic and for visiting the homes of tuberculous patients.

Treatment—Free institutional treatment of those for whom it is recommended and domiciliary treatment for other cases is provided as part of the National Health Service. Supervision by the Chest Physician is maintained so long as the disease is under any suspicion of remaining active, and for this purpose the tuberculosis patient is encouraged to attend the local clinic. An endeavour is also made to get all contacts of the patient examined and kept under necessary supervision.

Medical Records

10.28 Every tuberculosis patient treated in hospital or sanatorium has at least two personal medical records (1) the *hospital* record which is a fairly complete account of all previous treatment—made complete by ready exchange of information, and records, between hospitals, (2) the *clinic* record (which includes a home visiting record and socio-economic information) kept for supervision purposes—so long as contact is maintained, this is a complete account of the environment and progress of the tuberculous person and of his contacts; its completeness depends on reports from hospitals. Contact coverage has improved tremendously.

Expansion of diagnostic services

10.29 In recent years greater public awareness of the tuberculosis problem and of the need for earlier diagnosis, and generally improved diagnostic facilities have combined to intensify case-finding. Much more extensive tuberculin sensitivity testing in children has played some part in drawing attention to sources of infection. A very important diagnostic advance has been due to the mass miniature radiography services. By conducting surveys in factories and offices and among the general public the radiography units have discovered many unsuspected cases of tuberculosis. Apart from mass surveys the units are sometimes made available to general practitioners under special referral schemes, to education authorities for school leavers, to hospital out-patient departments, and to mental hospitals. In 1965 some 3,826,000 persons were examined in England and Wales and 3,998 cases of tuberculosis requiring treatment or close supervision were discovered, i.e. about one-fifth of the total new cases of respiratory tuberculosis were discovered by miniature radioagraphy.

Defects

10.30 The main defects of notification are

(1) Lack of standard criteria for notification so that there may be local variation in the selection of cases for notification. The difficulties of

182

definition are formidable. The Ministry of Health have issued only a general note of guidance indicating that 'Tuberculosis is required to be notified in order to check the spread of infection and to bring about the proper management of the individual case and its immediate contacts. A person who should be notified as "suffering from tuberculosis", therefore, is a person who, because of tuberculosis infection may infect others; or a person who is suffering from an active tuberculosis lesion which calls for medical treatment or for some modification of the patient's normal course of living.' Interpretation varies throughout the country.

(2) The only registers which exist are the filed notes at chest clinics. These are not uniform either in mode of maintenance or in extent of reviewal. As sources of statistical assessment of the condition of the tuberculous population they have been practically neglected. For national trends it has been necessary to depend on the death rate which becomes less and less adequate as an index of a disease that is rapidly becoming less fatal.

(3) There is no attempt to integrate with the notification system a follow-up of cases referred to chest clinics from radiological surveys or to integrate with the notification and mortality statistics, the results of radiological surveys (of disease) or tuberculin surveys (of infection) or of the infectivity of treated patients in order to watch the total reservoir of infection.

The reservoir of infection

10.31 It is possible to use (Benjamin and Nash, 1952) a hydrodynamic model to describe the composition of the total reservoir of infection in the community. In this model (Fig. 10.1) the unknown infector pool is fed by new disease. Diagnostic channels transfer cases from the unknown infector pool to the known infector pool; the unknown infector pool may also lose cases by death or healing without prior detection of the tuberculous disease. From the known infector pool there may also be losses by recovery or death. The two pools serve as the total reservoir from which new infections are transmitted with the important distinction between them that in the case of the known infector pool the barrier of hygiene which surrounds the detected case serves to reduce the outflow of new infection. The new infections, in circumstances in which there are factors inimical to the forces of resistance, produce new disease and thus the cycle is completed.

10.32 To illustrate the measurement of the various components of this system we restrict consideration to respiratory tuberculosis partly because more complete information is available of the respiratory form and partly because the infectiousness of non-respiratory cases is much less than that of respiratory cases. The term 'infector' means potentially infectious rather than actually sputum postive.

The following estimates were made in 1956. They are out of date and serve only to illustrate the method. Current figures are not wholly available.

The unknown infector pool

10.33 The mass radiography service then revealed previously unsuspected active tuberculosis in $2 \cdot 2$ per 1,000 examinees (Ministry of Health, 1956). This led to an estimated total number of unsuspected cases in England and Wales of 75,000 of which approximately 25,000 would be sputum positive.

10.34 *New disease*. This was measured by the radiological attack rate over a defined interval in persons whose X-rays were clear at the commencement of the interval. In a survey of repeat radiography in the Civil Service (industrial and non-industrial), Springett (1951) found the following rates—

Primary lesions
Annual attack rates per 1,000

Ages	Males	Females
15–24	3·0	4·0
25–34	2·0	2·5
35–44	1·5	0·5
45–49	1·0	0·5

Applying these rates to the population of England and Wales yielded 45,000 new cases each year. This was an understatement since some of those attacked subsequent to a clear X-ray might have been diagnosed on symptoms *before* repeat radiography and thus would not come to miniature X-ray again, but in

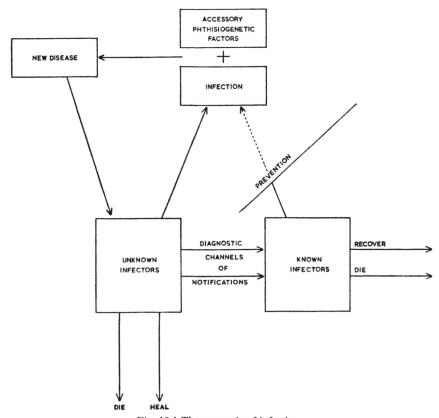

Fig. 10.1 The reservoir of infection.

184

view of the initially silent nature of many new lesions it seemed unlikely that the understatement could be greater than 20 per cent. This was the proportion of new cases diagnosed which were early and were detected otherwise than by mass X-ray (Lowe and Geddes, 1953). It was proposed, therefore, to assume a total of 55,000 cases of new disease each year.

10.35 *Notifications.* The numbers of new cases of respiratory tuberculosis notified in England and Wales in recent years had been (Ministry of Health 1956)

1950	42,435
1951	42,696
1952	41,904
1953	40,917
1954	36,973
1955	33,580

i.e. the current level could be taken as 35,000.

10.36 *Deaths prior to notification.* In addition there were the following deaths of tuberculous persons who were not notified before death.

1950	2,113
1951	2,067
1952	1,816
1953	1,751
1954	1,330
1955	1,224

These figures probably understated the true loss since they depended in part upon the extent of post-mortem detection of active lesions in persons dying from causes not primarily tuberculous and it was proposed to take a round figure of 2,000.

10.37 *Healing.* The numbers of new lesions which heal without becoming significantly active to an extent sufficient to promote symptoms and notification could be estimated from the rate of incidence of inactive post-primary lesions found by the mass radiography service (Ministry of Health, 1953). These proportions rose from $3 \cdot 7$ per thousand at ages 15–24 to $24 \cdot 6$ per thousand at age 60 and were equivalent to an annual healing rate of about $0 \cdot 55$ per 1,000 of the adult population, i.e. 18,900 each year. This took no account of those which healed and left a clear X-ray. An arbitrary addition of 1,100 could be made to bring the total to a round figure of 20,000. It was assumed that any case which had exhibited a radiological lesion had been at some time potentially infectious.

10.38 *Total movement.* It is thus seen that the unknown infector pool in 1956 was of the order of 75,000 persons, the annual movements then being:

	New lesions		55,000
Less			
	Healed lesions	20,000	
	Notifications	35,000	
	Deaths unnotified	2,000	
		———	57,000
	Net annual loss		2,000

185

10.39 Of the total unknown pool some 25,000 were infectious (sputum positive) and the net annual loss to this component would be only a fraction of the total outgo of 2,000 as most of the latter were likely to be minimal lesions. Thus the infectious component was then probably diminishing only slowly.

The known infector pool

10.40 At the end of 1955 there were 307,182 notified cases of respiratory tuberculosis on the clinic registers in England and Wales, of whom 19,323 were known to have had tubercle bacilli in the sputum in the preceding six months. The corresponding figure for 1954 was 297,153, and for 1953 283,601. The pool appeared to be increasing at the rate of about 11,000 a year. The average annual number of deaths from respiratory tuberculosis over the same period 1953-55 was 7,000 so that rather less than 20,000 cases must have been coming off the registers every year as recovered.

10.41 Deaths had been declining rapidly in recent years and might be expected to continue to decline. Whether or not this would be matched by increased recoveries was then not known. The numbers of patients on the clinic registers who have had a postitive sputum in the previous six months have been in recent years—

End of 1949	26,752
1950	27,139
1951	25,477
1952	25,947
1953	25,055
1954	21,655
1955	19,323

10.42 The number of infectious cases on the registers, had declined only slowly despite the effect of improved methods of treatment in prolonging life though the pace had quickened since 1953.

10.43 In England and Wales in 1956 therefore the population suffering from respiratory tuberculosis was of the order of 380,000 of whom perhaps 45,000 were sputum positive and therefore infectious.

10.44 The picture has changed dramatically. Diagnostic facilities have improved and the transfer from the unknown to the known pool must have been augmented. The flow of new infections whether to the unknown or to the known pool has diminished. At the end of 1965 there were 333,340 cases of tuberculosis under supervision of which only 9,928 had had positive broncho-pulmonary secretions during the previous year.

Prevention

10.45 The diagrammatic representation of the reservoir of infection indicates the salient features of the problem of preventing new disease. If cases can be transferred from the unknown to the known (notified) pool then a barrier may be interposed between them and their immediate contacts. Detection and supervision represent the twin objectives of the whole system of control. This picture also indicates the main statistical needs.

10.46 The barrier against the spread of infection consists in (1) educating the patient to reduce to a minimum the risk of transmitting bacilli to those with whom he may be in contact by practical measures of personal hygiene; (2) isolating the patient altogether during the most infectious phase of his disease; (3) gaining the co-operation of the patient in treatment so that conversion to a non-infectious condition can be speedily achieved; (4) observation of contacts and instruction in the risks they incur; (5) vaccination (BCG) of those close contacts who on the evidence of skin tests appear to have escaped infection at the time when the patient (referred to as the index case) is notified, on the assumption that if they are to continue to run the risk of infection they should gain immunity by inoculation of attenuated bacillus rather than by natural invasion. Vaccination has latterly been extended beyond such immediate contacts of infectious cases to special classes of persons who, possessing no acquired immunity by virtue of previous infection, are considered to be currently exposed to infection, e.g. nurses, school leavers.

Treatment

10.47 There are a number of aspects of treatment which are important to the successful conduct of a national anti-tuberculosis scheme, e.g. the adequacy of treatment facilities, the efficient selection of different types of patient for appropriate forms of treatment, the development of regimens of treatment which secure the highest possible degree of restoration of normal function. These aspects are not, however, germane to the discussion of statistical aspects of the control of tuberculosis. Here we are mainly concerned with the efficacy of treatment in reducing infectivity, i.e. with the speed and permanence of conversion from the sputum-postive to the sputum-negative state. In certain types of cases, e.g. young adult early cases of respiratory tuberculosis, conversion can be achieved by intensive chemotherapy. In more advanced cases much depends upon the successful closure of cavity by collapse therapy or its eradication by surgery and a time interval of many months may be involved. A good deal is known, from statistical reports of sanatoria and hospitals, of the proportion of sputum-positive patients who are discharged as sputum-negative (this requires definition, e.g. negative on three consecutive monthly tests, but there appears to be no accepted standard). Much less is known of the degree of permanence of this conversion or of the proportion of patients who though negative at the commencement and termination of active treatment nevertheless ultimately become positive. Such statistics depend upon pursuance of much more complete (though not complicated) systems of follow-up records than are generally adopted.

10.48 From statistics quoted by Snell (1951, 1953) it may be deduced that probably an average of 75 per cent of sputum positive tuberculosis patients were then converted to negative by institutional treatment of domiciliary chemotherapy.

10.49 In 1955 there were 33,580 notifications of respiratory tuberculosis in England and Wales of whom some 14,000 were sputum-positive. If 75 per cent of the latter were rendered negative by treatment, the addition to the known positive infector pool was 3,500. On the other hand, there were 5,837 deaths from respiratory tuberculosis during the year so that the number of sputum positive cases on the registers of chest clinics should have declined by about 2,300. In fact, as we have already seen, the number declined by 2,332 though the close agreement is probably fortuitous.

The statistical needs

10.50 The statistical needs of an effective system of control now become clear. These are—

(i) Knowledge of the degree of completeness of case-finding and the application of statistical methods to efficient deployment of case-finding resources.
(ii) Specificity in reporting and in maintenance of registers.
(iii) Analytical approach to local comparisons.
(iv) Follow-up records and effective national co-ordination.
(v) Integration of the statistical elements needed to enable the total problem of tuberculosis to be seen as a complete picture.

10.51 We may deal with these in greater detail.

(i) *Case-finding*

10.52 It is first necessary to analyse the source of new diagnoses and the following figures for Birmingham (Lowe and Geddes, 1953) are illustrative.

Source of new cases of respiratory tuberculosis
seen at chest clinic, 1952

Source	No.	Per cent
Notified by general practitioners	216	19·1
Referred to chest clinic as suspects	527	46·6
Examined as contacts	109	9·6
Referred from Mass X-ray	280	24·7
Total	**1,132**	**100·0**

10.53 We should consider the yield from each source in relation to the effort expended in order to decide which method is the most efficient. Typical figures showing the orders of relative yields are—

Source	No. of active cases of tuberculosis per 1,000 examinations
Mass radiography	
(a) examinations of volunteer members of the public	2
(b) routine referrals from general practitioners of cases with mild symptoms which simulate commoner complaints (colds, coughs, loss of weight, etc.)	20
Examinations of known contacts by chest clinics	20
Examinations of cases referred to chest clinics by general practitioners and suspected to be tuberculous	150–200

10.54 The efficacy of a particular mode of case-finding cannot be judged only by the proportion of examinations which result in a confirmed diagnosis of tuberculosis; if this were so, chest clinic examination of referred suspects would be incomparably superior to all other methods while mass miniature radiography would appear to be extremely inefficient. In the context of the analogy drawn in an earlier section the overrriding criterion should be the contribution made to *increasing* the speed of flow from the unknown to the known infector pool. It is necessary to consider whether in absence of the method under test the unknown case would be discovered at all, and this means that the presence or absence of symptoms must be taken into account.

(ii) *Specificity in reporting*

10.55 The extent of disease should be known for all reported cases so that by comparison with past statistics a clear picture may be obtained of how much earlier (in the time-scale of disease development) cases are being diagnosed, whether some types of disease not previously recorded are being notified, and how the symptomless case may best be detected.

10.56 A classification for this purpose (shown on p. 197) was devised for the mass radiography service by Dr V. H. Springett and the late Dr Marc Daniels. Cases referred to chest clinics from mass radiography units are at present coded by reference to this classification by Chest Physicians.

10.57 The following is a sample percentage distribution of cases aged 25–44 notified in London in 1917–39, 1940–47, 1948–53 classified under axis B of the four digit code in the Appendix.

Character of lesion	1917–39	1940–47	1948–53
1. Pulmonary or hilar calcification	4	5	10
2. Enlarged hilar glands only	—	—	—
3. Enlarged hilar glands and pulmonary focus	—	—	2
4. Pleural effusion	7	8	2
5. Infiltration without cavity	67	51	46
6. Cavity suspect	—	—	—
7. Definite cavity, more than 1 cm. (tomogram)	—	1	—
8. Definite cavity, more than 1 cm. (straight film)	22	35	40
Total	100	100	100
Number of cases	27	97	42

10.58 This particular sample was too small to support any firm conclusion but similar distributions based on larger numbers would provide information to indicate whether there have been changes in the general character of the disease of new cases over a period of time.

(iii) *Local comparisons*

10.59 Comparison of local notification rates may be rendered almost impossible by wide differences in the criteria adopted for notification. These differences are at present only surmised from variations in the ratio of deaths to notifications between different areas; these variations do not follow any recognizable pattern. If greater specificity could be applied to notification this difficulty would be overcome. It would then be possible to make proper local comparisons and thus to discern areas with the highest prevalence of disease upon which preventive resources might be concentrated. Intensive field surveys could be organized in the worst areas to raise the level of case-finding and to make such local epidemiological enquiries as would identify principal sources of infection, and would promote action to reduce spread. As examples, we may quote the comb-out of the boot and shoe industry in Northampton (Stewart and Hughes, 1951) and the Rhondda Fach Survey carried out by the M.R.C. Pneumoconiosis Unit (Cochrane, Cox and Jarman, 1952).

(iv) *Follow-up records and national co-ordination*

10.60 An attempt has been made in earlier sections of this chapter to indicate the meaning, in practical terms, of the phrase 'control of tuberculosis'. It involves a detailed knowledge of the tuberculous population as a distinct community, of changes in the size of that population in pace and direction, of sources of replenishment and modes of depletion. The structure of this population—age, sex, occupation—its infectivity, its invalidity and its expectation of survival are important components of the analytical picture. Nationally, the picture may be seen only when local knowledge is pooled on a uniform basis. Local records thus become of vital importance.

10.61 Two main records are created in respect of each patient under supervision by a Chest Clinic—the clinical record maintained by the Chest Physician and containing the full history of the patient and summaries of institutional treatment, and the home record maintained by the Tuberculosis Health Visitor containing reports of home conditions and tracing of contacts; the latter record is, of course, directly accessible to the Chest Physician.

10.62 The average chest clinic has under its care at any one time a large number of tuberculous patients. It is therefore impracticable to produce adequate surveys of the tuberculous population without the aid of card indices which lend themselves to statistical procedures either by straightforward manual sorting or by means of needle and edge-perforation or by full-scale punched card sensing machinery. Such a card must satisfy two requirements: (*a*) it must carry all the basic information arranged in such a way as to facilitate classification and enumeration and (*b*) it must be up-to-date, i.e. means must be found so to organize the management of the clinic records that new information is automatically added to the cards as soon as it is included within the case-history. So far as (*b*) is concerned the simplest process is for the cards themselves or an intermediate transcript document to be inserted in the case-folder prior to each clinic attendance (this presupposes an adequate appointment system). The chest physician or his clerk may then transfer new information on to the card or the transcript document at the end of the consultation or session. The cards are then immediately restored to the main file.

10.63 With regard to (*a*), what are the basic items of information? The following minimum list is suggested; further addition being subject to the research requirements of individual physicians.

(1) Identification particulars—serial number, name, address.
(2) Date of birth—it has been submitted that a direct coding of quinary age group should suffice but date of birth is preferred as allowing age at any other date to be computed and as being no more difficult to classify since the year of birth in fact forms an age code.

(3) Sex, marital condition ⎫
(4) Occupation   ⎬ These factors have a bearing upon exposure
(5) Birthplace   ⎭ to infection, susceptibility and prognosis.

(6) Source of patient—

1. General practitioner
2. Contact of index case
3. Transfer in   Important in
4. Mass miniature   relation to
    radiography   (i) above
5. School clinic   (para. 10.52)
6. Armed services
7. Other

(7) Presenting symptoms—

1. Cough
2. Pain   A great deal still remains
3. Haemoptysis   to be discovered of fre-
4. Loss of weight   quency distributions of
5. Lassitude   combinations of symp-
6. Anorexia   toms and of their possible
7. Other   relationship to activity.
8. Nil

(8) Antecedent condition of tuberculosis significance or association (and interval of time prior to first attendance).

1. Primary complex
2. Pleural effusion
3. Erythema nodosum   It is important to fix the
4. Other primary manifestation   probable age of infection
5. Pneumonia   and to resolve the prob-
6. Whooping cough   lem of the alleged exacer-
7. Measles   bating influence of other
8. Other   infections.
9. Nil

(9) Tuberculin sensitivity.

1. Patch   1. Positive
2. Mantoux   2. Negative
                        3. Not done

(10) Diagnosis

1. Non-tuberculous

International Statistical Classification of Diseases, Injuries and Causes of Death.

2. Tuberculosis

*Code shown in Appendix for Respiratory Disease. International Statistical Classification for Non-Respiratory Disease (include a category 'not yet diagnosed').

*Note—the code embraces extent of disease (area), character of disease (primary, infiltration, cavity, etc.), sputum state, and degree of activity.

(11) Date notified.

(12) Family history—state relative.

(13) Probable contact (especially to give a lead to industrial sources), viz.
    1. Home.
    2. Workplace.

(14) Home conditions affecting prognosis or spread to others (e.g. housing defect).
    1. No separate bedroom.
    2. Sanitary defects in house.
    3. Nursing deficiencies.
    4. Nutritional deficiency.

(15) Treatment given, with dates and site where relevant.
    1. Chemotherapy

Collapse therapy
    2. A.P.
    3. P.P.
    4. Phrenic crush

Major surgery
    5. Lobectomy
    6. Pneumonectomy
    7. Thoracoplasty
    8. Other
    9. Awaiting hospital admission

(16) Follow up at successive anniversaries of notification recording
    1. Active
    2. Arrested
    3. Died
    4. Transfer out
    5. Lost sight of or discharged

Work capacity—
    6. Not working—unfit
    7. Not working—fit—part-time
                    —full-time
    8. Working—original job
    9. Working—other—part-time
    10. Working—other—full-time.

(17) Date of last positive sputum.

10.64 The practicability of a scheme of abstraction of this type has been demonstrated by Stradling (1952) and similar schemes are known to be used by other chest physicians; the details vary especially in relation to coding of diagnosis where physicians tend to use short lists of clinical types (round focus, tension cavity, atelectasis, etc.) and in relation to changes in sputum state The difficulty about using descriptive clinical terms in relation to diagnosis is that such terms do not lend themselves to statistical classification; the range of terms and the meaning attached to them vary with the individual interest of the physician and comparability is often difficult to achieve.

10.65 Standardization of terminology for radiological description has been approached in this country with the publication of the report of a joint committee of the Joint Tuberculosis Council, the Faculty of Radiologists and the Society of Thoracic Surgeons (Ministry of Health, 1952), but the meaning of other clinical terms has not been standardized. The real difficulty is 'reproducibility', i.e. to ensure that the same case will be classified by different workers in the same way and that the use of the classification to specify a type of case, will yield always the kind of case that is coded by the same specification.

10.66 Statistical analysis of this form of record would enable chest physicians to prepare at regular intervals a complete survey of the tuberculous population under his care, classifying by age, sex, source, extent of disease, sputum state, treatment given, current working capacity, etc. At any time he could produce a qualitative as well as a quantitative assessment of the problem of tuberculosis as it confronts him.

10.67 The following tabulations are suggested as appropriate—

Returns I and II show what kind of disease is being notified and in what kind of people, for each locality. Returns III and IV similarly analyse the standing tuberculous population. Return V provides the basic information required for the actuarial calculation of survival factors—it is necessary to have a precise measure of the population at risk of death in each interval. It will be noticed that only cases notified within ten years are to be included; this restriction is necessary, in view of changing methods of treatment, to preserve some degree of homogeneity and to keep the measurements reasonably up to date.

It will be necessary from time to time for the cases shown on I-IV to be analysed locally

(*a*) to indicate industrial location
(*b*) to indicate source of case, viz., which method of case-finding was responsible.

Chest Clinic..............................

I. New cases of respiratory disease notified during the period ended..............................

Initial Assessment	No. cases	Extent of disease	Character of lesion							Sputum + ve	Total cases
			Pulmonary or hilar calcification	Hilar Glands	Hilar glands and focus	Pleural Effusion	Infiltration without cavity	Cavity Suspect	Cavity Definite		
Males 0–14											
Presumed healed healed		Unilateral— less than 2 interspaces									
Suspect—not confirmed		2–4									
		4+									
Occasional supervision		Bilateral— less than 2 interspaces									
Close clinic supervision		2–4									
Immediate											

II. New cases of non-respiratory disease notified during the period ended.............

Sex	Age	Site of lesion							Total
		Meninges and Central Nervous	Intestines and Peritoneum	Spine	Other bone joint	Disseminated (not lung)	Other		

III. and IV. Similar schema to I. and II. indicating the number of cases under supervision at the

V. Respiratory tuberculosis only—survival data

Notified within last ten years

Sex	Age	Extent of Disease	Alive at anniversary after notification					Removal prior* to anniversary				Lost sight of prior† to anniversary				Died prior* to anniversary			
			1	2	3	4	...	10	1	2	...	10	1	2	...	10	1	2	...	10
		Unilateral—less than 2 interspaces																		
		2-4																		
		4+																		
		Bilateral—less than 2 interspaces																		
		2-4																		
		4+																		

196

APPENDIX

Tuberculous Conditions

Classification under four headings:

A. *X-ray. Extent of lesion*
(1) No pulmonary lesion.
(2) Unilateral. Covering an area not greater than that equal to 2 interspaces.
(3) Unilateral. Covering an area greater than 2 but not greater than that equal to 3–4 interspaces.
(4) Unilateral. Covering an area greater than 2 but not greater than that of 4 interspaces.
(5) Bilateral. Covering an area not greater than that equal to 2 interspaces.
(6) Bilateral. Covering in all an area greater than 2 but not greater than that equal to 3–4 interspaces.
(7) Bilateral. Covering an area greater than that of 4 interspaces (including miliary).

B. *X-ray. Special characters of lesion*
(1) Pulmonary and/or hilar calcification, without lesions of other character.
(2) Enlarged hilar glands only.
(3) Enlarged hilar glands plus pulmonary focus.
(4) Pleural effusion.
(5) Infiltration without cavity (some calcification or fibrosis might be present).
(6) Cavity suspect.
(7) Definite cavity, more than 1 cm. diameter diagnosed by tomogram only.
(8) Definite cavity, more than 1 cm. diameter, on straight film.

C. *Tubercle bacilli*
(1) Only one direct smear taken, result negative.

(2) More than one direct smear, all negative.
(3) Laryngeal swab or gastric lavage, culture negative.
(4) Sputum culture negative.
(5) Laryngeal swab or gastric lavage, culture positive.
(6) Sputum culture positive.
(7) Only one direct smear taken, result positive.
(8) More than one direct smear taken, result positive once only.
(9) More than one direct smear taken, result positive more than once.
(10) No sputum, no laryngeal swab or gastric lavage done.
(X) Pleural fluid, culture positive.
(V) Pleural fluid, culture negative.

D. *Assessment not later than 6 months*
(1) Tuberculosis. Presumed healed. No further action needed.
(2) Suspect tuberculosis, not yet confirmed.
(3) Tuberculosis. Occasional supervision only needed.
(4) Tuberculosis. Close clinic supervision needed (not off work entirely, but may be on reduced hours or modified work, and receiving food supplements).
(5) Tuberculosis. Requiring immediate treatment (off work and/or needing collapse therapy or chemotherapy).
(6) Case notified.
(7) Not notified.

REFERENCES

ASPIN, J. (1952) *Lancet*, i. 502.
BENJAMIN, B. (1953) *Brit. Journ. of Tub.*, 47.4
BENJAMIN, B., and NASH, F. A. (1952) *Tubercle*, 33, 73
BRADFORD HILL, A. (1927) M.R.C. Industrial Fatigue Research Board Report No. 48.
BRADFORD HILL, A. (1929) M.R.C. Industrial Fatigue Research Board Report No. 54.
BRADFORD HILL, A. (1930) M.R.C. Industrial Fatigue Research Board Report No. 59.
CAIRNS, M., and STEWART, A. M. (1951) *Brit. J. Soc. Med.*, 5.73.
CAPLIN, M. GRIFFITHS, J. J., and SILVER, D. M. (1956) *Tubercle*, 37.233.
COCHRANE, A. L., COX, J. C., and JARMAN, T. F. (1952) *Brit. Med. J.*, ii. 843.
COLLIS, E. L., and GREENWOOD, M. (1921) *Health of the Industrial Worker*, Churchill, London
DANIELS, M., RIDEHALGH, F., and SPRINGETT, V. H. (1948) *Tuberculosis in Young Adults;* Report on the Prophit Tuberculosis Survey 1935–44, London. H. K. Lewis.
DAW, R. H. (1950) *J.I.A.*, 76, 143.

FOSTER CARTER, A., MYERS, M., GODDARD, D. L. H., YOUNG, F. H., and BENJAMIN, B. (1952) 'Results of Collapse and Conservative Therapy in Pulmonary Tuberculosis'. Brompton Hospital Report, Vol. XXI. p. 1.

FROST, W. H. (1939) *Amer. J. Hyg.* A. 30, 91.

GENERAL REGISTER OFFICE (1936) Decennial Supplement 1931 Part IIa, Occupational Mortality, H.M.S.O.

HART D'ARCY, P. (1932) Med. Res. Council. Spec. Rep. Series No. 164, H.M.S.O.

HART, D'ARCY, P., and PALING WRIGHT, G. (1939) *Tuberculosis and Social Conditions in England*, N.A.P.T.

LOWE, C. R. (1954) *Brit. J.. of Prev. and Soc. Med.*, 8, 91.

LOWE, C. R., and GEDDES, J. E. (1953) *Brit. J. of Prev. and Soc. Med.*, 7, 227.

Medical Research Council (1952) *Lancet*, i. 775.

Ministry of Health (1952) Standardization of Radiological Terminology in Pulmonary Disease. Memo 323/Med. H.M.S.O.

Ministry of Health (1954) Report of Chief Medical Officer for 1953, H.M.S.O.

Ministry of Health (1955) Report of Chief Medical Officer for 1954, H.M.S.O.

Ministry of Health (1956) Report of Chief Medical Officer for 1955, H.M.S.O.

NASH, F. A., BENJAMIN, B., and LEE, T. (1953), *Brit. Med. J.*, i, 304.

NEWSHOLME, A. (1899) 'The Prevention of Phthisis', paper read to Incorp. Soc. Med. Officers of Health. January 1899.

SCADDING, J. G. (1953) *Brit. Med. J.*, ii. 716.

SNELL, W. E. (1951) *Lancet*, ii, 415.

SNELL, W. E. (1951) *Lancet*, i. 1309.

SPICER, C. C. (1954) *J. Hyg.*, 52, 361.

STEWART, A. M., and HUGHES, J. P. W. (1949) *Brit. Med. J.*, i. 926.

STEWART, A. M., and HUGHES, J. P. W. (1951) *Brit. Med. J.*, i. 899.

STOCKS, P. (1949) *Stud. Pop. Med. Subj.*, No. 2. General Register Office, H.M.S.O.

STOCKS, P., and LEWIS FANING, E. (1944) *Brit. Med. J.*, i. 581.

STEIN, L. (1952) *Brit. J. Soc.*, 6, 1.

STRADLING, P. (1952) *Tubercle*, 33, 266.

SPRINGETT, V. H. (1951) *Brit. Med. J.*, ii. 144.

SPRINGETT, V. H. (1952) *Lancet*, i. 521.

CHAPTER 11

MATERNITY AND CHILD WELFARE

11.1 The care of expectant and nursing mothers and for their babies forms one of the most important branches of preventive medicine. Childbearing is a physiological process and maternal morbidity must be regarded, fundamentally, as preventible by efficient medical and social care. This task is more difficult in the face of pre-existing disease or pelvic abnormality but even then much can be done and has been done to reduce risks. The newly born infant faces a hostile environment of potential infection and injury which once took a heavy toll; in birth there is also risk of injury which may be functional or anatomical; and before birth, maternal disease may cause foetal mortality or such damage as impairs life from the outset. Careful nursing and feeding is essential to the health of the baby and mothers often need advice. The efficiency of these services must therefore be constantly tested.

11.2 In terms of mortality alone, apart from disablement, a sufficient indication of progress may be given by comparing 1901, when in England and Wales about five per thousand of mothers died from pregnancy, or childbirth and 15 per cent of infants died in their first year of life, with 1961, when the corresponding proportions had been reduced to $0 \cdot 3$ per thousand and 2 per cent respectively.

11.3 These gains can only be maintained if the maternity and child welfare services are sustained at full strength. Infant mortality in England and Wales began to decline rapidly at the turn of the century. The first health visitors were appointed in Liverpool in 1897 and Birmingham in 1899, and some voluntary visiting had taken place in Salford as early as 1862 though trained nurses were not employed in that town until after 1905, and rapid progress was thenceforward made in health education among nursing mothers. Infant welfare clinics and schools for mothers began to operate from a little before 1907, having been pioneered by Budin in Paris, and provided to an ever increasing extent free medical consultations for infants; later they were developed to care for all children under school age.

11.4 About the commencement of the century a number of towns had milk depots for the provision of clean cow's milk for poor mothers unable to breastfeed their infants. All these agencies formed the foundation of the maternity and child welfare service as we know it today. The first adoptive Notification of Birth Act was passed in 1907 to ensure that the Medical Officer of Health should get early intimation of births in order to institute visiting as early as possible. (It became compulsory in 1915.) The first National Conference on Infantile Mortality was held in London in 1906, and an International Conference was held in Germany in 1911. Despite wars and economic depressions there has been in this century and especially in the last two or three decades a continuous improvement in social conditions. Infant mortality is highly sensitive to changes in social conditions since a substantial part of the risk is of exogenous character, i.e. a product of environment. This is true in the sense that the mortality is to a large extent of infective origin, viz. pneumonia, enteritis or the common fevers or due to accidents, e.g. suffocation or burns. The remainder is endogenous and arises from congenital handicap or damage—malformation, birth injury or pre-maturity. Improved social conditions have also contributed to the reduction in maternal mortality. The training of midwives improved from the passing of the first Midwives Act in 1902. This act set up the Central Midwives Board which regulates the practice of midwives and whose capacity for maintaining high standards has become stronger with the passing of years.

11.5 Following the impetus given by the Maternity and Child Welfare Act of 1918 which strengthened the powers of local authorities, extensive investigations into maternal mortality were carried out by the Ministry of Health. A Departmental Committee was appointed in 1929 to advise upon the application to maternal mortality and morbidity of the medical and surgical knowledge available, and their final report issued in 1932 did much to encourage improved teaching of antenatal and obstetric care, and the better organization of maternity services. The greatest contribution to progress has been made by the introduction of sulpha drugs and antibiotics. These together with improved obstetrical and nursing care have greatly reduced mortality from puerperal sepsis which once formed the major component of maternal mortality. Higher standards of medical care have also produced striking reductions in other sources of maternal mortality, e.g. deaths from haemorrhage and shock have been considerably reduced by prompt blood transfusion, and toxaemia is now subject to more successful control as a result of prompter recognition of symptoms.

11.6 The trends of maternal and infant mortality rates are still, therefore, very important indices of the efficiency of local maternity and child welfare services; though the general levels through which these trends pass are largely conditioned by the average social conditions of the local area.

Maternal Mortality

11.7 The phrase 'maternal mortality' may be used in a number of different senses. It may include all deaths in women in whom pregnancy was a current or antecedent condition, or it may be restricted to those cases in which death was directly attributed to childbirth. In the first instance a pregnant woman dying from heart disease from which she had always suffered would be included; in the latter case she would be excluded on the grounds that the death was merely 'associated'* with but not directly due to her pregnant condition. Maternal mortality also may either include or exclude deaths due to abortion; such deaths are sometimes excluded on the grounds first, that the number at risk is less well established than for pregnancies which run to term and secondly, that it is a risk of a different quality from that associated with childbirth (partly as a result of the element of criminal, i.e. non-therapeutically, induced abortion). It is therefore necessary to make quite

---

* The official description is 'deaths of women not classed to pregnancy or childbearing, but certified as associated therewith'.

clear what the rate is intended to cover. Usually, but not invariably, it may be safely assumed that 'associated' deaths are excluded and it is usual to describe the rate as 'maternal mortality (excluding abortion)' or 'maternal mortality (including abortion)' as the case may be.

11.8 It is an important condition of any rate that no unit should be included in the numerator which would not also be covered by the definition of the denominator. The denominator of the maternal mortality rate for a particular period of time should therefore include all those women who are at risk of death from pregnancy and childbearing, viz. all those who are pregnant at any time during the period in question. This number is not known however since miscarriages (under twenty-eight weeks' gestation) are not reportable and many pregnancies are terminated without the knowledge of the registration or health authorities. It is necessary to use as a base the number of live and still births, a figure which can at least be obtained from registration data and which probably bears a reasonably constant proportion to the number of women pregnant during the interval of measurement.

11.9 The maternal mortality rate (excluding abortion) is therefore conventionally defined as the number of women dying from delivery, or complications of pregnancy, childbirth or puerperium during an interval of time (commonly a calendar year) per 1,000 live or still births occurring during the same period. (If actual occurrences are not available, it is permissible to use registrations especially if conditions are stable so that the two numbers are unlikely to differ by a significant quantity.) Mortality from associated causes (i.e. not directly due to childbirth, etc.), is also expressed in the relation to the same denominator but as a separate measure of associated mortality.

11.10 Abortion is commonly excluded. The number of women exposed to risk of death from abortion (especially if the incidence of abortion is changing) is less definitely related to birth registration than other maternal deaths. It is preferable to regard the incidence of abortion as proportional to the number of women of reproductive ages in the population and to express mortality from abortion as a death rate per 1,000 (or million) women living aged 15–44.

11.11 The statistics for 1964 for England and Wales were as in Table 11.1.

TABLE 11.1 *Maternal Mortality* (*excluding abortion*)
(*International classification rubrics in brackets*)

Cause	No. of deaths	Rate per 100,000 total births
Puerperal phlebitis, thrombosis and embolism (682, 684)	22	2·5
Puerperal sepsis (640, 641, 681)	10	1·1
Antepartum haemorrhage (643, 644, 670)	7	0·8
Post-partum haemorrhage (671, 672)	12	1·3
Toxaemia (642, 685, 686)	34	3·8
Prolonged labour (673, 675)	13	1·5
Trauma, shock, other complications of delivery (676–678)	26	2·9
Other causes (Rem. 640–648, 660–689)	53	5·9
Total maternal causes	177	19·8

11.12 The principal elements in this now very much reduced risk of mortality are toxaemia, haemorrhage, sepsis and pulmonary embolism, and the movement of the rates of mortality from these causes requires to be closely watched from year to year.

11.13 There are some cases of deaths of women who have some pre-existing disease of such severity that pregnancy produces an additional strain or exacerbation sufficient to cause death; there may be others where death was inevitable and pregnancy merely coincidental. In the cases where pregnancy, abortion or childbirth is mentioned as a secondary cause, the precise contribution to the fatal result is naturally difficult to evaluate. In England and Wales, in 1964, there were fifty-five such deaths not assigned to pregnancy or childbearing but certified to be *associated* therewith. Of these five were due to mitral valve disease and in total, heart and circulatory disease accounted for fourteen or 25 per cent of the deaths. The rapid decline in recent years in the number of these 'associated' deaths is evidence of the better care of pregnant women with health impairment; some part of the decline may also be due to preventive medical advice to avoid the special risks of pregnancy, resulting in a reduction of the number of such women becoming pregnant.

11.14 Mortality in abortion is very largely of septic origin and it is especially difficult to control this risk owing to the still significant number of criminally induced abortions where the methods used enhance the chances of sepsis intervening and where medical assistance is not sought until the condition has become serious. Recent statistics in England and Wales are shown in Table 11.2.

TABLE 11.2 *Mortality from abortion, England and Wales*
Rate per million women aged 15–44

Year	Sepsis (*Int. list* 651)	Other causes (650, 652)
1956	4	4
1957	4	3
1958	4	3
1959	3	2
1960	4	4
1961	4	2
1962	3	3
1963	3	2
1964	3	2

11.15 Deaths from abortion have been declining as rapidly as those attributed to other maternal causes.

Local variations

11.16 All the mortality elements are now small and for this reason figures for local authorities are subject annually to fairly wide chance fluctuations as a result of the small numbers involved. Maternal mortality tends to be above the average for England and Wales as a whole in the Northern and South Western Regions of England and in Wales; and it is generally higher in rural areas and small towns (urban areas with population under 50,000) than in the larger towns.

Age and parity

11.17 The figures in Table 11.3 have been taken from the *Registrar General's*

TABLE 11.3 *Deaths per* 100,000 *maternities in* 1948–49

Cause of death	Under 20	20—	25—	30—	35—	40—	45 and over	All Ages
146. Haemorrhage	8	8	8	19	27	30	168	14
(a) Placenta praevia	—	0	1	4	8	19	72	3
(b) Premature separation	—	0	—	1	2	2	—	1
(c) (d) Other haemorrhage	8	8	7	14	17	9	96	10
147. Infection	2	7	11	14	23	25	48	12
(a), (b) General and local	—	2	3	7	6	5	—	4
(c) Thrombophlebitis	—	1	4	4	9	7	24	4
(d) Embolism, sudden death	2	3	4	3	9	12	24	4
148. Toxaemia	14	12	15	23	38	60	264	21
(a) Eclampsia	10	6	6	8	13	19	72	8
(b) Albuminuria, etc.	3	3	5	9	15	28	144	7
(c) Acute yellow atrophy	2	2	3	3	6	5	—	3
(d) Other toxaemia	—	1	1	3	4	7	48	2
149. Other accident of childbirth	14	8	17	23	35	65	168	20
150. Other puerperal conditions	—	1	1	1	1	2	48	1
146–150. Total complications of childbirth and puerperium	38	36	53	79	124	180	696	68
Ratio of rate to that for ages under twenty	1·0	0·9	1·4	2·1	3·3	4·7	18·3	

Statistical Review (Text) for 1948–49. More recent figures are not sufficiently large to permit analysis.

11.18 The risk of dying from a complication of childbirth or the puerperium is extremely low at young ages—in 1948–49 at ages under 30 it was only 4 in 10,000—and then increased with advancing age at first slowly and then more rapidly; at ages 30–34 it was twice as great as at ages below 20, at 35–39 three times, at ages 40–44 nearly five times and at ages above 45, eighteen times as great.

11.19 Age and parity are highly correlated—the older mothers have, on the average, had more pregnancies than the younger mothers and the increase in mortality with age may merely conceal an increase of mortality with parity. Mortality rates specific for parity as well as age are not generally available but the figures in Table 11.4 were provided by the General Register Office.

TABLE 11.4 *Maternal mortality per* 1,000 *live and still births—England and Wales,* 1950

Previous children	Age groups				
	16—	20—	25—	30—	35–44
0	[0·45]	0·47	0·89	1·42	3·58
1	—	[0·30]	0·41	0·53	1·77
2	—		[0·42]	0·75	0·99
3	—	[0·39]	[0·72]	[0·69]	[1·08]
4	—		[0·41]	[0·99]	[1·07]
5—9	—	—	[1·61]	[1·54]	1·73
10—14	—	—	—	—	[2·88]
15+	—	—	—	—	—

[The figures in brackets are based on less than twenty deaths so must be regarded as subject to a fairly wide margin of error as indications of underlying risk.]

11.20 In each age group the risk is probably highest at the first maternity and lowest at the second and third maternities and then increases with increasing parity until at very high parity orders it is as great as at the first maternity. There is some suggestion for the older women that they are an exception to this general statement insofar as the second maternity as well as the first may be subject to higher than average risk.

11.21 An important test of the efficiency of the maternity services is provided by an examination of the preventability of such maternal deaths as do occur. Under arrangements made by the Ministry of Health in England and Wales, the Medical Officer of Health of a local health authority initiates a confidential enquiry by advising a local consultant obstetrician of the occurrence of a maternal death and supplying such initial information as is available to him, especially about domiciliary midwives or local authority ante-natal clinics involved in the case. It is intended that the consultant obstetricians should be invited to then obtain full information of all the circumstances, hospital or domiciliary, as far as possible by personal enquiry from those who have been in attendance on the woman. The obstetrician's report, with comments by the Medical Officer of Health, is then sent to a Regional Assessor, a senior obstetrician of high standing in the area. The Regional Assessor is asked to make an assessment of avoidable factors in the case and to forward a report to the Chief Medical Officer of the Ministry of Health. The report is treated as strictly confidential at every stage.

11.22 Regular reports analysing these records are published. That for 1961–63 relates to 692 deaths ascribed to pregnancy or childbirth and in 262 or 38 per cent avoidable factors were present. The reports show that the risk of death is higher in certain well defined groups of women, which include:—

(1) Women who have an obstetric or general medical abnormality either at the time of booking or developing during pregnancy.
(2) Women who are 35 years of age or more who are expecting their fifth or subsequent child or whose previous obstetric history has not been normal.
(3) Primigravidae who are 30 years of age of more.

Maternal morbidity

11.23 Deaths attributed to complications of pregnancy, childbirth and the puerperium are now so infrequent that local rates fluctuate from year to year in an irregular manner; in a single town with only two or three thousand births a year the chance occurrence of one or two additional deaths may double the mortality rate and it is not possible therefore to measure the efficiency of local maternity services by reference only to the mortality rate. It is necessary to attempt the more difficult task of assessing morbidity, i.e. the incidence of non-fatal abnormalities, with all the more detailed case-records that are necessarily involved.

11.24 In England and Wales the rules of the Central Midwives Board require that certain minimum standards of recording shall be maintained. Detailed records are important for a number of reasons. A fundamental need is to establish what is *normal* for the individual woman. In one case a rise in blood pressure may be very significant; in another patient such rises may have occurred in previous pregnancies without any unfavourable consequences and may be safely tolerated. This difficulty of establishing normality can clearly be met only by thorough and complete records of previous pregnancies and their incidents and outcome. The significance of an abdominal scar can similarly be interpreted only in relation to pelvic measurements and the size of the previous baby; was a Caesarean section performed because the baby was too large or the mother too small?—the latter condition is a permanent hazard and not an accident of a particular pregnancy producing an exceptionally large foetus unlikely to recur. There is some evidence (Gemmell, Logan, Benjamin, 1954) that women with a previous history of toxaemia are more likely to develop the condition in the current pregnancy than those without such a history. A similar 'proneness' appears to apply to premature delivery and stillbirth (not wholly because of the frequent association with toxaemia). The effect of **parity** itself has already been stressed. A precise account of antecedent pregnancies is obviously of vital importance.

11.25 In the current pregnancy close observation is necessitated by the insidious onset of certain abnormal conditions especially toxaemia or anaemia —in the one case requiring regular measurements of blood pressure and in the other a watch for symptoms and where necessary confirmatory blood counts. The detection of urinary abnormalities is also a matter of continuous observation. There is also the need to make careful records of blood tests— Kahn, Wassermann and Rhesus factor. It is no less important to have complete details of all the emergencies that may arise such as sepsis, shock, haemorrhage; not the least because in the event of serious outcome it will be necessary to assess preventability.

11.26 The Royal College of Obstetricians and Gynaecologists in England and Wales have recommended a standard form of report for individual centres or agencies administering a maternity service. The following groups of conditions are to be specially distinguished—

      Pre-eclamptic toxaemia
      Eclampsia
      Hypertension
      Hyperemesis gravidarum
      Heart disease
      Antepartum haemorrhage—accidental placenta praevia
      Postpartum haemorrhage
      Manual removal of placenta
      Breech presentation
      Laceration of perineum
      Retroversion of gravid uterus

11.27 For each group the individual cases are to be listed with supplementary details appropriate to the group. For example the classification of toxaemia cases will show age, number of pregnancies to date, gestation period, blood pressure (highest/lowest), presence or absence of albuminuria, oedema and other symptoms, whether specially treated, type of delivery (e.g. normal, forceps, breech, etc.) and the result for mother and child. Following the listed cases in each group there is a summary showing the number of maternal deaths (if any), the number of stillbirths, abortions and infant deaths with rates (per cent of mothers and babies respectively).

11.28 The report form also provides summaries (with clinical details) of different types of presentation (occipito-posterior, face, brow, transverse lie, multiple pregnancy); of cases of prolapsed cord; and of contracted pelvis. Summaries are also made of different types of induction, of breech deliveries, versions, Caesarean sections, embryotomies, forceps deliveries, and of cases of uterine inertia. In cases of Caesarean section for example the important details would be those relating to the indication (toxaemia, contracted pelvis, etc.), duration of labour, previous history, anaesthetic, type of section, weight of baby and survival, There is also a summary of all abortions; and of all cases with intercurrent disease.

11.29 A general assessment of the results of the service over the period surveyed may be obtained from statistics of the following type:

TABLE 11.5 *Statistics taken from the 1960 Clinical Report of Queen Charlotte's Maternity Hospital*

	Hospital cases		District cases	Totals
	Booked	Emergency		
Total maternities	2,563	197	588	3,348
Deaths	1	—	—	1
Stillbirths—number	58	6	3	67
rate*	22·2	30·5	5·1	19·7
Live births	2,616	197	588	3,401
Total morbid cases				
Infant deaths	46	6	2	54
Neonatal death rate†	17·9	31·4	3·4	16·2

* per thousand total births
† per thousand live births

11.30 The clinical summary for the same hospital in 1960 is—

Total number of deliveries	2,760
Abortions admitted	46
Eclampsia	3
Antepartum Haemorrhage—Accidental	21
Placenta Praevia	12
Unknown Cause	64
Uncomplicated breech delivery	42
Complicated breech delivery	44
Postpartum haemorrhage	75
Manual removal	42
Caesarean section	142
Caesarean section rate	5·1%
Forceps delivery	200
Forceps delivery rate	7·2%
Maternal mortality (per thousand)	0·36
Stillbirth rate (per thousand total births)	22·8
Neonatal death rate (per thousand live births)	18·9

11.31 Comparison of such figures as between successive years in the same maternity unit or as between different units in the same year provides a general indication of relative efficiency; important differences would then require to be investigated by reference to more detailed statistics of particular causes of morbidity and particular groups of women in which an exceptional incidence of morbidity was experienced. It has to be borne in mind that different units have different catchment areas and that the populations covered may vary in social conditions and therefore in general wellbeing or in their degree of co-operation with medical care.

Antenatal and postnatal clinics

11.32 Pregnancy is not a morbid condition but there are special risks, and preventive medicine has an important role to play in ensuring that the mother (and the baby) survive these risks. An expectant mother may seek to be confined in hospital or at home; the choice is not entirely free since her physical condition may be such as to make hospital attention imperative, or hospital beds may be so short that some selection of the more difficult cases has to be made. In both cases, however, after an initial examination by the obstetrician, the woman will be advised to attend for antenatal care regularly, so that any abnormal condition can be detected as soon as possible after onset and so that advice can be given to ensure that the woman takes proper care of her own health and is fully prepared for her nursing responsibilities. Such care may be given by the hospital or general practitioner or midwife and both hospital and domiciliary cases may be referred for intermediate care to clinics provided by local health authorities. These clinics are under medical supervision with the nursing assistance of health visitors; midwives who are booked to take domiciliary cases attend to see their own patients at frequent intervals, not only for the purpose of proper observation but in order to establish an atmosphere of mutual confidence. The figures in Table 11.6 indicate the extent of antenatal care in Birmingham in 1953 (taken from the City of Birmingham Abstract of Statistics, 1952–54).

TABLE 11.6 *Antenatal care in Birmingham*

Number of Visits or Attendances	Responsibility for Antenatal Care					Totals
	Hospital	Private Doctor	Maternity Service General Practitioner	Midwife and Antenatal Clinic	Not known	
1 or 2	106	10	75	89	—	280
3–5	670	68	537	383	—	1,659
6–8	1,939	196	1,641	742	1	4,519
9 or more	4,974	159	2,105	1,144	—	8,382
All with known amount of care	7,689	433	4,358	2,358	1	14,839
Amount of care unknown	1,716	217	1,547	71	132	3,683
Total	9,405	650	5,905	2,429	133	18,522
No antenatal care			80			80

11.33 The distribution of these same confinements (to Birmingham residents) by attendant at birth was as in Table 11.7.

11.34 In Birmingham such statistics as these are derived from the record compiled by the health visitors who call upon the nursing mother immediately after the birth notification has been received in the Public Health Department (Charles E.[1951]).

207

TABLE 11.7 *Distribution of births by attendant*

Attendant at birth	No.	Per cent
Domiciliary confinements		
Midwife only	2,330	12·5
Booked doctor	3,750	20·2
Midwife + medical aid	163	0·9
Ambulance nurse	106	0·6
Born before arrival of attendant	317	1·7
Attendant not known	96	0·5
All domiciliary confinements	6,762	**36·4**
Institutional confinements		
Hospital or maternity home	11,615	62·4
Private nursing home	225	1·2
All institutional confinements	11,840	**63·6**
Total	18,602	**100·0**

11.35 Two alternative procedures may be adopted. It is possible, and easier, to compile a history of the confinement after the event (as in Birmingham) by reference to the mother, midwife and medical attendant; this requires a degree of persistence, care and enthusiasm on the part of the health visitor (whose main focus is the infant). Alternatively an attempt may be made to bring together in one file (1) the clinical record maintained at the antenatal clinic, (2) the record of the confinement on a summary thereof, (3) a record of the attendance at postnatal clinic (to which mothers are referred for examination and advice after the confinement). (1) and (2) are, in a high proportion of cases, already in the possession of the Local Health Authority as the source of the clinical services. (3) is in the possession of the Local Health Authority if the confinement was domiciliary, and if the confinement took place in hospital a summary may usually be obtained in the form of a discharge notice from hospital (the hospital usually prefers to design its own discharge notice but co-operation between the hospital obstetrician and the local Medical Officer of Health secures that the minimum essential data can be provided including details of the antenatal care if provided by the hospital). Clearly this alternative procedure presents a problem in organization but it is possible that a greater degree of accuracy may be achieved since more direct records are involved; and certainly more work is thrown on clerks and less upon health visitors.

11.36 The need for this integration is stressed since the efficacy of preventive medicine cannot be assessed without knowledge of end results, and it is sheer frustration for the medical officers of antenatal clinics not to know what has happened to expectant mothers in their care.

11.37 In England and Wales the Ministry of Health requires the Local Health Authority to make an annual return of its services (Form L.H.S.27) and part of this return is devoted to the part played by the Local Health Authority in the maternity services. The Return (in its relevant sections) first calls for a statement of the number of live and still births notified (see p. 52) in the Authority's area (as adjusted by transferred notifications) separating domiciliary from institutional births.

11.38 Certain basic tables covering antenatal and postnatal clinics have to be completed. These show the number of sessions, new cases, and total attendances at both Local Authority and voluntary organization clinics.

11.39 These statistics show how far the Local Authority is supplementing other services. For example first attendances when taken in relation to the number of women becoming pregnant during the year (roughly equal to the number of births under stable conditions) indicates the proportion of expectant mothers who use the service. In Birmingham in 1952 there were 6,299 first attendances at municipal antenatal clinics, and the total confinements in the year (of Birmingham residents) was 18,602 indicating that about a third of mothers attended the clinics prior to confinement; in the County of London in the same year the proportion was a little higher (about forty per cent); for the balance of the expectant mothers in both cases, antenatal care is provided by hospital clinics or general practitioners. Statistics of hospital antenatal care are provided on separate hospital returns (p. 255).

Domiciliary midwifery

11.40 Where the Local Health Authority is responsible for the supervision of practising midwives under the Midwives Act, 1951, it is required to furnish in the same return statistics of (1) the numbers of midwives employed by the Local Authority, voluntary organizations, or hospital authorities, and whether domiciliary or institutional, (2) the numbers of deliveries attended by these different classes of midwives with and without the presence of doctors, (3) the number of cases where the midwife, working in the absence of a doctor, had to summon emergency medical aid, (4) the numbers of cases in which gas and air analgesia was administered, and whether or not in the presence of a doctor.

11.41 The object of these statistics is to enable the Ministry of Health to examine changes in the supply of midwives and the relative demands made upon their services by the various authorities and the balance of demand as between domiciliary and institutional confinements.

Infant mortality

11.42 The risk of death is greatest at the two extremes of the normal span of life. The very high risk in infancy actually begins at conception, for the implanted ovum is dependent upon maternal resources and the development of the foetus is affected by the mother's mental and physical health and her environment; inimical factors here, if not lethal, may produce congenital malformations or premature birth. At birth the foetus is subjected to physical stresses which, in certain circumstances, are capable of producing brain injury or asphyxia. After birth the infant's circulatory, respiratory and digestive systems are put to the test, and infections are encountered for the first time against which there is little natural immunity. These risks which the baby has to face may clearly be enhanced by a poor environment—insufficient food, insanitary housing, lack of warmth, inefficient maternal care—and it is not surprising that infant mortality has been found to be a sensitive index of the general level of living of the community, and, of the efficacy of public health measures to mitigate the effects of the existing social conditions. For this reason Medical Officers of Health have traditionally taken a great interest in infant mortality as one of the most important of vital statistics.

The infant mortality rate

11.43 Traditionally infant mortality has always been expressed as the number of registered deaths (in the particular year of measurement) of live born infants under one year of age for every 1,000 live births registered during the same year, e.g. for England and Wales in 1964

Deaths of infants under one year—17,445
Live births—875,992
Infant mortality rate = 19·9 per 1,000 live births

11.44 In more recent times it has been recognized that the numerator and denominator of the rate, as calculated above, are not strictly related. The registered deaths under one year include those of some births registered in a previous year; while some of the current year's births which do not survive the first of life may be registered as deaths in the following year. If fertility and mortality are stable these two errors tend to compensate but, since at times both factors have been undergoing fairly rapid change, various methods have been adopted to ensure that in the calculation of the rate, the numeraor includes only deaths of infants whose births are included in the denominator and conversely the denominator (the number 'at risk') includes only infants who if dying before the first birthday would be counted among the deaths in the numerator. This may be done by adjusting either the numerator or the denominator to bring it to consistency with the other.

11.45 The methods include (1) separating the infant deaths of one calendar year according to whether or not they were of births of the current year or of the previous year. The first part when divided by the births of the year gives mortality from birth to the end of the calendar year. The second part when divided by those of the previous years' births which *had* so survived (as estimated by the first type of mortality rate) provides the mortality up to the end of the first year of life, (2) adjusting as in (1) but for each quarter of the calendar year separately, (3) making the split of the deaths not exactly, but by the use of approximate proportions based on grouping by age within the first year of life, (4) splitting the deaths in narrow intervals of age and estimating the periods of births from which they must have emerged.

11.46 In conditions of stability the refinements, though logical, have little numerical effect and may safely be ignored especially when as in England and Wales the rate is based upon occurrences rather than registration of live births.

Neonatal mortality

11.47 Even within the first year of life there is considerable variation in mortality; not only do the risks vary in severity but they vary also in quality. In the very early weeks of life the predominant risks are those associated with the uterine development of the foetus and the birth process itself—congenital malformation, prematurity and birth injury. Later, risks of infection or accidents predominate. The figures in Table 11.8 for England and Wales in 1964 are illustrative.

11.48 These two groups of causes which account for over 90 per cent of all deaths in the first year differ widely in their age gradient. For the first group of constitutional and non-infective diseases more than three-quarters,

TABLE 11.8 *Infant mortality by cause of death*

Cause of death		Infant mortality per 1,000 related live births in age period				
		under 1 week	1 week and under 4 weeks	4 weeks and under 3 months	3 months and under 6 months	6 months and under 1 year
Immaturity, birth injury, postnatal asphyxia, atelectasis, erythroblastosis, congenital malformations and ill defined diseases peculiar to early infancy	M.	12·60	1·17	0·76	0·39	0·33
	F.	9·75	0·99	0·71	0·38	0·36
Pneumonia, bronchitis, gastro-enteritis, other infective diseases, accidental mechanical suffocation and lack of care	M.	0·57	0·68	1·69	1·63	1·08
	F.	0·44	0·50	1·19	1·29	0·91

of the deaths are in the first week; for the second group of infections and accidents, only a tenth of the infant deaths are in the first week, and four-fifths occur after the first four weeks.

11.49 Partly from consideration of these differential age gradients and partly on grounds of simplicity it has become customary to separate deaths in the first four weeks of life as attributable to *neonatal* mortality as distinct from later deaths which are classed as *postneonatal*. The neonatal mortality rate is calculated in the same way as the infant mortality rate, viz. per 1,000 live births. The tremendous reduction in infant mortality since the turn of the century has been more attributable to post-neonatal mortality (infections, diarrhoeal or respiratory, and accidents) than to neonatal mortality. Mortality from prematurity, congenital malformations or injury at birth has been more resistant to improvement.

TABLE 11.9 *England and Wales—rates per 1,000 live births*

	Neonatal mortality (under 4 weeks)	Postneonatal mortality (over 4 weeks and under 1 year)
1906–10	40·2	76·9
1964	13·8	6·1
Per cent reduction	66	91

11.50 In England and Wales the neonatal mortality rate per 1,000 live births from prematurity fell from 17·4 in 1921 to 14.5 in 1938, a comparatively slow rate of progress. This was followed by a temporary rise during the war, but when in 1944 the rate was 11·2, the Ministry of Health called attention to the need for special emphasis on the care of the premature baby by the provision of special hospital units, the loan of special nursing equipment, special health visiting and other services, and by 1950 the rate had fallen to 5·8. This indicates how much a determined effort can achieve against a hitherto intractable cause. Less progress has been made against the other important elements in neonatal mortality, birth injury and congenital malformation. Too little is known of the aetiology and indeed of the incidence of congenital

211

malformation and the General Register Office have instituted a system of notifications as from 1964. (General Register Office 1967.) The incidence of birth injury has been reduced by raised standards of obstetric management but the statistical effect cannot be clearly demonstrated because standards of diagnosis have also been rising leading to the increased allocation to birth injury of deaths which were formerly classed to less definite causes.

Stillbirth rate

11.51 The registration of stillbirths has been discussed elsewhere (p. 46). Stillbirths represent not only personal tragedies but also a significant source of wastage of life, and therefore the object of serious attention by public health authorities. The stillbirth rate for a given period is defined as the number of stillbirths (as defined for registration purposes, viz. of twenty-eight weeks or more gestation, in England and Wales) per 1,000 births (live and still) in the period. The form of certificate asks for an opinion as to cause. Table 11.10 shows a distribution of causes for 1961.

TABLE 11.10 *England and Wales* 1961—*Stillbirths per* 1,000 *births*

Maternal conditions	
Diabetes, circulatory disease	0·4
Diseases of pregnancy	3·4
Difficulties in labour	1·5
Placental and cord conditions	4·9
Foetal conditions	
Birth injury	0·5
Congenital malformation	3·7
Other and illdefined causes	4·3
Total	**19·0**

Other rates

11.52 There is a tendency to distinguish even more clearly the true natal deaths from those attributable to post-natal environmental influences by reference to deaths in the first week of life, and such deaths per 1,000 related live births provide an *early neonatal mortality rate*. These deaths combined with stillbirths and rated to 1,000 total births can be regarded as measuring mortality at a period of time surrounding birth and may be described as *perinatal mortality*. It is clear that perinatal mortality is likely to be a sensitive index (under standard social and climatic conditions) of the efficiency of obstetric services.

11.53 The perinatal mortality rate has the advantage that unlike its components, the stillbirth and early neonatal rates, it is not likely to be disturbed by variations in the practice of recording or in the actual timing of foetal deaths. If a foetus is regarded as surviving beyond intra-uterine existence a death is transferred from the stillbirth to the early neonatal category though the actual reality of the situation—death *around* the point of delivery—is unaffected. This is quite an important point as the precise fixation of the time of foetal death is often difficult. The following figures indicate that the perinatal rate is relatively less subject to year to year variation than the component rates.

England and Wales 1950–55

	1950	1951	1952	1953	1954	1955	Standard deviation	% of mean rate
Stillbirths (per 1,000 total births)	22·6	23·0	22·7	22·4	23·5	23·2	0·41	1·8
Deaths under 1 week (per 1,000 live births)	15·2	15·5	15·2	14·8	14·9	14·6	0·33	2·2
Perinatal mortality (per 1,000 total births)	37·4	38·2	37·5	36·9	38·1	37·4	0·49	1·3

Total wastage

11.54 The Medical Text of the *Registrar General's Annual Statistical Review* for 1950 provides an interesting attempt to estimate the total loss of life during pregnancy and labour and the first year of life, by bringing into account the loss among embryos and foetuses prior to the twenty-eighth week of gestation which is not covered by registration data. It may be estimated from various sources, reviewed by the Medical and Biological Committee of the Royal Commission on Population (1949) and the Interdepartmental Committee on Abortion that, roughly, 9 per cent of pregnancies in England and Wales are terminated by spontaneous abortion and a further four per cent are terminated by induced abortions, i.e. the total live and still births form 87 per cent of the total pregnancies. The following statement may then be prepared for 1950.

Total pregnancies (713,181 live and still births $\div$ 0·87) = 819,748.

	No.	per thousand
Abortions	106,567	130
Stillbirths	16,084	20
Neonatal deaths	12,917	16
Post-neonatal deaths	7,900	10
Total reproductive wastage	**143,468**	**176**

Factors influencing foetal mortality

11.55 In an important series of papers (Heady, Daly and Morris, 1955) giving the results of comprehensive studies carried out in England and Wales by the Medical Research Council Social Medicine Unit (with the help of the General Register Office) it has been demonstrated that the stillbirth rate rises with age for mothers of a particular parity while the post-neonatal rate decreases with age (except for mothers over thirty-five). The stillbirth rate for mothers of a given age is high for first births, falls for second and third births, and rises thereafter; the post-neonatal rate for mothers of a given age, rises steadily with increasing parity. The neonatal rate varies less than the other two rates and appears to occupy an intermediate position. These results indicate, for post-neonatal mortality, the increased opportunity for infection (the principal cause) in larger families and the strain on economic resources and parental care of the larger family. Three 'vulnerable' groups are picked out—

(1) Mothers over thirty-five, bearing first babies have a high risk of stillbirth
(2) Mothers over forty of any parity have a high risk of stillbirth.
(3) Babies of young mothers with large families for their age have a high risk of death in the post-neonatal period.

These findings have been confirmed and extended by Butler and Bonham (1963).

11.56 Economic conditions play an important part in determining mortality levels. Generally infant mortality is two and a half times as great in Social Class V (unskilled workers) as in Social Class I (professional and administrative workers); the gradient is more marked for post-neonatal mortality than for stillbirths and neonatal mortality.

11.57 Foetal mortality is higher for illegitimate births than for legitimate births, as can be seen from the following figures.

England and Wales 1964

	All infants	Illegitimate
Stillbirth rate (per 1,000 total births)	16·3	20·2
Early neonatal rate (per 1,000 related births)	12·0	17·2
Late neonatal rate (per 1,000 related births)	1·8	2·2
Post-neonatal rate (per 1,000 related births)	6·1	6·8
(4 weeks and under 1 year)		

11.58 It will be seen that the excess is mainly in the perinatal period. As to the cause of this excess it has to be borne in mind that the social factors referred to above operate adversely in that section of the population in which illegitimacy tends to have a higher incidence.

11.59 But it is not only a question of social conditions. The level of living will be generally lower for those bearing illegitimate babies. No direct comparison is possible as the father is not frequently recorded at registration of illegitimate births, but of mothers of illegitimate infants born in 1951 in England and Wales 23 per cent were in occupations of Social Classes IV and V, and 49 per cent were unoccupied, while 26 per cent of legitimate births were to women married to husbands in Social Classes IV and V or unoccupied. (General Register Office, 1957.) If only a fraction of the 49 per cent unoccupied were living in conditions appropriate to Social Classes IV and V, this makes the comparison unfavourable to illegitimate babies. Nevertheless, other factors are involved. We are dealing with a less responsible section of the community. The level of intelligence and standards of prenatal and maternal care tend to be lower, there is more likelihood of reluctance to seek medical care at an early stage or to co-operate with such medical care, and general standards of hygiene will be lower. The result is that even for the same social class the illegitimate births are subject to higher mortality rates.

England and Wales 1949–53

	Social Class (of mother for illegitimate and father for legitimate births)				
	I	II	III	IV	V
Stillbirth rate (per 1,000 total births)					
legitimate	16·3	19·9	22·5	24·5	27·4
illegitimate	(46·8)	31·1	32·4	35·5	37·8
Neonatal mortality (per 1,000 live births)					
legitimate	14·0	15·6	18·3	20·0	22·8
illegitimate	(13·3)	34·9	28·9	31·0	38·2

The bracketed figures are based on small numbers and are unreliable.

Health Visitors and Child Welfare Clinics

11.60 A key figure in the system of observational care which has done so much to improve the health of children in this century and to enhance the standing of preventive medicine is the health visitor (in America, she is called a Public Health Nurse). When a birth is notified to the Local Health Authority in England and Wales under the Public Health Act, 1936, the name of the infant is added to a birth register maintained by the authority and is also added to a health visitor's record card which, passed to the health visitor for the appropriate district, serves as a notice of addition of a new infant to her district list. The mother is visited as soon as possible after the departure of the midwife and is invited to avail herself of further periodic visits by the Health Visitor and of attendance at the child welfare clinic for the area (there may be one clinic for several health visitors' districts). The advantage of clinic attendance lies in the fact that not only is the health visitor herself present to give advice but a medical practitioner is also available for consultation where necessary; and facilities are also available for baby weighing (an important guide to progress of the infant as well as a factor of great psychological importance for the mother) and informal lectures and demonstrations (e.g. of food preparation or clothes making, etc.).

11.61 For those infants who are brought to the clinic a medical record is maintained, usually apart from the health visitor's record, in which a proper account of medical observation and consultation is given.

11.62 These records provide a fund of information about the activities of the health visitors and the clinic services and about the health of the infants within their field of supervision. Considering that almost all infants are visited at least once by the health visitor and that the great majority of babies are brought to the clinics at least during the early months of life. these records cover a very high proportion of the pre-school child population. The process of deriving useful statistics from them presents a problem of organization far from easy to solve. There are not only the usual difficulties associated with long-term follow-up records, viz. that the subjects are continually passing into and out of observation and the records are in continuous use so that they cannot all be made available except for a short period of time; further difficulties arise in that (1) the children are all at different stages of a continuous process of development. It is more than a matter of reviewing patients at fixed anniversaries, e.g. of hospital discharge; (2) a large part of the record is in narrative form relating to conditions seen or reported by nursing mothers and advice given. A large number of nurses and doctors are involved and it is impracticable to impose either a rigid pattern of arrangement or a standard range of language. In consequence it is difficult to summarize the record for statistical purposes; (3) normally there is a large number of records scattered over many centres. Sampling is indicated but not easy to accomplish in the absence of skilled supervision—nurses are not always aware of the need to adhere strictly to prescribed sampling procedures. It seems likely that the choice is between two alternatives (i) to so restrict the scope and manner of reporting that the documents are almost entirely on a self-coding 'check list' basis, i.e. items are numbered and the answers are of the 'yes/no' type, with ticks or the ringing of numbers as the indication. This facilitiates periodical statistical analysis, either manually or by punched cards; and such an analysis may be made at intervals, say over a year, when the records are least likely to be disturbed (e.g. during holiday periods); (ii) to provide an independent statistical summary form to be completed currently (or at a specified stage in the 'life' of the main record) by clerical assistance provided from the central office to which such forms would be passed for analysis. Such a method does not in any way inhibit the work of the medical or nursing staff and is to be preferred if sufficient clerical assistance can be made available.

Surveys of child health

11.63 Analyses of these records as a routine would provide the Medical Officer of Health with valuable information about the current health of the child population. A number of special surveys have been made, using records of the same type modified for the *ad hoc* purposes of the research project, notably those carried out by the Institute of Social Medicine at Oxford (A. M. Stewart and W. T. Russell, 1952), and under the joint auspices of the Royal College of Obstetricians and Gynaecologists and the Population Investigation Committee (J. W. B. Douglas, 1951). A study of growth records has been made in London in 1948 (A. T. Gore and W. T. Palmer, 1949), in Oxford (J. Parfitt, 1951) and in Sheffield (R. S. Illingworth *et al.*, 1949); such studies have provided much needed standards against which to compare the records of infants at clinics. Generally speaking, the records have not yet been properly utilized (or adequately designed) except in certain special instances and there is scope for considerable experimentation particularly in the derivation of indices of child morbidity.

Administrative statistics

11.64 Apart from the clinical content of the records it is necessary for administrative purposes, i.e. for the efficient utilization of manpower and equipment, to measure the activity of health visitors and clinics. The kind of analysis which should be made is indicated by the following statistics for London for a typical quarter in 1962. (Table 11.11).

TABLE 11.11 *Health visiting—visits paid during quarter*

	First visits		Subsequent visits
Type of visit	No.	Per cent of related births*	
Children—			
Under 1	16,402	97	47,484
1—4	—		97,328
Old people	4,455		
Miscellaneous	28,026		6,513
Unsuccessful	31,087		
Total	**79,970**		**151,325**

Number of Health Visitors 444 (whole time or equivalent)

11.65 It can be seen from these figures that 97 per cent of new babies were visited. By comparing such indices for smaller subdivisions of the area, a picture of relative effectiveness of coverage can be obtained. It can also be computed that the 444 health visitors made an average of eight home visits per working day in addition to their clinic duties; and that one in every seven visits was unsuccessful (in most cases because the mother was not at home).

11.66 Typical figures for welfare centres, again for the same quarter of 1962 in London, were—

216

| Sessions | First attendances | | Total attendances |
	No.	Per cent of related population	
Children			
0—1	11,447	76	137,381
1—2			21,486
2—5			14,618
Special toddlers	(a)		8,532

(a) These children in most cases have already made a first visit but have been recalled by special 'birthday' invitations.

11.67 Here again we see that 76 per cent of the babies born in London attended a welfare centre during their first year of age. For every first attendance in the first year of age there were twelve total attendances, i.e. on the average every child attending in the first year did so twelve times before the first birthday. In the second year of age we have to remember that the total attendances relate to infants who began to attend in the previous year of age, so that on the average, attendances per child in the second year of age numbered only two.

11.68 The Ministry of Health in England and Wales require figures similar to those shown above in relation to health visiting and for child welfare. The need for statistics of child welfare clinic attendances renders it advisable to institute sessional returns (compiled weekly) from centres giving particulars of numbers of children attending in the different age groups distinguishing those attending for the first time. Alternatively or in supplementation, the health visitor could make an annual 'stocktaking' review of all case records that have been current during the year; this would have the advantage of bringing to her attention the names of the very frequent attenders as well as those of the non-attenders.

REFERENCES

BUTLER, N. R., and BONHAM, D. G. (1963) Perinatal Mortality. E. and S. Livingstone.
CHARLES, E. (1951) Brit. J. Soc. and Prev. Med., 5. 41.
City of Birmingham (1955) Abstract of Statistics 1952–54.
DOUGLAS, J. W. B. (1951) Population Studies, 5, 35.
GEMMELL, A. A., LOGAN, W. P. D., and BENJAMIN, B. (1954) J. Obstet & Gyn. 65. 458.
General Register Office (1953) Registrar General's Statistical Review of England and Wales, 1948–49 Text, Medical.
General Register Office (1954) Registrar General's Statistical Review of England and Wales, 1950 Text, Medical.
General Register Office (1957) Registrar General's Decennial Supplement. Occupational Mortality II, Vol. 2.
General Register Office (1967) Annual Statistical Review 1964 Pt. III p. 171.
General Register Office (1967) Regional and Social Factors in Infant Mortality. Stud. Med. Pop. Subj. No. 19, H.M.S.O.
GORE, A. T., and PALMER, W. T. (1949) Lancet, ii. 385.
HEADY, J. A., DALY, C., and MORRIS, J. (1955) Lancet, i. 343, 395, 445, 499, 554.
ILLINGWORTH, R. S., et al. (1949) Lancet, ii. 598.
Ministry of Health (1953) Report for 1952 Part II.
PARFITT, J. (1951) Brit. J. Soc. Med., 5, 1.
Queen Charlotte's Maternity Hospital (1960) Clinical Report.
STEWART, A. M., and RUSSELL, W. T. (1952) Medical Officer, 88, 5.

CHAPTER 12

STATISTICS OF THE HEALTH OF THE SCHOOL CHILDREN

12.1 An early result of the recognition of the association between poverty and ill health, and equally of an appreciation of the futility of attempting to teach children handicapped by poor physique and minor ailments, was the institution of a regular and compulsory system of medical inspection in schools and of free treatment centres for dental caries, eye disorders, and other minor ailments especially skin diseases and infestation which at the time were rife among elementary school children. This obligation was placed upon local education authorities by the Education Act of 1907 which created what has become known as the School Health Service. Much of the treatment organization which was formerly an integral part of the School Health Service has been replaced by the more comprehensive facilities of the National Health Service with the family doctor as the focus, but the school medical officer still plays an important part in the maintenance of health in school children and of healthy conditions in schools.

12.2 Compulsory 'periodic medical inspections 'of pupils attending maintained primary and secondary schools (including special schools) take place in accordance with Regulation 10 (1) (a) of the School Health Service and Handicapped Pupils Regulations 1953 which requires 'a general medical inspection of every pupil on not less than three occasions at appropriate intervals during the period of his compulsory school age and other medical inspections of any pupil on such occasions as may be necessary or desirable: provided that there may be fewer than three general medical inspections for any pupil who attends schools maintained by the Authority for less than the period of his compulsory school age or, if the Minister approves, for all pupils'.

12.3 These medical inspections are cursory to a degree because of limitations of time and they have been criticized on this account by Gordon who pointed out (1947) that in the short time available 'nothing not immediately apparent to the head, eye, and ear will be noticed, and, unless the doctor is especially aware and trained, not even those'; moreover they do not embrace children who are absent from school because they are ailing. Nevertheless despite inherent defects in the system the statistics derived therefrom do provide an index of school health, comparable year by year. Gordon himself admits that 'statistics of the incidence of school age complaints are hard to come by, and school inspection is one of the main ways of obtaining them'.

12.4 In addition to the 'periodic' examinations, there is an oral inspection by a dental surgeon every year, or as often as staff permits if not annually. If teachers express a desire to have a doctor's opinion at any time as a matter of urgency without waiting for a routine age group examination a 'special'.

inspection may be arranged; such non-routine 'special' examinations include also inspections for employment certificates, for school journeys and holiday camps, and periodical inspection of pupils who have been 'ascertained' to be handicapped by a special defect (physical or mental). 'Reinspections' are made of pupils who at any earlier medical inspection have been referred for treatment in order to check that such treatment has been sought. The school nursing sisters carry out routine hygiene inspections to detect cases of head or body lice, scabies, impetigo or ringworm, now much more rare than in former times when poverty and ignorance combined to produce lower standards of hygiene than those which are general at the present time.

The main school medical record

12.5 The system normally operates in the following way. For each child attending school there is maintained a standard medical record designed and supplied by the Ministry of Education. This forms a permanent dossier of the pupil's medical history throughout school life; indeed if, on the attainment of school entry age, the local health authority transfers child welfare records (see p. 215) for filing with the school medical record, the medical history extends back to birth. The main school record may be filed at the school as in London or at a district or central offices as in smaller urban areas. If a child moves from the area to that of another education authority it is customary to transfer the record cards to the receiving authority.

12.6 When a medical or dental inspection session has been arranged the school nursing sister makes a prior selection of the cards for the children who are to be reviewed. These are then made available to the clinician for recapitulation of previous history and for the recording of current findings. At the end of the session the records are collected for statistical processing.

Statistical analysis

12.7 The method of analysing the results of school medical inspections will depend upon the size of the authority and on whether the school medical records are kept at a central or district office or at the schools themselves. In a relatively small town with centralized records it would be possible normally to schedule the current year's inspections directly on to specially columnized stationery. In a larger authority the numbers of inspections may be so large and the records so scattered that it is necessary to use some intermediate form of return which can be completed after each inspection session and can be processed by machine methods. Gore (1948) has given an account of the method used by the London County Council (replaced in 1965 by the Inner London Education Authority); essentially this consists in the use of a self-coding form on which the school nursing sister lists the children examined in a particular sex age group during the session and for each line of which a punched card is prepared from the coded information.

Total coverage

12.8 In 1964 in the then County of London there were 414,598 on school attendance rolls. During the year there were 155,273 routine (detailed) inspections and 122,191 other inspections, a total of 277,464 inspections. Allowing for some degree of duplication between routine and other inspections it is clear that a large proportion of children are seen by a school doctor during a typical year of school life. The routine inspections alone represented 37 per cent of the school roll.

Referrals for treatment

12.9 An immediate index of the comparative state of school health is provided by the proportion of children who were referred to their family doctor as in need of treatment. In calculating this proportion it is customary to exclude dental treatment and treatment for infestation; in the latter case because it is a condition of a different quality from the other disorders recorded and is becoming increasingly rare; in the former case because the provision of a separate system of detailed dental inspections renders the dental component of routine medical inspections incomplete. Thus we find on referring to the same year 1964 for the County of London that, with the above exclusions, 9·3 per cent of entrant boys were referred for treatment compared with 18·7 per cent in 1949; and 13·8 per cent of boy leavers were referred for treatment in 1964 compared with 14·4 per cent in 1949.

Principal groups of defects

12.10 Serial figures for the County of London for specific groups of ailments found at routine inspections and referred for medical care are shown in Table 12.1.

12.11 Such figures as these can throw light upon the way in which the health of school children reacts to external conditions (especially when the rates are calculated for specific age groups so as to avoid the effects of changes

TABLE 12.1 *Defects found on medical inspection of school children, per cent incidence*

	1938	1942	1950	1961	1964
Number examined (excluding special schools and training colleges)	*	*			
	169,995	88,325	169,742	163,598	155,273
			percentages		
Skin diseases	1·0	2·0	0·97	1·19	1·18
External eye diseases	1·7	1·9	0·57	0·54	0·41
Defective hearing	0·2	0·3	0·44	0·90	1·15
Otitis media	0·6	0·4	0·69	0·51	0·54
Enlarged tonsils and adenoids	9·2	7·3	8·98	3·59	3·57
Defective speech	no figures available		0·60	0·87	1·00
Enlarged cervical glands	1·5	1·2	1·38	0·63	0·60
Heart and circulation	1·4	0·8	0·69	0·87	1·00
Lung disease (not tuberculosis)	1·5	1·1	1·62	1·21	1·46
Orthopaedic defects	⎫		4·84	3·52	3·00
Defects of nervous system	⎬ no figures available		0·33	0·43	0·56
Psychological defects	⎭		0·70	1·08	1·42
Anaemia	0·4	0·2	0·36	0·12	0·13

* Figures for these years include cases not specifically requiring medical action.

in the age distribution of the children being examined). Thus, during the early years of the Second World War when schools were closed by air raids or evacuation movements, children were herded in classrooms to a much less extent with the result that the transmission of infection was restricted; this was reflected in a decline in the incidence of enlarged tonsils, enlarged glands, otitis media, and respiratory disease. On the other hand if children were more in the open air they were less subject to supervision and it was difficult to maintain standards of hygiene; in consequence the incidence of skin disease rose.

Defective vision

12.12 An important function of the school medical inspection is the detection of errors of refraction. Since this normally depends on the Snellen tests the records are naturally restricted to children old enough to read letters. In 1964 in the County of London 76·7 per cent of boy leavers and 77·3 per cent of girl leavers had visual acuity 6/6 (children not wearing spectacles). The proportion requiring spectacles for the first time remains steady at about 6 or 7 per cent in each age group but the proportion already possessing spectacles but requiring adjustment of lenses with the passage of time rises from 1 per cent at age seven to 6 per cent at age fifteen. The figures show a remarkable stability from year to year; a constant feature is the slight excess of recorded defect of visual acuity in girls as compared with boys.

General condition

12.13 The Ministry of Education at one time required examining medical officers at periodic inspection to classify the pupils on a relative scale of general physical condition, viz. 'good', 'fair', 'poor'. The following are the figures for London from 1947 to 1952—

	Percentages		
	Good	*Fair*	*Poor*
1947	42·0	54·3	3·7
1948	40·8	56·0	3·2
1949	41·8	55·1	3·1
1950	46·3	50·9	2·8
1951	47·6	49·8	2·6
1952	50·5	47·1	2·4

12.14 The terms 'good', 'fair', 'poor' are purely subjective and relative; it is possible for the conception of 'normality' to undergo changes from year to year as the general level of health improves and for the distribution to remain comparatively unaffected by the improvement. Nevertheless this is hardly likely to affect short term comparisons and the favourable trend shown by the above figures is probably valid despite the fact that for each of these years the proportion of children actually referred for treatment for nutritional disease was about 1 per cent. Since 1956 the classification has been reduced to a simple dichotomy: (1) physical condition, satisfactory; (2) physical condition, unsatisfactory. In London the per cent unsatisfactory fell from 1·0 in 1960 to 0·6 in 1964.

Personal hygiene

12.15 In 1921 nurses' rota visits to schools in London revealed that 20·5 per cent of children were verminous; in 1952 the corresponding figure was 2·2—an eloquent testimony to health education, improved social conditions, and rising standards of parental care. The price of protection of the individual child is still 'eternal vigilance' and though these statistics show that the problem is of small dimensions, nevertheless the figures are kept under close observation by the school medical officer. Indeed though comprehensive surveys in London in 1964 showed an incidence of only 0·97 per cent, the rate for selective surveys (for schools with a 'history') was 2·0 per cent compared with 1·2 per cent for such surveys in 1960. This led to a special investigation as to whether the rise was real or due to improved case finding.

Employment

12.16 Where necessary, school-leavers with adverse medical records are advised that their physical defects represent contra indications against specific types of employment; in 1964 about one-eighth of London school-leavers were so affected. The actual figures were as shown in Table 12.2—

TABLE 12.2 *Contra-indications for employment*

	Boys	Girls
Contra-indications	*No.*	*No.*
Heavy manual work	248	128
Sedentary work	12	6
Indoor work	3	–
Exposure to bad weather	108	102
Wide changes of temperature	61	144
Work in damp atmosphere	77	73
Work in dusty atmosphere	151	103
Much stooping	46	36
Work near moving machinery or vehicles	116	80
Prolonged standing, much walking or quick movement from place to place, heights	248	175
Normal colour vision	334	2
Normally acute vision	1,246	960
Normal use of hands	32	12
Work requiring freedom from damp hands or skin defects	22	27
Handling or preparation of food	51	24
Normal hearing	71	39
Other forms of unsuitable work	28	10

Heights and weights

12.17 As a control upon the subjective impression of nutritional state gained from the physical appearance of children, many authorities arrange for the weighing and measuring of children at the time of routine inspection and for the progressive plotting of such measurements on a chart (usually weight against height for age) so that the medical officer can see any tendency to depart from normality. The main focus is not so much on the absolute deviation from 'normal' measurements, since children vary in their physical 'types' from the lean to the chubby without there being necessarily any variation in healthiness, but on any tendency for the deviation to increase over time (especially when this is a rapid increase). The physical measurement controls and supplements the clinical assessment but does not and cannot supplant it.

12.18 Jones (1938) tested the efficiency of various physical indices on 2,000 Liverpool school boys in two ways—

(1) By determining the percentage of boys who must be selected by the index in order to ensure that those selected include at least 80 per cent of the boys already diagnosed as ill-nourished. The lower the percentage the better the index.

(2) By determining the proportion of the ill-nourished boys among the lowest 30 per cent of boys when ranked by the physical indices. The higher the proportion the better the index.

12.19 A selection of the results (those for the twelve-year-old age group) is given below—

Index	Percentage of group screened to secure 80% of ill-nourished	Ill-nourished among lowest 30% of boys, as percentage of all ill-nourished in group
Weight	40·5	61·0
W/H	31·0	74·0
W/H²	31·0	74·0
Ht. × constant = Wt.	31·0	74·0
Wt. for Ht.	31·0	74·0
Wt. for Ht. and Age	30·5	78·0
(W/H) × (381—months)/54	29·0	82·5
W/HC	48·0	65·0
HC/constant = Wt.	48·0	65·5
Wt. for Ht. and Chest	60·5	39·0
Wt. for Ht. and Hip	42·5	60·5

12.20 The best result (for all age groups) was given by Tuxford's index (1917)—

$$(W/H) \times (381 - \text{age in months})/54$$

with [Wt. for Ht. for age] as the next best index.

12.21 Tanner (1952) has reminded of the dangers of a standard of 'normality' in the hands of those who do not appreciate that the 'normal' is merely the centre of a natural distribution and that a large proportion of children even within a population of homogeneous standards of nutrition naturally deviate substantially from the average. 'When standards were first published what is implied by "the spread of the normal"... was not generally understood. Anxious parents consulting the oracular weighing-machine, plagued their practitioners with complaints of their children being five pounds under- or over-weight for their height and age, and this despite both mother and father being miracles of thinness or rotundity.' He points out that the distributions of 'healthy' and 'unhealthy' children overlap and that a rule for excluding from the 'healthy' extreme values which represent the beginning of the distribution of the 'unhealthy' must also exclude some children who are healthy—the object is therefore to separate the distributions as much as possible and to choose a dividing line in which errors of omission are minimized for the maximum screening of the 'unhealthy'.

12.22 Tanner (ibid.) favours percentiles as being more suitable than standard deviations for describing distributions which, as is usually the case, are not symmetrical and Normal, and suggests that increments of growth (velocity) are to be preferred to attained growth (distance) as the measurement to be tested.

12.23 In Tanner's opinion the most reliable standards of attained height and weights in England and Wales were:

Ages 1–4. Gore and Palmer (1949) took a cross-sectional sample of children in London child welfare centres; 5,684 children were weighed but unfortunately only 921 had their length (or height) measured. Mean weights and standard deviations are given weekly to three months, monthly to one year and three-monthly thereafter.

Ages 5–17. Daley (1950) has reported the height and weight measurements in 1949 of 21 thousand London school children, with means, standard deviations, 10th, 50th and 90th percentiles and the complete frequency distributions for the two sexes separately. [Since 1949, there have been further surveys to update these tables.]

Other measures

12.24 In America, Stuart and Meredith have recommended that in addition to height and weight, other measurements should be taken (and would take but little extra time), viz. hip width and chest circumference (as a guide to shape), calf circumference (for muscular measurement) and subcutaneous tissue thickness under the scapula and above the crest of the ilium. They give (1946) percentile standards for boys and girls from five to eighteen years based on Iowa school children of the professional and managerial classes measured between 1930 and 1945. These data are probably not applicable to British children.

Multiple measurements

12.25 The use of multiple measurements for screening introduces the problem of their combination into a single index (Tuxford's index above, is a simple example where only two measures are involved). The problem is an exercise in discriminant analysis, i.e. in the determination of a function combining these measurements such that the relative weight given to each achieves the maximum separation of healthy and unhealthy. Where the measures are correlated with each other one can use all except one in a regression formula to predict the remaining measurement, i.e. to provide a standard against which to test the actual measurement. A simple example in school health practice is the use of correlation between height and weight within age intervals to make weight prediction from height and age against which to test the actual weight of the individual child. If charted against age for the individual child successive predictions and deviations also indicate progressive falling off or recovery in the rate of growth and the chart can be channelled to set limits to the falling off (or conversely, excessive growth) beyond which the child is treated as requiring medical care.

Treatment statistics

12.26 The responsibility for treatment of illnesses in school children is shared between the three branches of the Health Service, viz. the general practitioner, the hospital and the local authority, with the latter playing a much diminished part. The local education authority still has the duty of making arrangements for free medical treatment of school pupils but the parents have complete freedom of choice and it is natural and proper that they should select the agency in which they have greater confidence or with which they have had closer association. The result however is that constant liaison is necessary to ensure that, in total, treatment facilities are both comprehensive and efficient. Complete statistics of treatment represent an ideal not yet achieved. Many hospitals do send reports on children they have treated for inclusion in the school medical record and if the system becomes comprehensive it may eventually be possible by sample analysis of the school records to obtain statistics of hospital treatment. Since the family doctor is now the focus, general practitioner statistics, not yet sufficiently extensive, appear to hold the key.

12.27 The local education authority does still maintain clinics for the treatment of minor ailments, defective vision, dental disorders, and for special investigations, e.g. enuresis, deafness, child psychiatry and maladjustment and the demands made upon these clinics themselves provide rough indices of the trend of incidence of the defects treated. In addition through the follow-up of children referred for treatment from routine and other medical inspections, the school medical authorities do become informed of the character of the treatment carried out. At present, therefore, the statistics of treatment are based on numbers 'known to local education authorities to have received treatment'. If the intensity of follow-up and the completeness (or incompleteness) of reporting from hospitals and other centres remains constant, year to year comparisons can be made; but there is no way of knowing how incomplete the figures are and of whether the degree of completeness is varying and in the circumstances it seems dangerous to draw any inferences from the figures.

Dental services

12.28 Subject to the availability of staff every endeavour is made to maintain a systematic system of regular dental inspection in schools. The statistics of interest are (apart from the statistics of the total volume of work), the proportion found to require treatment (in London this has in recent years been stable at just over 60 per cent); the number of attendances per treatment (about three); and the ratio of permanent teeth restored to permanent teeth extracted—typical figures for the County of London are—

1945	4·04
1950	3·29
1960	7·57
1964	12·6

12.29 The decline in this ratio after 1945 reflects a severe shortage of staff and as a consequence a reduction of capacity to provide ameliorative treatment. Since then there has been a massive improvement in the extent of conservative treatment partly due to greater accessibility of dental care (outside the school service) and partly due to the increased demand for care consequent upon improved education. Total neglect is now seldom seen.

Dental surveys

12.30 As a check on the general effectiveness of total facilities for dental care—school health service, National Health Service and private treatment facilities—and of parental co-operation therefore, the Ministry have encouraged and co-ordinated the carrying out of local surveys of the incidence of dental caries. A 'DMF' method of assessment is employed, viz. the numbers of *d*ecayed, *m*issing and *f*illed teeth in each child are aggregated and the results expressed in two ways:

(*a*) the percentage of children with no DMF teeth; and
(*b*) the average number of DMF teeth per child examined.

Other special surveys

12.31 There is a limit to the medical information that can be collected routinely and where it is required to measure the extent of a particular problem (e.g. in order to decide whether some special service is required) without any implication of the necessity for observation (in the same form) it is clearly more economical to proceed by field survey. Apart from the dental surveys referred to above there have been a number of surveys of other diseases and investigations of which the following are but a few examples.

12.32 Craigmile (1953) made a survey of foot defects in 12,765 Middlesex school children and found, for example, the following percentage incidence of defects in children aged twelve and over.

	Percentage	
Defect	*Boys*	*Girls*
Proximal Hallux Valgus	4·0	22·4
Varus 1st Metatarsal	8·7	8·0
Cramped toes	14·5	24·1
Valgus ankles	3·9	5·2
Pes Cavus	0·44	0·02
Unsatisfactory footwear	21·5	35·0

12.33 Henderson (1949) reports a survey in several parts of England and Wales to assess the incidence of diabetes mellitus. Of 1,307,000 children under sixteen years of age living in sixteen English cities and towns and five counties, 183 (1 in 7,000) were known to have diabetes (about one-third of the incidence in children in the United States as revealed by a United States Public Health Service Survey [Joslin, 1946]).

12.34 Benjamin and Pirrie (1952) investigated the effect on growth and health of a dietary supplement of Vitamin B.12 administered to children in day open air schools. The results were negative (though this was important in itself) but the investigation also served to show that a properly controlled investigation could be carried out within the ordinary school medical organization given adequate co-operation from teaching and nursing staff.

12.35 Sorsby, Benjamin and Yudkin (1955) carried out a survey of the incidence of defects in visual function (convergence, accommodation, hetero-phoria, binocular vision, colour vision, dark adaptation) and found that though 75 per cent of all children had normal visual acuity, only 70 per cent of these were normal when other visual tests were considered. However they came to the conclusion that there was no case for extending the routine medical examination at school to cover visual functions other than central acuity.

12.36 Hughes and Cooper (1956) have investigated the incidence of head-ache and eye pain in school children in Northumberland and especially its relationship to tenderness of the first tip of the central tranverse process in the neck. In ten-year-old children 2 per cent complained of headaches of sufficient severity to have 'reduced the child to tears or bed'.

12.37 On grounds of economy it is generally necessary to use sampling methods. The object here should be to draw a sample which is both representa-tive and appropriate to the type of enquiry and it is worth stressing that strict theoretical considerations of random sampling often have to give way to considerations of practicability. For example bias may be introduced by the fact that selection is dependent upon reporting by hospital treatment centres or upon voluntary co-operation of parents and children in undergoing certain tests or upon the accessibility of homes to a single medical officer with limited scope for movement. It is often much better that the survey should be attempted with knowledge of the source of bias (and with such steps as are possible to reduce its influence) than that it should not be attempted at all.

Ministry of Education returns

12.38 In order to provide statistics of the operation of the School Health Service for inclusion in its own Annual Report the Ministry of Education and Science requires the Local Education Authority to complete a series of returns including the following information—

Numbers of medical inspections, by type (periodic or special) and by age group showing the number of children referred for treatment (vision defects being treated separately).

Numbers of defects found at inspections by disease group and severity (i.e. whether for treatment or observation).

Classification of children by physical condition (satisfactory, unsatis-factory).

Numbers of hygiene examinations by nurses and cases of infestation found.

Numbers of pupils whose treatment has been 'brought to the Authority's notice' by disease and whether treated by the Authority or otherwise.

Numbers of dental inspections with detailed analysis of treatment given.

Infectious disease

12.39 It should be borne in mind that a primary consideration of the school medical officer is the prevention and control of infectious disease, the transmission of infectious disease being facilitated by the herding together in classrooms of susceptibles and infectors. Statistical aspects of infectious disease are covered in Chapter 9.

REFERENCES

BENJAMIN, B., and PIRRIE, G. D. (1952) *Medical Officer*, 87, 137.
CRAIGMILE, D. (1953) *Brit. Med. J.*, ii. 749.
DALEY, A. (1950) Report on Height and Weight of School Pupils in the County of London in 1949. L.C.C.
GORDON, I. (1947) *Brit. J. of Soc. Med.*, 1. 238.
GORE, A. T. (1948) Medical Officer, 80. 123.
GORE, A. T., and PALMER, W. T. (1949) *Lancet*, i. 385.
HENDERSON, P. (1949) *Brit. Med. J.*, i. 478.
HUGHES, E. L., and COOPER, C. E. (1956) *Brit. Med. J.*, i. 1138.
JONES, R. H. (1938) *J. of Roy. Stat. Soc.*, 101.1.
JOSLIN, E. P. (1946) *The Treatment of Diabetes*, London.
Ministry of Education, Chief Medical Officer (1954) Report for the years 1952 and 1953, H.M.S.O.
SORSBY, A., BENJAMIN, B., and YUDKIN, J. (1955) *Brit. J. Prev. and Soc. Med.*, 9, 1.
STUART, H. C., and MEREDITH, H. V. (1946) *Amer. J. Publ. Hlth*, 36.1365.
TANNER, J. M. (1952). *Arch. of dis. child.*, 27.10.
TUXFORD, A. W. (1917) *School Hyg.*, 8, 656.

CHAPTER 13

OTHER PUBLIC HEALTH STATISTICS

13.1 There are a number of sources of statistics which bear some relationship to measures of public health which do constitute in themselves major aspects and these are described in the following notes.

Accident statistics

13.2 In England and Wales in 1964 there were 534,737 deaths registered of which 18,727 were assigned to accidental causes (excluding homicide and suicide). Of these 7,256 were of persons under the age of forty-five. The toll of accidents even in terms of deaths is serious enough but these figures do not reveal the greater dimensions of the problem of incapacity arising from non-fatal accidents.

13.3 Among a total insured male population in Great Britain of 15,080 thousand at risk between June 1960 and June 1961, there were 552·9 thousand spells of certified incapacity attributed to accidents, poisonings and violence, of an average duration of about two weeks (Ministry of Pensions and National Insurance, 1963). For females the corresponding figures were, 4,947 thousand at risk and 118·1 thousand spells. Apart from these spells of incapacity which form the subject of ordinary sickness insurance there are the statistics of industrial injury insurance. These show that among populations of the same order of size (males 13,971, females 7,499, thousands) there were, for males, 686,460 and for females 77,740, spells of absence arising from industrial accidents, in the same year.

13.4 Clearly, accident prevention is just as much a public health (or ill-health) problem as any other aspect of disease prevention.

13.5 No comprehensive system of accident records exists. Industrial accidents may form the subject of reports to the Chief Inspector of Factories and of claims under National Insurance legislation from which as an administrative by-product statistics are derived; some figures have already been quoted. Non-industrial accidents do not come to official notice unless they cause the sickness of an insured person or cause hospital admission or, if road accidents, are covered by such records as are maintained by police. The criteria of severity and causation vary so much between these sources that it is difficult to achieve adequate integration. If there were comprehensive general practitioner records it would be possible to obtain complete coverage of accidents requiring medical care. For example in the ten general practices co-operating in the General Register Office Survey (1956) the incidence of accidents may be assessed from the statistics in Table 13.1.

13.6 Unfortunately, no classification by *cause* of injury is available but these figures serve to underline the dimensions of the problem in so far as they reveal that (in these practices) one-tenth of male patients and one-twelfth of

TABLE 13.1 *Patients consulting per* 1,000 *population: Average annual rate*
1951–54

Disease	Males					Females				
	0–	15–	45–	65+	All ages	0–	15–	45–	65+	All ages
Fractures	5·1	9·3	11·0	8·2	8·4	4·7	2·7	9·2	13·6	5·8
Dislocation without fracture	0·3	0·8	1·1	0·5	0·7	0·4	0·4	0·5	0·8	0·5
Sprains and strains, joints and muscles	12·0	29·5	16·0	8·8	19·9	13·4	18·9	16·5	10·8	16·3
Head injury (excl. skull fracture)	9·4	3·3	2·1	2·5	4·7	5·7	1·5	2·1	4·9	2·9
Internal injury of chest, abdomen and pelvis	0·1	0·2	0·2	—	0·1	0·2	0·1	0·1	0·2	0·1
Laceration and open wound	20·0	17·3	10·6	9·5	15·9	12·2	7·8	7·0	4·4	8·2
Superficial injury	13·9	8·5	4·6	8·6	9·2	12·7	9·6	9·4	6·5	9·9
Contusion and crushing	17·6	16·6	14·4	13·0	16·1	12·1	9·7	15·4	22·1	12·8
Effects of foreign body	3·9	3·9	3·3	1·3	3·6	3·5	2·3	2·6	0·7	2·4
Burns	7·6	4·1	3·1	4·2	4·9	7·0	6·0	5·2	5·2	6·0
Injury to nerves and spinal cord without bone injury	—	0·3	—	—	0·1	—	0·0	0·1	—	0·0
Effects of poisons	1·9	1·5	0·6	0·5	1·3	2·1	2·1	1·5	1·0	1·8
Effects of weather, exposure, etc.	1·2	0·9	0·7	1·1	1·0	1·2	1·5	0·8	0·5	1·2
Other injuries and reactions	17·6	23·1	17·0	11·8	19·3	12·0	12·5	16·4	15·7	13·6
Total	110·6	119·3	84·7	70·0	105·2	87·2	75·1	86·8	64·4	81·5

female patients consulted their doctors each year for conditions arising from external causes.

13.7 Some special surveys have been carried out. In the United States, accident recording was included in the morbidity study of the Eastern Health District of Baltimore where sample households were visited at monthly intervals over a five-year period ending in 1943 to obtain records of all illnesses and incapacity (Collins, Phillips and Oliver, 1953). A total of 2,690 accidents were recorded for 21,505 full-time person-years of observation for

TABLE 13.2 *Accident rates—Baltimore*

External cause of accident	Annual rate per 1,000 population	
	Total	Disabling
Fall	37·2	16·1
Handling or striking object	12·7	3·3
Motor vehicle	7·4	5·4
Other transportation	1·5	0·8
Sports and recreation	5·2	2·5
Animals and insects	4·5	0·4
Hand tools	3·9	1·3
Falling objects	3·7	1·9
Machinery	1·4	0·7
Other miscellaneous causes	47·6	19·1

Nature of injury	Annual rate per 1,000 population	
	Total	Disabling
Laceration	32·7	9·4
Superficial injury	32·5	9·0
Miscellaneous other injury	15·5	8·0
Dislocation and sprain	15·0	9·3
Burn	9·7	2·6
Fracture	9·7	7·8
Poisoning	4·2	2·8
Foreign body	3·2	0·9
General effects	2·7	1·9

the canvassed (white) households. Of the total accidents 1,110 were disabling in the sense of causing a loss of one or more days from work or other usual activity, whether or not the person was gainfully employed. The total amounted to an annual rate of 125 accidents per 1,000 population, 52 of which were disabling for one day or longer and 73 did not cause any loss of time from work or other usual activities. The statistics in Table 13.2 are illustrative of the type of information obtained.

13.8 This information was sub-divided according to sex and age—for example the annual rate of disabling accidents from falls for males was 16 for ages under 5, 21 for ages 5–14, 5 for ages 15–24, 8 for ages 25–64 and 30 for 65 and over; the corresponding figures for females being 15, 16, 8, 26 and 29; and by site of injury—head and face injuries constituted 16 per cent of the total, eye 4, mouth and teeth 1, arm 11, hands and fingers 22, trunk and vertebrae 7, lower extremities 27, multiple sites 5; and by duration of disability and income levels.

13.9 The statistics in Table 13.3 show that among adults the home and public places together are more 'dangerous' than workplace.

TABLE 13.3 *Accident rates by place of accident—Baltimore*

Place and cause of accident	Age adjusted rate—persons 15 and over—all accidents per million person-hours in specified place
Home	
All causes	13·15
Falls	4·42
Handling or struck by object	2·18
Other	6·52
Public Place	
All causes	26·93
Falls	9·26
Motor vehicle	5·35
Sports	2·21
Handling or struck by object	1·27
Other	8·84
Work	
All causes	27·86
Falls	2·85
Handling or struck by object	6·02
Other	18·52

Accidents in the home

13.10 The problem of home accidents had become so disturbing that in 1947 the Home Secretary set up a Standing Interdepartmental Committee on Accidents in the Home 'to co-ordinate departmental action in connexion with the prevention of accidents in the home, and to maintain contact with unofficial organizations interested in the subject'. This Committee reported in 1953. An appendix quotes the following revealing and eloquent figures for deaths in England and Wales:

	1949	1950	1951
Domestic accidents	4,891	5,086	5,483
Road accidents	4,103	4,523	4,698

231

13.11 Apart from figures of deaths and of hospital cases, i.e. of severer cases however, the Committee was able to furnish very little statistical information of the *total* problem. The report quotes an inquiry made by the Domestic Accidents Panel of the Scientific Advisory Committee to the Ministry of Works in 1946–48, which was directed to ascertaining how far building design was responsible for domestic accidents. Reports on accidents were obtained from health visitors and housing managers. 'Eight per cent of the accidents covered by the inquiry were primarily due to faulty design (through such factors as the design of stairs including handrails, single steps between different floor levels and the position of light switches on stairs and in passages) and a further 20 per cent to poor maintenance, particularly of flooring, stair treads, handrails, and to inadequate lighting. But the majority of accidents seemed clearly due to the risks inherent in ordinary domestic activities, especially during busy periods. In the study of some hundreds of accidents, mostly non-fatal, reported by hospital almoners and home visitors 60 per cent happened in the kitchen or living-room, while cooking or clothes washing was being done, or when tea had just been made. It is in conditions such as these that children are most easily burned or scalded.'

Traffic accidents

13.12 Traffic has become one of the most intractable problems of modern urban development and injuries from road accidents its most distressing byproduct. The main sources of information are the reports on accidents made by police authorities on a standard form. These are processed nationally by the Ministry of Transport and Scottish Development Department. The basic measure is the casualty rate per hundred million vehicle miles. The figures for 1964 for Great Britain were:

Casualty rates per 100 *million vehicle miles*

	Killed	Seriously injured	Total casualties
Pedal cycle	12·3	169	792
Two-wheeled motor	30·9	555	1,953
Other vehicles	3·2	45	203

13.13 The analyses extend to the factors of age, day and time of accident, and class of road user. The Metropolitan Police publish their own annual analyses in even greater detail.

Industrial accidents

13.14. Considerable information is available about industrial accidents. Any accident which occurs in a factory, within the meaning of the Factories Act 1961, and which is either fatal or disables an employee to the extent of preventing him from earning full wages for more than three days must be reported to the District Inspector of Factories. Consolidated statistics appear in the *Annual Report of the Chief Inspector of Factories*.

13.15 This permits the calculation of a frequency rate for 100,000 hours worked

$$= \frac{\text{Total number of accidents} \times 100,000}{\text{Total man-hours worked}}$$

13.16 On this basis the frequency in 1965 varied from $0 \cdot 86$ in clothing and footwear and $1 \cdot 55$ in vehicles to $3 \cdot 26$ for bricks, pottery etc. and $3 \cdot 95$ for shipbuilding and marine engineering, the average for all industries being $2 \cdot 38$.

13.17 The report gives information of the incidence of accidents in different types of industrial processes, e.g. steam plants, building sites, foundries, cranes, electrical work, etc. Accidents are classified not only by industry but under sex and age, primary cause, and nature of injury.

Accidents, and morale

13.18 Reference must be made to the use of accident statistics taken together and in proper balance with statistics of absenteeism and disputes and against the background of an intimate knowledge of working conditions, as a pointer to morale and to the efficiency of managements. Revans (1955) showed that in the major coalfields in Great Britain there was a tendency for attendance to be worse in the larger pits; that the mean accident rate averaged over size groups of mines was proportioned to the logarithm of the number of men in the size group (and this was independent of such factors as mechanization and depth); and that the tonnage lost in disputes was greater in the larger mines. He came to the conclusion that 'one of the principal disabling causes of the large pit is the relative dilution of its management, particularly in its higher ranges'. In a more general discussion (1956) Revans has shown that these influences are not confined to coalmining. Accident, sickness absence, and associated statistics bearing on morale can thus be used to throw light upon defects in the structure of industrial management.

Home nursing

13.19 Under the National Health Service Act, 1946, a Local Health Authority is empowered to provide a home nursing service on demand by general practitioners and hospitals and subject to the availability of resources and agreement as to medical need. The Authority often provides this service through the agency of voluntary district nursing associations and organizations, to whom it makes a grant for approved expenditure. There was already a widespread provision for home nursing by voluntary organizations.

13.20 In recent years the service has been subjected to increasing pressure owing to the greater numbers of aged and chronic sick patients being nursed at home.

13.21 Two types of statistical information may be regarded as essential—

(i) A general measure of work done. For this purpose bare numbers of cases treated (new cases taken and total case-load), visits made and staff employed would suffice without details of names, addresses or diagnoses, etc.

(ii) A detailed picture of the clinical pattern of the demand placed upon the service, i.e. how many cases of a particular disease in a particular age group, the normal period of treatment and frequency of visit for this disease. A complete account of the treatment of individual patients can only be given at the termination of treatment and such details are, therefore, not required for the entire case-load but only for those cases discharged during the period of the return.

H*   233

PUBLIC HEALTH DEPARTMENT

(fig. 13.1)

Division No. .... District Association.................... Month .... 196 ....

PART I—TOTAL PATIENTS AND STAFF

(a) Total patients nursed at beginning of month ....

New series of visits commenced during month ....

Treatments completed during month ....

Total patients nursed at end of month ....

(b) Grand total of visits paid during month ....

(c) Number of nurses at end of month—
(a) Whole-time ....

(b) Part-time .... (Whole-time equivalent = ...

(c) Students ....

PART II—TREATMENTS COMPLETED DURING MONTH

Ref. No.	Initials	Age	M or F.	Nursing ordered by	Date of commencement	Completion		Suffering from	Total visits in whole series
						Date	Reason		

13.22 In London these and other considerations led, after some experimentation (MacGregor and Benjamin, 1950), to the drafting of a simplified return (Fig. 13.1), which provides a summary of activity, in general, in the form of numbers only (Part I) and details of treatment for completed cases only. These completed cases, shown in Part II, form only about one-third of the total numbers treated in any one month. A plan of organization is shown on the diagram (Fig. 13.2) which includes a basic index card. This procedure, if closely followed by the district associations, enables them to satisfy any inspection for the purposes of local supervision, to answer any individual inquiry and to prepare the monthly return without difficulty. It should be noted that the return does not call for the insertion of addresses of patients nor for a description of the nursing treatment given.

13.23 At the time this return was instituted it was felt that the limited value of description of treatment given, difficult to describe and interpret and even more difficult to classify, did not justify the extra work entailed in supplying the information. However, some areas do collect statistics of treatment given and a possible classification (not mutually exclusive) would include injections, blanket baths, enemas, dressings, changing of pessaries, washouts, douches or catheterization, etc. as common items.

13.24 The following information has been mainly taken from the *Annual Report of the County Medical Officer for London for* 1964.

Visits

13.25 The principal details of work done in the year were as follows:

Population	Nursing treatments completed	No. of completed treatments per 1,000 population	Total visits paid during year	Total visits per 1,000 population
3,185,000	36,464	11·4	1,576,008	495

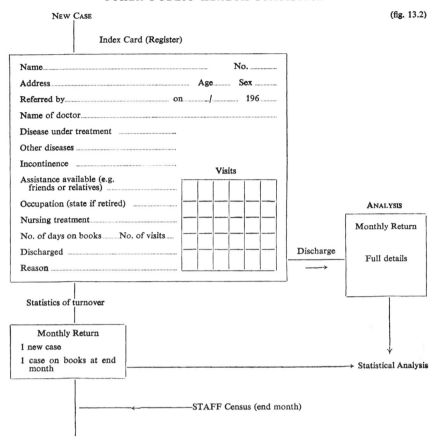

13.26 The county totals only are shown, though it should be understood that in relation to total volume of work and all other aspects it is the practice to take out separate figures for local areas within the county in order to measure local variations in the nature of the service.

Clinical analysis

13.27 During the year there were 36,464 nursing treatments (series of visits to individual patients) completed, leaving 11,414 patients on the case-load at the end of the year. Disregarding students, the average case-load for each of the 449 full-time (equivalent) nurses was 25 patients. Each nurse made an average of 35 visits to each patient.

13.28 The analysis of completed treatments enables tables to be prepared showing the incidence of different conditions treated by diagnostic group and by age and sex of patient treated. Salient features were—

(i) 57 per cent of all cases were over sixty-five years of age.

(ii) Females formed about two-thirds of the total number of patients treated, i.e. nearly twice as many as males.

(iii) the main conditions treated included respiratory, skin, circulatory and digestive diseases.

Duration of treatment

13.29 The length of time and the frequency of visits involved in any treatment varies considerably with the nature of the disease. Rheumatic patients are nursed for three months at a time with two or three visits a week. At the other end of the scale, respiratory conditions, the most common of all diagnoses, are nursed on the average for a fortnight only, but with almost daily visits. Digestive diseases (other than cancer) are normally of short duration. Tuberculous patients, as might be expected, require prolonged nursing as also do patients with heart disease—about nine weeks. Cancer and cerebral haemorrhage cases extend over about six weeks.

The value of the statistics

13.30 The main value of the statistics lies in the way in which they help to fill in the picture of chronic sickness in the population, a problem of growing dimensions as the structure of the population grows older. (See Chapter 2.)

Domestic help service

13.31 Some light on the problem of infirmity among the aged population is thrown by the statistics of the domestic help service provided by the Local Health Authority though these are not the only types of case assisted.

Immunization and vaccination

13.32 These statistics are referred to in Chapter 9.

Blindness

13.33 It has already been noted that attempts to gather information about the incidence of infirmities at population censuses have not proved successful. At least on one infirmity however there is now a useful alternative source of statistics. Under the National Assistance Act 1948 those who register with local authorities and are certified as blind* (by qualified ophthalmologists) are entitled to supplementary financial assistance at any age and some domiciliary assistance. Not every blind person registers since there is no compulsion to do so and there are an appreciable number whose financial and social circumstances are so favourable that they can ignore the financial inducement to register. Sorsby (1950, 1953) made a review of the statistics and estimated that the register may be deficient by 15 to 20 per cent. Nevertheless, it seems likely that stable conditions have been reached and that the statistics are comparable from one year to another and are representative of the blind population as a whole; they enable the trend of prevalence of blindness to be observed both in total and for different causes of blindness and permit some degree of assessment of the efficiency of treatment.

13.34 Thus in the *Annual Report of the Chief Medical Officer of the Ministry of Health for* 1965 it was reported that at December 31, 1964 the Blind

---

*(1) 'So blind as to be unable to perform any work for which eyesight is essential.'

(2) A blind person can take a contributory pension at age forty instead of at age sixty-five, but national assistance is usually more favourable.

Register for England and Wales stood at 98,512, the age and sex distribution being as follows:

	0–1	1–4	5–15	16–20	21–49	50–64	65 and over	Not known	Total
Males	4	176	1,062	556	6,467	8,400	22,628	12	39,305
Females	9	153	840	395	4,596	8,541	44,664	9	59,207

13.35 The excess of females in the blind population is confined to the higher age groups and merely reflects the marked excess of women in these age groups in the general population. If adjustment is made for this factor it is found that the overall risk of blindness is substantially the same for both sexes (though the causes of blindness involved are slightly different).

13.36 New registrations in 1964 amounted to 13,088. As to causes of blindness, among those aged less than 65 years, the main causes were: Retrolental fibroplasia (14 per cent), myopic chorioretinal atrophy (13), diabetic retinopathy (15), optic atrophy (12), and retinitis pigmentosa and allied abiotrophies (8).

REFERENCES

Chief Inspector of Factories (1966) Annual Report for 1965 Cmnd. 3080.

COLLINS, S. D., PHILLIPS, F. R., and OLIVER, D. S. (1953) United States Department of Health, Education and Welfare. Public Health Monograph 14, U.S. Government Printing Office.

Department of Scientific Research (1963) Research on Road Safety, H.M.S.O.

General Register Office (1956) *Studies on Medical and Population Subjects, No. 9;* General Practitioner Records.

MACGREGOR, M., and BENJAMIN, B. (1950) *Medical Officer*, 84, 227.

Ministry of Pensions and National Insurance (1963) Digest of Statistics Analysing Certificates of Incapacity.

Ministry of Health (1965). Annual Report of Chief Medical Officer for 1965 H.M.S.O.

REVANS, R. W. (1955) *Oper. Res. Quarterly*, 6, 91.

REVANS, R. W. (1956) *Pol. Quarterly*, 27, 303.

SORSBY, A. (1950) Causes of Blindness in England and Wales, M.R.C. Memorandum No. 24. H.M.S.O.

SORSBY, A. (1953) Causes of Blindness in England 1848–50. Ministry of Health. H.M.S.O.

CHAPTER 14

INDUSTRIAL AND GENERAL INCAPACITY

14.1 We have already seen (p. 135) that sickness in any exact sense of departure from normal well-being is difficult to measure and that it is easier to adopt a more practical if more selective concept of sickness which might be more capable of objective recording.

Recording difficulties

14.2 At first sight absence from work or (if not employed) inability to participate in the daily activities normally undertaken, appeals as a elear and unequivocal indication of sickness and on the whole this is true but there are two important reservations:

(1) Sickness absence for employed persons is often associated not only with the payment of National Insurance benefit but with benefits from private insurance with a Friendly Society and in many cases with maintenance of part or full wages by the employer. The point of time at which an employed person 'goes sick' will depend not only on the absolute fact of feeling unwell but on whether there is any loss of income involved, and if so, upon what degree of incapacity at which any financial pressure to remain at work ceases to operate. The same factors operate to determine the point of time at which he returns to work. Sickness absence becomes therefore a relative measure and may mean different degrees of illness for different groups of workers. Even for non-employed persons a similar difficulty arises; a housewife with a large family and unable to afford assistance may struggle to carry on longer than those with less responsibility and more domestic help.

(2) Not all sickness absence is medically certified and even where it is so certified the administrative arrangements for the disbursement of sick pay may mean that the medical certificates cannot be made directly available to those who are concerned with statistical analysis and the quality of the data may suffer in this respect if recording has to be left to works officials whose interests are naturally more in factory administration than in medical statistics and who do not appreciate the problem of classifying diagnoses. Furthermore the need to submit the medical certificate to any employer may tend to make the medical practitioner circumspect in his description of the condition causing incapacity, if only that in the interests of the patient, he may have to be definite about a diagnosis before he is certain (which means that subsequent certificates for the same absence may bear different diagnoses as he becomes more certain) or he may consider it necessary to conceal a condition which is likely to jeopardize the continued employment of the patient. Persons not gainfully employed, e.g. housewives, are less likely to consult doctors for minor degrees of incapacity and even where the conditions

are serious it is unlikely that they would voluntarily produce medical certificates to satisfy the needs of any survey of incapacity; such surveys therefore are only likely to elicit information about the conditions they 'complain' of rather than precise diagnoses. (This is not to say that statistics of 'complaints' are without value.) Generally therefore practical conditions militate to weaken the validity of the diagnostic classification of sickness absence records.

Development of measures of incapacity

14.3 The earliest measures of sickness absence of the kind we are considering were developed by the Friendly Societies—organizations for medical insurance against the economic effects of sickness, which in some form or another go back to antiquity. The Friendly Societies as such developed out of the Guilds of the thirteenth and fourteenth centuries which were formed (as distinct from protective trade guilds) for charitable purposes, and approached their modern form towards the end of the eighteenth century. Occasionally limited in membership as to numbers, and sometimes restricted to specific occupations, these societies provided, for a uniform premium, benefits in sickness and at death. From the earliest times, and certainly in their later development, differences existed between one type of society and another in financial organization, in the relationship between premiums and benefits (some were no more than savings banks) and in the general degree of solvency and permanency of activity. Those who were concerned to apply proper actuarial principles for ensuring that the premiums charged from entry provided, on the average, the cost of the benefits paid out, soon found it necessary to analyse their experience statistically as a basis for the premium calculation.

14.4 The earliest recorded attempt to construct what became known as a table of sickness was made by the Highland Society in 1820 and was based on data voluntarily contributed by seventy-three societies in Scotland, the number of years of life observed being over 104,000. Further tables were produced by Ansell in 1835 based on the experience of various societies for the five years 1823–27. In 1845 Neison published tables based on Government returns from societies from 1836–40 and embracing 1,147,000 years of life. It is believed that these tables were the first to differentiate the experiences of rural, town, and city districts, which was common to all subsequent investigations. In 1854 further tables based upon Government returns were published by Finlaison; these tables are of interest for their selective character arising from Finlaison's restrictive view of sickness—'Nothing but sickness in the true sense of the word, that is, sickness incapacitating from labour and requiring constant medical treatment, and of limited duration, as distinguished from chronic ailment and mere decrepitude, was considered to be sickness. For instance, slight paralysis, blindness, mental disorder, or senile infirmity was not included.' Thus chronic sickness of a superannuating character was not covered by these tables. [This exclusion serves to emphasize that the tables of sickness of Friendly Societies were not designed to measure morbidity as such but sickness as it affected the financial administration of the societies; they were concerned with the periods of time during which members were making claims upon the funds.] The best known tables were those of the

Manchester Unity of Oddfellows which were produced for 1866–70 and for 1893–97; the latter especially (the work of Alfred [later Sir Alfred] Watson who became the first Government Actuary) became established as a standard and as a classic analysis of sickness experience.

14.5 Watson emphasized (1930) that sickness benefit as provided by Friendly Societies and by the original compulsory system of National Health Insurance of 1911* was strictly associated with suspension of earning capacity attributable to disability, and was not primarily concerned with the underlying cause of the disability itself. In such circumstances the establishment of medical diagnosis was less important than the practical difficulty of establishing loss of earning capacity, with the immediate problem of deciding whether inability to work is to be assessed in relation to usual occupation, any alternative employment which might normally be available, or in more absolute standards. The danger of confusing this concept with true morbidity can be emphasized by the fact that even in times of improving hygiene and falling mortality, sickness claims were often found to increase substantially if economic incentive to claim were provided by unemployment or by any relaxation of the rules of the Friendly Societies.

14.6 From the earliest times therefore the actuary concerned with sickness insurance has been accustomed to measure sickness in terms of the 'average number of weeks of sickness (claim) experienced by each individual between ages x and $x+1$'. This measure was represented by the symbol z_x and because it was calculated like a death rate (except that the numerator referred not to deaths within the year of age but to total weeks of sickness) it was called a 'sickness rate'. An important difference between a sickness experience and a mortality experience is, of course, that one person may receive sickness benefit several times and does not necessarily pass out of observation after once receiving benefit, i.e. the denominator of the sickness rate z_x is the average number alive between ages x and $x+1$ over the period of time to which recorded weeks of sickness within these ages relate in the experience under review.

14.7 The Statistics Sub-Committee of the Registrar General's Advisory Committee on Medical Nomenclature and Statistics (1954) have issued a report on the measurement of morbidity in which the term 'sickness rate' is not used. One of the rates defined is 'the average duration of sickness per person' [the term 'sickness' being used in a generalized sense without any attempt at specificity.] This is effectively the same as the actuarial rate of sickness but the Sub-Committee propose only the short title 'average duration per person'.

14.8 Actuarial rates of sickness in Great Britain relating to persons covered by National Insurance are prepared by the Government Actuary and published in his reports on the operation of the National Insurance Acts. There are a number of special features of this experience which must be borne in mind such as the exclusion of non-contributing employed married

* The Friendly Societies survived the introduction of a national system of sickness insurance in 1911 and many of them, known as Approved Societies, while providing supplemental insurance for additional benefits, co-operated with the Government by acting as agencies for the collection of contributions and payment of benefits for the National Health Insurance Scheme.

women, and exclusion of the armed forces; and in particular it must be remembered that sickness benefit is not paid for the first three days of a spell of sickness which does not last at least twelve days and that there is evidence that most illnesses lasting less than four days are not reported to the Ministry of Social Security; further, the statistics are slightly deficient in long term sickness mainly in the younger age groups, because persons who suffer prolonged illness before they have paid 156 contributions have their sickness benefit limited to one year in any unbroken spell—for this purpose spells separated by less than thirteen weeks are aggregated—but the numbers affected are small. The sickness dealt with is 'sickness or accident involving incapacity for work and certified as such by medical practitioners for the purpose of the National Insurance Acts'.

14.9   Table 14.1 shows a selection of the rates for 1962–63—

TABLE 14.1 *National Insurance Experience*

Weeks of sickness benefit per annum per insured person in each age group, in 1962–1963

Ages last birthday at beginning of year	Employed men	Self-employed men	Employed unmarried women (Spinsters, widows and divorced)	Employed married women	Self-employed unmarried women (Spinsters, widows and divorced)
15–19	0·81	0·35	1·00	1·79	0·20
20–24	0·88	0·53	1·18	1·53	0·20
25–29	0·98	0·67	1·44	1·66	0·89
30–34	1·22	0·62	2·06	2·45	1·38
35–39	1·47	0·69	2·67	3·43	1·14
40–44	1·77	0·78	3·66	4·30	1·67
45–49	2·05	1·06	3·72	4·97	3·21
50–54	2·83	1·67	4·98	5·84	3·90
55–59	4·28	2·67	5·81	7·03	4·16
60–64	7·07	4·85	—	—	—

14.10   These rates were obtained from an effective 5 per cent sample of National Insurance records.

14.11   The rates quoted show the rise in sickness incidence with age, the heavier claims of women as compared with men (especially married women), and the lighter claims of the self-employed.

Comparison with other experiences

14.12   In using ordinary Friendly Society data it has to be borne in mind that although like National Insurance data they relate to claims for benefit, it is a common practice in Friendly Societies to reduce the scale of benefit after certain periods of 'linked up' sickness. The tables therefore give rates for different durations, e.g. 'first six months', 'second six months' sickness according to the method of reduction of benefit, as well as for all durations combined. The deterrent effect of a reduction of benefit in long term sickness is likely to render such tables non-comparable with rates for National Insurance where there is no such reduction in benefit.

14.13 As a matter of interest the following rates may be quoted for the Manchester Unity (Whole Society) experience of 1893–97—

Age	All sickness per person (weeks)
30	1·01
40	1·45
50	2·38
60	5·20

14.14 As it happens although the circumstances are different these rates do not differ very much from those given above for employed men in the National Insurance experience.

14.15 It should be noted that the Manchester Unity Experience of 1893–97 was the first to provide reliable data on occupational variation in the incidence of sickness claimed. The following groups were distinguished:

(A) Agriculture.
(B) Outdoor building trades, brickfield and clay workers, masons and stone workers, dock labourers, canal banksmen and bargemen and unskilled labourers employed as a rule in outdoor occupations.
(C) Railway service.
(D) Seafaring, Fishing, etc.
(E) Quarry workers.
(F) Iron and Steel workers (skilled and unskilled) engaged in such branches of industry as involve heavy labour and exposure to great heat.
(G) Mining occupations, chiefly underground but including some on the pit brow.
(H) Remainder (Rural)
(J) Remainder (Urban)

14.16 In final comparisons groups A (agricultural) and H–J (general) were combined as a 'non-hazardous' group; B, C, D and also E, F were found to be closely allied with respect to sickness liability. The following figures are illustrative of the occupational variation—

All periods of sickness

Percentage of Actual Sickness to Standard Expectation (1865–70 Table)

Age	Group A.H.J.	Group B.C.D.	Group E.F.	Group G.
16–44	109	131	162	207
45–64	116	144	157	214
65 and over	137	157	181	212

Analysis of the sickness rate

14.17 The average number of weeks of sickness per person in a year of age may be regarded as the product of the proportion falling sick in a year of age and the average duration of sickness per person falling sick or, since separate spells of sickness of the same person are distinguished, as the product of the number of spells of sickness current at some time in the year of age per person and the average duration of sickness per spell. [For the first element in this product, the term 'rate of prevalence of spells of sickness in a period' or 'period prevalence rate (spells)' has been suggested; and for the second, 'average duration per spell' (General Register Office loc. cit.).]

14.18 In the National Insurance experience 1962–63 the breakdown for employed males 1962–63 was as in Table 14.2.

TABLE 14.2 *National Insurance duration rates* 1962–63

Ages last birthday at beginning of year	Number of spells per insured person	Weeks of sickness benefit per spell	Weeks of sickness per insured person i.e. (2) × (3)
(1)	(2)	(3)	(4)
15—19	0·45	1·8	0·81
20—24	0·40	2·2	0·88
25—29	0·42	2·3	0·98
30—34	0·45	2·7	1·22
35—39	0·44	3·3	1·47
40—44	0·46	3·8	1·77
45—49	0·44	4·7	2·05
50—54	0·50	5·7	2·83
55—59	0·55	7·8	4·28
60—64	0·64	11·0	7·07

14.19 These figures demonstrate that the increase in cost of sickness benefit at older ages is not so much due to the greater risk of falling sick as to the longer time taken for recovery; it is not the frequency of sickness but the quality of sickness which changes—there is relatively less acute and relatively more chronic sickness at older ages.

14.20 It is often of value to analyse rates in this way in order to see whether differences in sickness rates arise from more people falling sick or the same number of people falling sick for longer periods.

Distribution of spells of benefit by duration

14.21 The figures in Table 14.3 for employed men, also taken from the 1962–63 experience illustrate the increasing length of spells of sickness with advancing age—

TABLE 14.3 *Distribution of spells of sickness by duration*
Percentage of spells of duration (weeks)

Ages	1 or less	1—	2—	4—	13—	26—	52 or more	All durations
15—29	37	34	18	9	1	1	0	100
30—44	29	32	24	12	2	1	0	100
45—59	19	27	29	19	4	1	1	100
60—64	12	22	32	25	5	2	2	100
15—64	26	29	25	15	3	1	1	100

243

Current spells of sickness

14.22 The figures in Table 14.4 show the distribution of the employed men who were sick at June 1, 1963 according to the length of time they had been receiving benefit.

TABLE 14.4 *Distribution of men sick at June 1, 1963 by duration*

Ages	Proportions sick— all durations	Percentage of current illnesses of duration (years)					All durations
	per cent	*Under 1*	*1—*	*2—*	*4—*	*6 or more*	
15—29	1·7	94	6	—	—	—	100
30—44	2·8	82	4	4	3	7	100
45—59	5·5	64	9	9	5	13	100
60—64	13·4	47	14	16	9	14	100
15—64	4·1	69	7	10	5	9	100

14.23 These figures illustrate graphically the heavier toll of sickness as the normal retirement age is approached. The proportion actually sick rises from 1·7 per cent at 15–29 to 13·4 per cent at 60–64 and at the latter ages one-fifth of the sickness had already lasted four years.

Industrial injury

14.24 The figures quoted above exclude incapacity for which injury benefit is payable under the Industrial Injuries Acts during the first six months after an industrial accident or the onset of an industrial disease, but they do include sickness benefit which is payable in the normal way during receipt of a disablement pension. The rate, in terms of weeks of benefit for employed males at risk, rises only gradually from 0·16 at ages 15–19 to 0·22 at ages 60–64. The initial industrial injury benefit is a much more level risk with advancing age than the payment of sickness benefit.

Other National Insurance Statistics

14·25 A more detailed breakdown of National Insurance statistics is given in the *Digest of Statistics Analysing Certificates of Incapacity* which is produced regularly by the Ministry of Social Security. This digest is a collection of basic facts and is an extremely valuable reference source. Over and above the range of statistics referred to above in connection with the *Government Actuary's Report* the main interest in the digest lies in the extensive analysis of spells of sickness by certified medical diagnosis and by industry and occupation.

14.26 The tables all relate to Great Britain, and are mainly based on a 5 per cent sample of the records. Comprehensive notes on definitions, etc., are provided with the tables. For example it has to be noted that benefit is not paid for Sundays and durations are measured in terms of a six-day week.

14.27 The figures in Table 14.5 have been extracted from the digest for 1960/61 for illustrative purposes—

TABLE 14.5 *Sickness claims certified as due to Bronchitis—Males*

Age	Spells commencing in year 1960–61 per 1,000 at risk	Claimants incapacitated at 3/6/61 per 1,000 at risk
15—19	16·0	0·7
20—24	16·4	0·7
25—29	17·5	0·9
30—34	21·2	1·0
35—39	26·2	1·4
40—44	30·9	2·1
45—49	41·6	3·4
50—54	54·1	6·2
55—59	78·6	11·8
60—64	106·1	25·3
All ages	40·9	4·8

14.28 These figures show the rapid increase with advancing age, not only of new spells of sickness from bronchitis but also of the prevalence of the disease at any one point of time. Of the 199·9 million days of incapacity in the year 1960–61 for males, 26·1 or 13 per cent were attributable to bronchitis. No other cause contributed so large a proportion.

Survey of sickness

14.29 Between 1944 and 1952 the Social Survey (an organization instituted by the British Government for carrying out sampling surveys of the population) interviewed at the beginning of each month samples of the civilian population of ages sixteen and over and recorded the illnesses and injuries said to have been experienced during each of the two calendar months preceding. The size of each monthly sample throughout England and Wales was about 3,000; it was drawn from local card indexes of the National Register and was representative of all areas, urban and rural [Slater 1946, Box and Thomas 1944]. An account of some of the results of this survey has been given by Stocks (1949) and routine tables were published in the *Quarterly Returns of the Registrar General* from 1947 up to the end of the survey.

14.30 Stocks (loc. cit.) tested the adequacy of the sample and found it sufficiently representative and large to support the calculation of incapacity rates by diagnostic group and by age and sex and for quarter to quarter comparisons of sickness incidence. He also examined the 'memory factor', i.e. the tendency for people to post date the inception of an illness to a date nearer the date of interview or to forget the more remote illnesses. For 'new and recurrent illness starting' the rate (all ages combined) in the more recent month of the interview period was 109 per cent of that for the two months combined for males, and 107 for females; hence the decision to base rates on the two months combined.

14.31 Several different rates were calculated for routine publication, e.g.

Prevalence rate, i.e. number of illnesses present in the population at any time during the period, regardless of when they began, per stated number of population.

Sickness rate, i.e. number of persons who were ill at any time during the period, regardless of when they began to be ill, per stated number of population.

Inception rate, i.e. number of illnesses which began during the period, per stated number of population.

Incapacity rate, i.e. total days of incapacity (away from work, or for those not working prevented by illness from going out of doors) per stated number of the population during the period.

14.32 Rates were calculated in denary age groups for each sex for different medical cause groups, and for all causes combined for different industrial groups and for different income groups (i.e. income of the principal wage earner in the family). Frequently, rates of medical consultation were also recorded. The survey of sickness provided a general indication of the level of morbidity in the population at a time when other sources of information were not developed. A possible criticism of the survey is that it was elevated to a more precise objective than that originally intended. A more modest classification of what people complained of, e.g. backache, sore throat, depression, tiredness, etc. (the variety of these symptomatic categories is not as wide as may be generally imagined) might have been more meaningful in terms of how the population 'felt', than a seemingly precise and detailed categorization of diseases obtained by forcing such general statements of symptoms (made by the patients themselves without medical certification) into the International Statistical Classification of Diseases, Injuries and Causes of Death. A survey of complaints related strictly to what the people interviewed actually said would provide a valuable supplement and counterpart to analyses of medically certified sickness.

14.33 The figures in Table 14·6 are taken from the *Quarterly Returns of The Registrar General* for the quarter ended March 31, 1952, the last in which routine figures appeared. The survey was terminated at March 1952 as an economy measure.

14.34 It is clear from these figures that there is much less variation between occupational and income groups in the proportion of people complaining of having been ill than in the extent to which they are actually incapacitated.

Health surveys in the U.S.A.

14.35 Since 1963 the National Centre for Health Statistics has set up a continuing National Health Survey. This takes a number of different forms; (1) using the field force facilities of the Bureau of the Census to interview sample households of the population. This was proved to be an important source of statistics of illness, accidental injuries, disability, use of hospital, medical, dental and other services in the general population; (2) direct examination, testing and measurement of national samples of the population to obtain estimates of the medically defined prevalence of specific diseases in the United States; (3) collection of statistics based on a national sample of

246

TABLE 14.6 *Sickness in December, 1951 (January and February Interviews)*

Occupation and Income Group	No. of persons	Persons with illness or injury		Days of incapacity		No. of persons	Persons with illness or injury		Days of incapacity	
		No.	per cent	No.	per person		No.	per cent	No.	per person
Professional and Managerial	660	412	62	417	0·63	138	99	72	95	0·69
Clerical	154	105	68	70	0·45	163	108	66	130	0·80
Operatives and other grades:										
Manufacturing	691	462	67	750	1·09	266	191	72	251	0·94
Transport and Public Services	302	181	60	358	1·19	15	10	67	7	0·47
Mining and Quarrying	141	92	65	343	2·43	2	2	100	—	—
Building and Roadmaking	178	116	65	162	0·91	—	—	—	—	—
Agriculture	128	78	61	174	1·36	16	9	56	3	0·19
Distribution	200	132	66	113	0·57	99	67	68	99	1·00
Other industries	284	188	66	289	1·02	213	154	72	139	0·65
Housewives	—	—	—	—	—	2,706	2,121	78	3,036	1·12
Retired, part-time, unoccupied or unstated	458	397	87	777	1·70	240	199	83	557	2·32
Weekly Income of Head of Household:										
Nil	16	15	94	28	1·75	28	20	71	17	0·61
Up to £3	465	368	79	1,087	2·34	874	728	83	1,439	1·65
Over £3 and up to £5	239	185	77	434	1·82	388	307	79	374	0·96
Over £5 and up to £7 10s.	1,129	731	65	930	0·82	1,067	798	75	959	0·90
Over £7 10s. and up to £10	615	408	66	426	0·69	471	358	76	499	1·06
Over £10 and up to £20	292	191	65	300	1·03	182	133	73	261	1·43
Over £20	57	36	63	35	0·61	31	21	68	25	0·81
Not ascertained	383	229	60	213	0·56	819	595	73	743	0·91

medical care institutions of various kinds; (4) analysis of discharge records of a national sample of hospitals; (5) mortality studies. Reference should be made to the considerable volume of publication in the Report Series for Vital and Health Statistics which have an international reputation for their high standard both of basic methodology and presentation. A noteworthy feature of the approach of the organization is the way in which sample results are, whenever possible, validated against other sources of information.

Sickness absence records in industry

14.36 Early in World War II concern about the effects of the heavy demands of the war production drive upon human physique (intensified by the fact that many men and women were drawn into employment after long periods of not having been gainfully occupied) led the Industrial Health Research Board to encourage the adoption of a uniform system of recording sickness absence throughout industry. In a report issued in 1944 they suggested that a day by day record of all absences with reasons should be kept for each employee together with sufficient identification details (age, sex, marital status, occupation, etc.) to permit adequate statistical analysis. The report further suggested that the record should summarize absences under two headings (1) long sickness absence of four consecutive working days or more which should be medically certified, (2) short sickness absence of less than four consecutive days (not including absences of under one day) and that there should be a yearly analysis of the amount of medically certified sickness absence in broad disease groups (which were specified). It should be noted that it is sometimes difficult to separate from staff absence records the absences which are due to medical certified causes and those due to social or domestic reasons, e.g. to attend to urgent private business. For this reason crude absence records may not be a satisfactory guide to sickness incidence.

14.37 A number of industrial concerns did set up records of the character suggested by the Industrial Health Research Board. A notable example is the system of records set up by the London Transport Executive in 1949 (Lloyd and Spratling 1951). For each London Transport occupational group records are kept on punched cards of (a) the staff employed. The card for each employee shows, *inter alia*, the date of birth, the dates of commencement of service and of employment in the particular occupation. The file of cards is kept continually up to date as wastage occurs and new entrants are admitted, (b) sickness absences. A separate card is provided for each spell of sickness showing personal details of the employee, the dates and days of the week of commencement and termination of the spell of sickness absence, the duration of the spell, and the diagnosis (three digit code to provide ultimately for some twenty main disease groups for tabulation purposes). These cards provide therefore the denominators and numerators respectively of the various rates of sickness which are required. For reasons of irregularity in the incidence of rest days the durations of spells are recorded on the basis of a seven-day week.

14.38 Three statistical indices are used: (1) the average annual duration per person, (2) the annual inception rate (spells), i.e. the average number of spells commencing in a year per employee, (3) the average length of a spell, i.e. the ratio of (1) and (2).

Industrial sickness absence in the U.S.A.

14.39 The Division of Occupational Health in the United States Public Health Service (Gafafer 1950) regularly presents data on sickness absenteeism among male and female employees. The data are obtained from 'a group of reporting organizations comprising mutual sick benefit associations, group health insurance plans, and company relief departments and are limited to sickness and non-industrial injuries causing absence from work for eight consecutive calendar days or longer'. The published reports which provide a continuous series from 1921 quote frequency rates, i.e. absences (as defined) per 1,000 persons beginning within the specified period, separately for males and females for a short list of causes. Ten-year average rates are given as a basis of comparison.

Comparability of statistics

14.40 It is important, in making comparisons between different sources of industrial sickness absence statistics to check on the following points

(1) inclusion or non-inclusion of absence without medical certification,
(2) whether all absences or only those after a certain time-lag, e.g. after four days, are included,
(3) whether all employees or, for example, only those entitled to sickness benefits are covered,
(4) the conventions used (a) for dealing with rest days, (b) for dealing with sickness absences which commenced in a previous period and were still current at the beginning of the period under review—it is usual to

count only sickness within the period but it may be convenient to count the whole duration of absence, balancing this by the exclusion of absences commencing in the period under review but still outstanding at the end of the period (on the grounds that the overlapping sickness is roughly the same from period to period provided there are no disturbing factors),

(5) inclusion or exclusion of absences from industrial injuries or sickness from prescribed industrial diseases where these are covered by separate sick benefit or insurance schemes,

(6) the nature of the rate presented, e.g. a duration rate or a frequency of commencement of sickness and the time interval of the rate.

REFERENCES

BOX, K., and THOMAS, G. (1944) *J. of Roy. Stat. Soc.*, 107, 151.

GAFAFER, W. M. (1951) Public Health Reports 66, 1550, U.S. Public Health Service, Washington.

General Register Office (1954) Measurement of Morbidity, *Studies on Medicine and Population Subjects*, No. 8, H.M.S.O.

Industrial Health Research Board (1944) 'Recording of Sickness Absence in Industry' Report No. 85.

London Transport Executive (1956), *Health in Industry—Sickness Absence Statistics*, Butterworths Medical Publications.

LLOYD, F. J., and SPRATLING, F. H. (1951) *Journal of Inst. Actuaries*, 77.196.

Ministry of Pensions and National Insurance (1956) Digest of Statistics analysing Certificates of Incapacity 1958/61 (stencilled).

SLATER, P. (1946) 'Survey of Sickness 1943–45', Social Survey.

STOCKS, P. (1949) 'Sickness in the Population of England and Wales in 1944–47', General Register Office. *Studies on Medical and Population Subjects*, No. 2.

WATSON, SIR A. W. (1930) *J. of Inst. Act.*, 62, 12.

CHAPTER 15

HOSPITAL STATISTICS

Hospital administration and the need for statistics

15.1 Statistical methods render information more intelligible and by assisting analysis ensure that the utility of the information is fully exploited; but the statistician neither creates the facts themselves nor the problems which call for the examination of facts. How then, does he assist in administration? Is administration dependent upon fact finding?

15.2 The task of the administrator is to design and co-ordinate manifold services to achieve a specific social objective with the minimum absorption of collective human effort. This is true of all social organization whether it be shipbuilding or large-scale agriculture or education or the Health Service. However, before the administrator can bring the complex resources to meet the complex need, both complexes must be examined and separated into component elements. Each element of need must be matched by a scientifically designed function or element of service. These functions may then be pieced together to form a coherent organization. Analysis must always precede synthesis. Both the precision of the design of the functions and the coherence of the organization are essential to efficiency. The phrase 'scientifically designed' was used advisedly partly to emphasize the essential foundation of knowledge, but partly also to attempt to correct the impression that administration is wholly an art. It is agreed that the humanities enter into administration, for we are dealing with human beings; it is true that the design of functions like any other design has an artistic significance; but fundamentally we are predicating policy upon knowledge. To this end statistics clearly make an essential contribution.

15.3 It is not suggested that administrators should become specialists in statistical technique or that they need necessarily employ more statisticians. It would profit them to interest themselves in elementary statistical methods; to encourage the statisticians to perfect methods particularly applicable to administrative ends; to learn themselves to recognize problems which are peculiarly statistical, i.e. to know when to consult the statistician; and to practise statistical judgment objectively, that is to do consciously what many now do intuitively.

15.4 Administration has been spoken of in general terms. It is now necessary to show how these general assertions are applied to the hospital service. The object of the hospital service is to remedy such sickness as may be more efficaciously treated by the hospital service than by other means. This implies first, identification of the patient specifically needing hospital treatment; second, designing clinical facilities for diagnosis and treatment of the disease pattern peculiar to the area, together with ancillary services of buildings, food, equipment, communications and secretarial assistance; third, welding these services together into an efficient organization.

Beds and bed usage

15.5 Suppose we begin at the beginning by assessing the demand for hospital beds. This depends upon the population served by the hospital group (this term is used loosely in the present context to identify any administrative unit), the incidence of illness severe enough to require hospital treatment, and the duration of hospital treatment. For example, if the average duration of hospital stay is twenty days, then one bed will be used eighteen times in a year and will support an annual admission rate of eighteen. If 9,000 people require treatment every year, then 500 beds will exactly meet the demand. If the 500 beds are not available then two things may happen; either a waiting list develops or the criteria for referral to hospital treatment change—for example the clinicians, aware of the limitation of resources, decide that only, say, 7,000 of the 9,000 really must have hospital treatment.

15.6 The estimation of local bed demand is not easily made. Even if the proportionate incidence of illness (so many per 1,000 per year) is known it is still necessary to ascertain the basic population to which to apply the proportion, i.e. the number at risk—the number of people who, if they were to need hospital treatment would come into the group. Reference is sometimes made to the 'catchment area' of the hospital group, but unfortunately it is not possible to fix any area such that the whole population and no other population is served by the hospital group; even a hospital region is not a watertight compartment in this respect. It is, however, possible to fix an approximate area surrounding the hospital group from which the bulk of the patients are drawn—that for example, the group serves mainly the administrative areas A and B, the populations of which add up to 200,000. Norris (1952) has suggested another method based on census of patients in hospital on a particular day (or discharged over a period). The method assumes that, if of all residents in area A in the aggregate hospitals (taking every hospital in the field surveyed) 10 per cent are in hospital X (or, in cases of discharges, were discharged from X), then 10 per cent of area A will always choose X and hospital X may be regarded as serving one-tenth of A. If 20 per cent of all hospitalized residents of B are in X, then X also serves one-fifth of B; and so on. The total population served by X is $\cdot 1A + \cdot 2B$, etc. The success of the method depends upon fixing the survey field so as to cover every hospital in which a significant number of residents from A, etc., may appear.

15.7 The rate of occurrence of illness requiring hospital treatment is not known, since the only reporting system available is that resulting from the referral to waiting list or the records of emergency admissions; and the criteria for hospital treatment have been constantly changing. However, either by reference to such records (and their importance is emphasized) or by local survey we might discover that $4\cdot 5$ per cent (say) of the population require hospital treatment every year which would yield 9,000 admissions a year and require about 500 beds.

15.8 The special needs of teaching hospitals would require more than such a simple calculation since it may be desirable to vary the criteria for the selection of patients and the policy with regard to length of treatment to suit teaching needs. Moreover the 'catchment area' of a teaching hospital is usually much wider than that of a non-teaching hospital. Equally the calculations should be made with reference not only to sex and age differentials, but

251

also to important disease categories and to the separate specialist departments of the hospital group, viz. ideally, it would be necessary to measure the proportion of the population in a given sex and age group who require treatment for a particular disease (say osteomyelitis) in a given department (orthopaedic) in a given period of time; to apply such rates to the population at risk and to produce estimates of bed needs which may be tabulated by disease group and hospital department.

15.9 These rates would vary with changes in clinical policy. For example the introduction of sulphonamide treatment rendered unnecessary the admission to hospital of patients suffering from erysipelas save in severe or complicated cases. From time to time there have been changes in the official policy with regard to the admission to hospital of uncomplicated pregnancies.

Clinical policy

15.10 As an outcome of this examination of resources, an approach might be made to the elucidation of an outstanding problem of considerable importance and difficulty. Given a limited number of beds, which is below the potential demand, how are these beds to be used? The manner in which beds have hitherto been used is hardly the result of any conscious policy. For different diseases there is a different waiting period, a different chance of admission to hospital based not on any rational policy, but upon the accident of circumstances, upon the interplay of outside pressure and the internal distribution of specialists, nurses and beds.

15.11 What should the rational policy be? Should it be directed to the maximum palliation of existing discomfort, e.g. concentration on disabling conditions; to the maximum suspension of mortality, e.g. concentration on fatal conditions; to the maximum prevention of ultimate disease, e.g. earlier operations in malignancy, or segregation of infectious cases; or to specialist diagnosis. It is not for a statistician to say or for any administrator; but the clinicians and administrators as a team have to produce a policy.

15.12 However, given a particular admission practice there is much that can be done statistically to ensure proper use of beds. As a result of concern about the possible wastage of beds the Hospital Administrative Staff College of the King Edward's Hospital Fund for London set up a Study Group on Hospital Bed Occupancy which reported in 1954. This group amassed a large body of information about the operation of hospitals in the London area and as a result made a number of suggestions to hospital administration as to ways in which they might improve bed usage.

15.13 Pressure on hospital beds had hitherto been measured by the average percentage occupancy of beds, i.e. the average number of beds occupied day by day divided by the average number of beds available day by day.

15.14 Average beds occupied in a quarter $= \dfrac{\Sigma_1^{91} x_r}{91}$

where x_r is the number of beds occupied on the rth day of the quarter and $\Sigma_1^{91} x_r$ is the sum of the values of x for each day, viz. the 'occupied bed-days'.

15.15 Average beds available $= \Sigma_1^{91}(x_r + y_r)/91$

where y_r is the number of vacant (and staffed available) beds on the rth day of the quarter, and $\Sigma_1^{91}(x_r + y_r)$ is the total available bed-days.

15.16 Hence the percentage occupancy $= \dfrac{\Sigma_1^{91}(x_r)}{\Sigma_1^{91}(x_r + y_r)} \times 100$

and it is thus only necessary to form a cumulative record of the daily bed state in the hospital (obtained from daily counts) in order to obtain the value of Σx_r and Σy_r.

15.17 The Group called for an index of bed vacancy on a departmental basis which would be more explicit than the average percentage of beds unoccupied, would be more readily visualized by the staff concerned, and more directly related to the turnover of patients and their length of stay.

15.18 They suggested the 'turnover interval', viz. the average number of days a bed lies vacant between successive patients. This is obtained by adding up for each day of the period the number of vacant (and available) beds in the department, i.e. the total vacant bed-days, and dividing this by the discharges and deaths in the department during the same period.

15.19 The turnover interval $(t) = \Sigma_1^{91} y_r \div \Sigma_1^{91} d_r$

where d_r is the total discharges and deaths for the rth day.

15.20 We may note that $\Sigma_1^{91} x_r \div \Sigma_1^{91} d_r$ is approximately the average duration of stay in hospital, n. [if the conditions are stable and admissions equal discharges daily with a constant length of stay of n days per patient, a constant population of $n.d_r$ would have been accumulated after which d_r would be discharged and d_r admitted daily so that total bed days $= (nd_r)91$ and total discharges and deaths $= 91.d_r$, and the ratio of the two numbers is equal to n].

Thus $t = \dfrac{\Sigma(x_r + y_r) - \Sigma(x_r)}{\Sigma d_r}$

$\qquad = \dfrac{\Sigma(x_r + y_r) - \Sigma(x_r)}{\Sigma x_r} \cdot n$

$\qquad = \dfrac{\Sigma(x_r + y_r) \cdot n}{\Sigma x_r} - n$

whence $\dfrac{n + t}{n} = \dfrac{\Sigma(x_r + y_r)}{\Sigma x_r}$

and $\quad 100 . \dfrac{n}{n + t} = \%$ occupancy

i.e. if the percentage occupancy is 85 and the average length of stay is 25 then $t = (0 \cdot 15)25 \div (0 \cdot 85)$ or $4 \cdot 4$ days, Alternatively $\dfrac{25}{25 + 4 \cdot 4} = 0 \cdot 85$ approximately.

15.21 The turnover interval is thus not so much a new measure as a new way of looking at the occupancy figures.

15.22 If in this particular case the turnover interval of $4 \cdot 4$ were regarded as too high and a figure of $1 \cdot 5$ were regarded as the minimum to permit of efficient nursing preparation it is clear that the occupancy could be increased to $\dfrac{25}{25 + 1 \cdot 5}$ or $94 \cdot 3$ per cent so that the total number of patients treated in any period, say a quarter, would have to be increased by about

$\dfrac{(94 \cdot 3 - 85)}{85} = 11$ per cent, i.e. if the total beds available (vacant and occupied) were 200 (average occupied $0 \cdot 85 \times 200 = 170$) this would mean increasing the present number treated from $\dfrac{91 \times 170}{25} = 619$ per quarter to 687 per quarter, i.e. by 68.

15.23 We could achieve the same result by estimating first that the vacant bed days were previously $91 \times 200 \times 0 \cdot 15 = 2{,}730$ and that it is intended to reduce these such that the new figure for vacant bed days divided by the increased number of patients $(619 + E)$ would give a t of $1 \cdot 5$.

$$\therefore \frac{2{,}730 - E.25}{619 + E} = 1 \cdot 5 \text{ whence } E = 68 \text{ as before.}$$

(Note: each extra patient increased the occupied bed days by 25 because an extra admission per day would increase the hospital population by 1 each day for 25 days after which the first extra patient will be discharged and thereafter additional discharges will balance additional admissions and thus $\dfrac{E}{91} \times 25$ is the increase in average beds occupied and $\dfrac{E}{91} \times 25 \times 91$ or $25E =$ the extra bed-days in the quarter.)

15.24 The Study Group also called for a more intensified study of the unavailability of beds and the reasons for beds being out of use. One of the difficulties hitherto has been a lack of precision in the measurement and indeed in the definition of available beds and occupied beds. Hospitals tended to retain a fixed 'complement' which was hallowed by constant repetition from one report to another but often bore no relation to the beds actually in use or the maximum which could be erected. For this reason the Ministry of Health in England and Wales who require annual statistical returns from hospitals within the National Health Service have laid down certain standard definitions.

Ministry of Health Returns

15.25 For hospitals within the National Health Service in England and Wales the Ministry of Health collect and publish statistics of departmental activity. These statistics are derived from annual returns of which the main form (S.H.3) requires for each hospital the following facts:

For the year ended December 31st

I. For financial purposes the average daily occupation in part payment or private accommodation has to be separated into that provided for paying patients and that provided for non-paying patients.

II. The return provides for the recording of the following figures for every department of the hospital (General Medicine, General Surgery, Staff Wards, Paediatrics, Dermatology, Radiotherapy, etc.)—

Inpatients

Number of staffed beds allocated (irrespective of actual use) at December 31st.

Average number of available beds (irrespective of actual use).
Average daily bed occupation during the year.
Discharges and deaths during the year.
Average duration of stay (in days) of patients discharged or died during the year.
Waiting list on December 31st.
Outpatients
New outpatients during the year.
Total attendances during the year (new and old patients).
Annual number of clinic sessions held.
III. For purposes of assessing the maternity service—
Number of births during the year (1) Live
(2) Still
Beds, if any, specifically set aside for ante-natal care.
IV. The pathological and radiological departments and the hospital eye service are required to assess the services they have rendered on the basis of certain prescribed units of value of work. The physiotherapy department must also state units of treatment and in addition the number of new patients and total attendances of all patients.
V. Numbers of new patients and total attendances of new and old patients (separating inpatients sent down from wards from outpatients) are required for all outpatient departments, viz.

Occupational therapy
Chiropody
Electro encephalography
Electro cardiography
Speech therapy
Hearing aids
Audiometry
Sight-testing (by hospital opticians)
Optical dispensing (by hospital opticians)
Orthoptics
Surgical appliances
Dietetics

[There are pitfalls in such departmental statistics in so far as there is overlapping. For example, children admitted for surgical treatment for paediatric diseases may appear under 'general surgery' not 'paediatrics' if there is no paediatric department. Nevertheless these statistics do provide a broad picture of selective departmental pressure; they indicate by the year to year movement in the figures the development of the different specialities in different parts of the country and give some indication (which can be confirmed by local analysis) of the adequacy of specialist services.]

15.26 The returns are centrally consolidated for each hospital group management committee through which the non-teaching hospitals are administered in addition to being provided for each individual hospital in the group. They are also consolidated for each Board of Governors of the thirty-six Teaching Groups. A few of the more important items (mainly relating to overall bed and clinic usage) on Form SH3 are called for on a quarterly basis (Form SBH.1).

15.27 A number of different types of returns are used to collect details of numbers of various grades of medical, nursing, orderly, maintenance, etc. and administrative staff employed by hospitals.

15.28 Despite the obviously large number of common factors hospitals vary appreciably in the general pattern of the work they perform and in the precise internal organization used to arrange for this work to be done. For this reason, what may appear to be a clear statistical category (of type of clinic, or patient) in one hospital, may be far from distinct in another. This not only makes it necessary to specify the content of any category very carefully but at the same time makes it difficult to frame definitions which will be meaningful and acceptable to all hospitals. Furthermore this is a field in which considerable development is taking place and where administrative organization is becoming more specialized. The Ministry of Health have had to face a major problem in supplementing their statistical returns with adequate notes on definitions and their application.

Statistical organization in the hospital

15.29 It will be clear that most of the figures required for the Ministry returns as well as others of local interest will be required by the local hospital authority itself and further that these figures involve the counting of patients' movements as they occur from day to day so that some permanent, though fundamentally simple, organization must be provided for their accumulation.

15.30 The principal documents for this purpose are:

Inpatients
  (i) Admission notice
  (ii) Ward return
  (iii) Admission and discharge register (or equivalent)
  (iv) Discharge record (for statistical analysis)
Outpatients
  (v) Appointments register
  (vi) Clinic return (or equivalent).

(i) *Admission notice*

15.31 There must be some means of notifying the ward to which the patient is allocated and other persons affected including the officer responsible for statistics, that the patient has in fact passed through the full admission procedure of the hospital. It is customary in most hospitals for the admissions office to use a duplicating pad with continuous stationery which allows several copies to be written in one operation; the copies are then torn off and distributed to various departments of the hospital. The admission notice will usually give such details as name, hospital registration number, home address, sex, age, occupation, next of kin, name of physician or surgeon to whose care the patient is admitted, whether emergency admission or from waiting list, and name and address of attending general practitioner.

(ii) *Ward returns*

15.32 Hospitals are often extensive in size and contain many departments not necessarily all contained in the same building. It is impossible therefore for any one person to be aware of all inpatient movements unless there is some machinery for conveying this intelligence to the administrative centre. Furthermore the occupation of beds can only be assessed by a 'count of heads' carried out at some fixed hour of the day (usually midnight because this is the time of day when movement is minimal and conditions are quiet), and it would not be practicable for a single person to make a physical count throughout the hospital in a sufficiently short time to approximate to an instantaneous enumeration. [The need for a 'fixed hour' arises from the need to work in terms of bed-days—a varying time would involve an interval of bed occupation of varying duration and would rob the statistics of any meaning. A daily count does imply the assumption that the number of patients occupying beds at the fixed time may be regarded as the average number occupying beds during the previous twenty-four hours. If there is any significant number of patients admitted and discharged during the same day and between counts, e.g. admitted for a few hours for shock recovery, then a separate record must be kept if this element of bed usage is to be taken into account; but often it is possible to ignore this.]

15.33 It is customary therefore for every ward in the hospital to make this count at midnight or some other fixed time and to record this number on a standard form which also shows admissions to and discharges from the ward during the previous twenty-four hours. The form must reconcile with other data. The total of patients shown must agree with the total of the previous day's number and the net movement during the day (excess of admissions over discharges). The number of admissions must agree not only with the ward record of new patients put into beds but also with the admission notices received from the admissions office.

(iii) *Admission and discharge register*

15.34 The ward returns when collected together form a *complete* account of the bed state and the total daily movement in the hospital, and in some hospitals no further register is considered necessary. In other hospitals it is considered more convenient to provide a register in which to list each day's movements. While this involves a certain amount of clerical labour it has the following advantages:

(a) it provides a vehicle on which to carry out a summation and reconciliation of the movements with explicit totals, for the day and for any longer period;

(b) it provides a reference book for checking records of admission and discharge dates and earlier periods of treatment;

(c) space can be provided for additional details to be recorded against each patient, viz. religion (for reference,) source of admission, specialty, diagnosis, duration of stay in hospital, etc.

15.35 The procedure is to list each individual movement, entering a single unit, code number, etc. in the appropriate columns. Most of these are then cast for the day. In turn the daily totals may be cast to a monthly or quarterly summary. International Statistical Classification code numbers would be ticked off on a frequency summary sheet for an appropriate period. In some cases the register does not provide for individual listing but only for ward or specialty totals.

(iv) *Discharge record*

15.36 While it is possible in many hospitals to assemble together the units of information recorded on ward returns or discharge registers (where they exist) into whatever statistical arrangement may be desired, e.g. tables of total movements by age, of diseases treated by specialties simply by counting or ticking off cases falling in particular categories, it is much easier to do this if the units of information are first entered on a summary record suitable for data processing especially when the numbers are large. The usual procedure in such cases is to enter the principal registration details on a record when the patient is admitted (the card may then be used as a ward index) and further details such as diagnosis are added upon discharge when the record passes to the office for statistical purposes.

(v) *Outpatient appointment register*

15.37 Where outpatient attendances are regulated by appointment a 'diary' type of register with provision for duplicates provides automatically a daily list of appointments for each clinic, separating new from old patients. If this list is checked at the clinic and non-attendances are deleted while emergency attendances are added, the lists may then be cast and the appropriate totals transferred to a cumulative register to provide weekly, monthly, or quarterly, etc. totals. Where no register exists a simple form (i.e. [vi] of 15.33) may be supplied to each clinic for ticking off totals of new and old patients attending. The same procedure would be used for casualty.

Local presentation of statistics

15.38 The actual form in which hospital statistics are presented to the local administrator of a group of hospitals (or a single hospital) will naturally depend upon his particular instructions based upon the special problems of administration with which he is currently concerned. A typical report would show for each hospital for the period under review (usually a quarter):

At end of period:
  (*a*) The bed complement
  (*b*) Beds available and staffed
  (*c*) Beds temporarily unavailable
  (*d*) Beds unused for lack of staff
  (*e*) Emergency fever reserve
  (*f*) Beds out of use for major structural alterations
  (*g*) Waiting list
During period:
  (*h*) Average daily number of beds occupied
  (*i*) Average daily number available
  (*j*) Percentage occupancy (i.e. [*h*] as a per cent of [*i*])
  (*k*) Total discharges
  (*l*) Total deaths
  (*m*) Average length of stay—
        maternity
        other acute
        other

258

(*n*) Units of work in department—
Pathology
Radiology
Physiotherapy
others (attendances)
(*o*) Maternity Department—
live births
stillbirths

15.39 In addition the following figures will usually be given for each specialty—

Inpatients:
(i) Number of beds allocated (irrespective of actual use)
(ii) Average daily bed occupation
(iii) Waiting list at end of period
Outpatients:
(i) New outpatients during period
(ii) Total attendances
(iii) Number of clinic sessions.

15.40 An accompanying commentary would compare these figures with those for the preceding quarter and (say) the corresponding quarter of the previous year in order to indicate trends in activity in the different specialties and departments. Has the occupancy kept pace with any increase in the availability of beds? What was the turnover ratio; can it be improved or are there staff difficulties preventing further reduction? Do the disparities between waiting lists or outpatient attendances for different specialties suggest that there should be some reallocation of beds? Is hospital mortality higher than normal?

15.41 It is important to stress that in drawing conclusions from these service statistics the hospital administrator will have recourse to medical opinion on aspects of *medical* efficiency. This is an important factor. While it may be ideal that more and more patients are using the same number of beds and staying an ever shorter time where will be a point reached at which further reduction in the duration of stay must result in inadequate treatment, prolonged invalidism and high readmission rates. While it may be desirable to reduce waiting lists to very low proportions there may be, for a particular specialty, a size of waiting list which best provides time for pre-admission procedures and the proper regulation of the flow of work into the department and associated surgical facilities in the interests of most efficient treatment. The medical staff will, for purposes of medical policy require a statistical service of this kind which Hospital Activity Analysis (see 15.58) is intended to provide.

Local studies

15.42 There are statistical comparisons which can and ought to be made between individual hospitals, but which are neglected. It might be very revealing to compare the average duration of treatment in different hospitals for the same disease with the same degree of severity in similar age and sex groups and to examine the reasons for differences. They might be due to differences in staff-bed ratios which clearly ought also to be compared; or to differences in the availability of surgical resources—hospitals have been known to outgrow their operating theatres; or to the creation of bottlenecks because patients wait for other procedures; or to differences in the arrangements for convalescence. It might be possible in this way to identify sources of unbalance in internal planning.

15.43 Similarly, comparisons of waiting list turnover would be worth while. The average wait for treatment X may be longer in hospital A than in hospital B while for treatment Y the reverse holds. It may be unavoidable; it may draw attention to the necessity for revising the allocation of beds; it may be evidence of differential 'cross-hauling', i.e. for treatment X patients may prefer to travel long distances to hospital A (because it has a 'good name' or because the family doctor has become associated with it) to inflate the waiting list while for treatment Y the movement is in a different direction.

15.44 'Cross-hauling' is a study in itself. From time to time hospitals should examine the places from which their patients are drawn, if not in relation to diagnosis at least in relation to a broad division between medical and surgical cases. There may be mal-distribution of facilities within the group; there may merely be misunderstandings among general practitioners or patients. Whatever the reason, the information should be sought.

15.45 How much time is spent on the average in the out-patient department: (a) by the patient arriving too early for an appointment? (b) in registration? (c) in waiting for attention beyond the appointed time? (d) in movement between registry and clinic? (e) in making reappointments, etc.? It is clearly unnecessary to make a routine analysis of these details, but there is scope for an occasional time and motion study of this kind. It is an important piece of research, especially if carried out in hospitals with differing routines and internal geography and it is not difficult to carry out where, as is usually the case, there is some control over the movement of patients.

Evaluating the need for clinical services

15.46 A working group of the Medical Section of the Royal Statistical Society reported in 1955 the results of their consideration of various methods of assessing the need for clinical services. The group drew attention to certain initial difficulties, e.g. ascertainment of catchment populations for particular services; and to the possibility that pent-up demand may be suppressed by the failure of general practitioners to refer cases when waiting lists are long thus rendering waiting lists misleading as indices of demand.

15.47 Various forms of assessment of demand were suggested, e.g. a field survey with each diagnostic group tabulated as follows:

Medical (Diagnosis) Demand	Bad*	Sociological Aspects (affecting urgency of admissions) Doubtful	Good	Total
Immediate	1	2	3	d
Non-urgent	4	5	6	e
No demand	7	8	9	f
Total	a	b	c	p = Population exposed

* Viz. admission socially highly desirable, e.g. infectious case in overcrowded home.

260

15.48 In Britain the values of d and e would have to be obtained by inquiry of general practitioners to assess the numbers of patients they would have sent to hospital for specified groups of diagnoses if complete facilities were available. Distinction of age groups and of urban as distinct from rural areas would be desirable. The values of a, b, c might be derived from census data or from *ad hoc* survey.

15.49 For groups of diagnoses in which risk is likely to vary with sociological factors the enquiry would have to be sufficiently detailed to enable the cells of the table to be separately completed for each such diagnostic group. Where the risk of the disease is not related to social conditions the cells could be filled in by applying marginal proportions, viz. $1 = \dfrac{da}{p}, 4 = \dfrac{ea}{p}$ etc. It might be possible for general practitioners to make a sociological grading at the time of listing cases of a particular diagnostic group with treatment need; they would also have to classify the remainder of the practice population in order to derive 7, 8 and 9.

15.50 The figures could be converted into bed requirements by multiplying the expected annual number of new cases, p, by the average stay in days (of similar cases), n, plus the turnover interval, t, and dividing by 365, viz. $\dfrac{365}{n+t}$ is the number of cases which can be treated in one year by one bed and $p \div 365/(n+t)$, i.e. $\dfrac{p(n+t)}{365}$ is therefore the number of beds required to clear p cases within the year. Alternatively if w is the total number of currently outstanding cases revealed by the survey then in addition the temporary provision of b beds will enable this list to be cleared in $\dfrac{w.(n+t)}{b.30}$ months.

[These relations apply generally and may be used apart from surveys involving social categorization, e.g. this kind of estimate of additional beds required to clear waiting lists may be part of the ordinary routine statistical reporting of hospital administrators.]

15.51 The working group considered various sources of existing statistics of use of clinical facilities which might be used to derive 'demand' rates or at least differentials (social or diagnostic) in such rates and these are included within the bibliography at the end of this chapter.

Hospital discharge studies

15.52 There have been attempts to use hospital inpatient statistics to obtain a measure of morbidity. In present circumstances this is not practicable. Morbidity implies a risk or a rate, and there is no population at risk to which tabulations of hospital clinical records can be related until 'catchment areas' can be more precisely defined. Morbidity implies sickness in its generalized connotation, while the enquiries based on inpatient records are directed, not to all sickness, or to all sickness serious enough to be treated in hospital, but only to those illnesses which, in the peculiar circumstances of present opportunity (waiting lists and priorities, etc.), are actually treated in hospital.

15.53 The attempt to use the analysis of case records for morbidity purposes distracts attention from more important uses. This is unfortunate, for the domestic uses of hospital records in indicating differential prognoses, the efficacy of various forms of treatment, and, indeed, the efficiency of medical work generally, need to be stressed. As McKinlay has said (1949): 'The main contributions of hospital information to the general requirements of a morbidity programme are quite other than as indicators of sickness prevalence. Initially, at least, we should look to them for knowledge, primarily, of the effects of therapy—the relative merits of the varying treatments at present in use with a view to choosing the best, and to provide the necessary and adequate background of data for the speedy assessment of any new methods which may be introduced.'

15.54 In 1949 the General Register Office began to analyse statistics of hospital discharge records. The large training hospitals and certain others agreed to provide summaries of inpatient treatments on a standard form which was used until the end of 1951. A preliminary study of the data derived by this means from the participating hospitals was published (MacKay, 1951). A more detailed study of the data covering the experience of the whole of 1949 was published as the *Supplement on Hospital In-Patient Statistics to the Registrar General's Statistical Review* for the year 1949; subsequent supplements have been issued.

15.55 During 1952 a trial was made of a new in-patient case summary form and of methods of selecting a representative sample of hospital patients. The enquiry was extended from the beginning of 1953 to cover, on the basis of a sample of one patient in every ten, some forty-one groups of hospitals from most of the hospital regions as well as nineteen groups of teaching hospitals. Further extension has since taken place to cover all NHS hospitals.

15.56 The form used asks for three classes of information—information about the patient himself, information about the administrative arrangements at the hospital for the particular case and information about the condition treated in the hospital and, for maternity cases, information about the children born. Information about the patient includes age, sex, marital status, area of residence and occupation. Information about administrative arrangements includes method of admission, e.g. from a waiting list or as an emergency, the length of time the patient had to wait for admission, the department in which he was treated, whether he was discharged direct home or was sent to a convalescent institution, and the length of time he was in hospital. Information about the condition treated in hospital includes in addition to main diagnosis, a statement of other diagnosis present and whether the patient underwent surgery or radiotherapy; a separate section for maternity cases provides for the particular character of such cases.

15.57 Each month the participating hospitals send to the General Register Office the forms relating to every patient who has been included in the sample and who was discharged or who died in hospital during the previous month. The information on the forms is coded and punched on to cards for data-processing.

Hospital Activity Analysis

15.58 There has recently been a reorientation of outlook involving an emphasis on local uses of hospital discharge analyses. For some time the General Register Office, on behalf of the Ministry of Health, has, as stated above, been collecting abstracts after the discharge of a 10 per cent sample of patients and processing these abstracts into annual tabulations. These tabulations, however, have been designed by the Ministry to meet its central administrative needs, they do not, in general, descend in detail to hospital management committee level. They have not been therefore of any real use to local management and there has been little or no local interest. For this reason, without diminishing central interest or requirements in any way, a considerable effort has been made to set up *local* hospital information systems based upon 100 per cent processing of patients records and on the accessibility of computers at Regional Hospital Boards to achieve rapid processing and feedback of information to individual hospital requirements. (The system has been called 'Hospital Activity Analysis'.)

15.59 Hospital activity analysis does not imply any essentially new elements in the hospital statistical system, only the rationalisation of the way in which they are brought together. It has long been recognized that the basic units for the measurement of in-patient activity have been fragmented in separate documents—a waiting list register, an admission and discharge register, supplemented by individual notices, and individual documents for post-discharge statistical analysis. It is desirable that for economy of effort and assurance of completeness all this information should be integrated into a single vehicle (summary sheet, manuscript card or dual-purpose punched card).

15.60 The in-patient summary for hospital analysis has to provide for three essential data requirements:

(i) Since it is fundamental to hospital activity analysis that a personal feedback of information is provided for the individual consultant, the latter must (within the reasonable bounds of practical data-processing possibilities) be allowed some discretion as to the scope of the flow of information. Over and above any data which may be common to all hospitals there may be certain details required routinely to satisfy particular local needs as determined by agreement among the consultants.

(ii) To permit the production of regional and national tabulations of hospital activity there must be a minimum degree of comparability in the record from one hospital to another. The minimum content for this purpose will include the following:

Patient's name and address
Sex, date of birth
Marital condition
Date of admission
Source of admission (waiting list, immediate, transfer, etc.)
Date of entry to waiting list
Type of bed (private pay bed, staff, preconvalescent etc.)
Type of medical care (specialty)
Name of consultant
Disposal (discharge to home, transfer, died, etc.)
Date of discharge or death
Service given (treatment, investigation, etc.)
Diagnosis (or diagnoses)

Surgical operations

Radiotherapy

(For obstetric cases this is extended to include type of medical care, previous pregnancies, antenatal abnormality, labour and delivery, puerperium, details of birth.)

(iii) Although most research requires an *ad hoc* prospective record, there will be occasions when to deal with a particular administrative or clinical enquiry it will be sufficient to add items to the routine record in order to accumulate sufficient data to deal with the enquiry. Such items must be scrupulously discarded as soon as the need has been met. It might be desirable to programme such special surveys one by one over a longer period so as to spread the recording burden.

15.61 Some of the main types of analysis which can be routinely prepared using the records described above are:

Waiting list distribution of patients on current list of each consultant by age, sex, priority, and duration, changes in waiting lists. *Also* distribution of time waited by patients who have been admitted to hospital.

The ward returns together with the patient cards give bed availability, bed occupation, turnover interval, length of stay, mortality, admissions and discharges (by type). Most of these can be analysed by ward, specialty or consultant, and also according to the sex or age of the patient.

Complete up-to-date tabulated diagnostic index. This can show in addition to patient reference and diagnosis, sex, age, etc.

Annual summary of discharges and deaths by diagnostic group, by sex and age and showing length of stay.

Analysis of hospital experience in specific common diseases—e.g. analysis of length of stay by consultant for different sex and age groups for peptic ulcer, hernia, cataract, etc.

15.62 This is a minimum list. It can be extended to meet administrative need and to the extent that information is added to the patient record. Examples of such extension are: coding of the patient's address to give the hospital's catchment area for different specialties; recording of date and type of operations; adaptation of cards and analysis for obstetric work. Ultimately the availability of computer facilities will permit the extension of the record to contain current clinical information for immediate analysis as an aid to the care of the patient (pathological laboratory tests, radiology, electrocardiograms, and other clinical measurements).

15.63 The term 'diagnostic' has been used here in a very general sense of referring to data analysed by disease entity. In speaking of computer applications one has to be careful to distinguish between this general use of the term and the more specific use of the word 'diagnostic' to describe the direct processing of data (often on-line) to assist in the *making* of a diagnosis. This of course is a later stage which will be reached only when adequate clinical data are added to the processable record.

15.64 The use of patient record cards together with a simple ward return can provide all the data required centrally or by regions on waiting time, bed use, patient treatment and diagnosis. Thus nearly all the data required for

S.H.3 and all data of a type now given by the General Register Office Hospital In-patient Enquiry will be covered. In the Birmingham region the discharge summaries are completed and diagnostically coded at the hospitals. The data are processed each quarter by the Birmingham Regional Hospital Board computer and are fed back to the hospitals. Once the local needs have been met, regional tabulations are prepared. Finally the computer produces a 10 per cent sample (as a punched card output) for national tabulations. These cards are punched in the same fields as other cards used centrally and local codes are automatically translated into those required for national purposes. Thus the central authority obtains a checked deck of cards compatible with other cards in the national pack. The hospitals are relieved of the need to produce separate forms for the General Register Office.

15.65 This use of the patient record is being developed in a major way in other regions. The important practical requisites for the development of this work generally are: co-operation of medical staff in prompt accurate recording of diagnosis and return of medical records; clerical staff, trained in diagnostic coding, to record data on the patient summary; access to punched card equipment or, preferably computer (guaranteed time). Once the importance of the proper recording and analysis of hospital data is recognized these practical problems are not formidable.

15.66 If the medical staff committee of a hospital is fed regularly with information of the use of beds (occupation, turnover interval and duration of stay for different specialties) the consultants are no longer dependent on impressions which, however based on acute observation, may be misleading. They become immediately aware of the precise dimensions of the individual pressures under which they are working and the implications of the individual clinical policies they are employing. Differences can be discussed in a purely professional atmosphere and any indicated adjustments in the allocation of beds can be made by mutual understanding.

15.67 Mutual discussion of the use of beds, operating theatres, or laboratories is only a beginning. Regular feedback of diagnostic tabulations provides the clinicians with an accurate measure of the local prevalence of diseases requiring hospital treatment, the diagnostic pattern of hospital morbidity of those segments of the population who are prone to these diseases (sex, age, social and geographical differentials) and of time trends that may be emerging. The correlation of the results of batteries of diagnostic tests with eventual diagnosis renders the diagnostic potential a self-improving mechanism; the profiles of disease become more sharply defined and procedures which are wasteful of diagnostic time, or resources, or not diagnostically efficient can be safely eliminated, and new procedures can be quickly calibrated. Another certain extension of the system will be in assessing the results of treatment. Hitherto, except for those conditions with prolonged follow-up arrangement (e.g. cancer, tuberculosis or diabetes) little has been done. It may ultimately be possible to bring the general practitioner into the system to give a record of the whole disease episode.

15.68 The principal value of in-patient analyses is in the picture they present of the contemporary clinical work undertaken by the individual hospital. Changes in this picture over a period of time provide the information which is essential to the proper allocation of beds, surgical facilities, ancillary

I*

diagnostic services and staff; to the arrangement of teaching programmes; to the design of selective admission policy. Statistics of outcome of treatment (recovery rates, incidence of complications, length of stay) for specific diagnostic entities, standardized for sex, age, and social conditions, can also provide an index of the efficacy of hospital care, improvement from year to year and of differences between hospitals subjected to different systems of direction and organization or adopting different treatment policies.

Hospital In-patient Studies in the USA

15.69 A pilot study of hospital in-patient records was undertaken in New York in 1954, jointly by the Department of Hospitals and Health of the City of New York in co-operation with the Russell Sage Foundation. An analysis of the statistics of 121,952 patients discharged from thirty-one municipal hospitals during a six-month experimental period was published (Fraenkel and Erhardt, 1955). This report gives tabulations by sex, age, condition on discharge, duration of stay, etc. for a large range of diagnostic groups and provides special studies of obstetric, traumatic, psychiatric, tuberculous, cardiac and malignant conditions treated in municipal hospitals. There are also special chapters on the hospitalization of children and of aged persons. More recently a service for analyses of discharges has been provided on a semi-commercial basis to any hospital in the United States wishing to take advantage of it. The service is provided by two organizations both subsidized by research grants, a general service under Dr Virgil Slee at Ann Arbor, and the other, for perinatal studies, under Dr Sidney Kane at Philadelphia. Mention has already been made of the national samples of the National Centre for Health Statistics of the Department of Health, Welfare and Education. There are many well developed projects associated with teaching hospitals and there is a particularly interesting attempt at the Henry Ford Hospital, Detroit, to use the system of compiling a summary to build up profiles (recognizably typical patterns of the characteristics of diagnosis, treatment and diagnosis) of specific clinical entities.

Comparative assessment of services

15.70 A further problem arises; the examination of the relative efficiency and cost of different clinical facilities. Is it possible, is it cheaper to give as effective geriatric treatment to the aged sick in their own homes as in hospital? Most people answer this question in the affirmative, subject to reservations about special circumstances, but before this belief influenced public policy statistical demonstration of its foundation was necessary. Cosin has shown that the aged and infirm need not be bedfast for long periods and that those cared for in long-stay annexes have only short terminal illnesses during which they need full nursing and medical care. Should we go on recruiting hospital midwives and opening up maternity beds for all those expectant mothers who prefer to be confined in hospital? Sometimes the preference is medically indicated, sometimes it is on the grounds of increased confidence conveyed by the proximity of specialist resources, but sometimes it is on personal grounds.

15.71 Sometimes considerations of cost are wholly outweighed by the contrast in efficacy. If a treatment produces a proportion of cures in a disease which was formerly invariably fatal then monetary considerations are relevant only to the extent that limited national resources may impose restrictions. No refined statistical tests are necessary to justify the use of streptomycin in tuberculous meningitis.

15.72 More often than not marginal cases arise where the assessment of the relative effectiveness of therapeutic or diagnostic services is a real statistical problem. The decision depends upon the carrying out of careful long-term follow-up of similar cases given different treatment and upon the tests of their relapse rates for significant differences. Much follow-up work may be wasted (in this respect, though not, of course, in relation to the well-being of the individual patient) either because it is not possible or no attempt is made to 'control' the investigation, that is, to provide comparisons with similar groups treated differently; or because no proper attempt is made to examine the records statistically. Nevertheless, follow-up studies, though they cost money, make a valuable contribution to the efficiency of the hospital service.

15.73 On the diagnostic side, it is vitally important that there should be statistical justification for the employment of expensive equipment and highly skilled staff in the place of less costly means of ascertainment. There is, perhaps, no basis for criticism when most observers are impressed by the contributions made by pathology and radiology to differential diagnosis and to the shortening of the interval between first symptom and final diagnosis. The problem may sometimes lie in the proper application of diagnostic services; for example to what population is it most productive to apply them? To the unsuspecting as a routine check or only to those selected on the basis of symptoms of disease?

Computers

15.74 There has been a computer explosion in medicine in recent years. There have been a number of serious misconceptions, the worst being to treat the computer as an end in itself rather than (as it should be) a *means* to an end. The *end*, in this context the statistical needs, is still a matter of prior judgment involving careful thought and is in itself unaffected by the computer though clearly the computer makes more of the desirable objectives attainable. There is now a considerable body of literature on computer appreciation in medicine and references are given at the end of this chapter.

Standardization of records

15.75 Hospital activity analysis (see 15.58) clearly requires some standardization of records and report forms used in hospital. Reference should be made to 8.13 p. 139 for some discussion of this. See also Benjamin (1966).

REFERENCES

BENJAMIN, B. (1966) Computers: their use in medical and health statistics, *J. Roy. Soc. H.*, 86.213.
COSIN, L. (1948) Proc. Roy. Soc. Med., 41, 333.

FRAENKEL, M., and ERHARDT, C. L. (1955) *Morbidity in the Municipal Hospitals of the City of New York*. Russell Sage Foundation, New York.

General Register Office (1955). Registrar General's Stat. Rev. 1950–51 Supplement on Hospital In-Patient Statistics. H.M.S.O.

Hospital and Specialist Services Statistics for England and Wales, 1953 (1955) H.M.S.O.

LEDLEY, R. S. (1965) Use of Computers in Biology and Medicine. McGraw Hill. New York.

LOGAN, W. P. D. (1953) General Practitioners' Records. General Register Office, *Stud. Pop. Med. Subj*. No. 7. H.M.S.O.

MACKAY, D. G. (1951) Hospital Morbidity Statistics. General Register Office, *Stud. Pop. Med. Subj*. No. 4. H.M.S.O.

Medical Research Council (1965) Mathematics and Computer Science in Biology and Medicine. H.M.S.O.

MCKINLAY, P. L., (1949) *Medical Record*, 1. 6.

NORRIS, V. (1952) *Brit. Med. J.*, i. 129.

TAYLOR, T. R. (1967) The principles of medical computing. Blackwell Scienitfic Publications.

CHAPTER 16

CANCER STATISTICS

Cancer mortality trends

16.1 In England and Wales the crude death rate from cancer has been rising for many years. In 1921 the rate per 1,000 was 1·24 and in 1964 the corresponding rate was 2·21, an increase of 78 per cent. Some part of this rise is due to the increased numbers of older people in the population, cancer being a disease of old people. For cancer (including Hodgkin's disease and leukaemia) the Standardized Mortality Ratio for persons rose only 4 per cent between 1950 and 1964 though the crude death rate rose by 12 per cent. Most of the real overall increase in cancer mortality can be attributed to the increase in the number of deaths attributed to lung cancer. Here again there is a difference between the apparent and the real, for it is since about 1920 that facilities for radiological examination have been developed and a part, though probably only a small part, of the increase in lung cancer is due to improved diagnosis.

Mortality rates by sex and age and for different sites

16.2 Discussion of crude rates of mortality leaves out of account important differentials in the trends both in relation to the two sexes and to anatomical sites. On the whole cancer mortality in females has been showing a tendency to remain steady. There have been slight rises in mortality from cancer of some sites of lesser importance, e.g. ovary and fallopian tubes, leukaemia, this has been more than compensated by declines in mortality from cancer of sites where treatment has a larger measure of success, notably stomach and intestine. For males the main site of cancer for which mortality has been rising is lung and bronchus though there have also been increases for pancreas, kidney, bladder and leukaemia. There has been a decline in mortality from cancer of the tongue and buccal cavity, oesophagus, stomach and intestine, and rectum. For a proper evaluation of the trend of cancer mortality it is desirable to examine age specific death rates for each site, separately for each sex. The main difficulty in the absence of reliable statistics of incidence is that it is not possible to analyse changes in mortality rates into that part which is due to variation in results of treatment and that which is due to variation in incidence.

Aetiological factors

16.3 A considerable amount of information has been gathered as to the effect of various environmental and other specific factors upon the causation of cancer.

16.4 There is an urban gradient for some sites, notably lung and stomach, as the figures in Table 16.1 show—

TABLE 16.1 *England and Wales—Standardized Mortality Ratios* 1964

	Cancer of bronchus and lung		Cancer of stomach	
	Males	Females	Males	Females
Conurbations	122	123	105	105
Urban areas with population				
100,000 and over	107	97	117	109
50,000–100,000	95	101	96	94
Under 50,000	88	82	98	98
Rural areas	75	79	86	91

16.5 In the occupational mortality study of 1930–32 (Registrar General 1938) cancer mortality was found to be higher in the lower social classes for many sites, the exceptions being intestine, rectum, breast and ovaries (females), thyroid, pancreas, kidney, prostate (males) and lung. Broadly, it was found that mortality for sites most exposed to external irritation increased continuously from Class I to Class V while mortality from cancer of the intestines and for most of the deep seated sites was almost uniform throughout the social scale. The same investigation showed a high mortality from cancer of the lung and pleura in certain occupations e.g. grinders, French polishers, metal moulders and casters, iron foundry furnacemen and labourers, dock labourers, messengers and porters, printing machine minders; from cancer of oesophagus and stomach in gas producer men, slate miners and quarriers in Caernarvonshire, stevedores, dock labourers, furnacemen, rollers and skilled assistants, messengers, barmen and certain other occupations; from cancer of the buccal cavity and pharynx notably in barmen, inn and hotel keepers, makers of alcohol drinks as well as some of the occupations with high mortality in other sites. These results were not entirely confirmed by the 1949–53 investigation (General Register Office, 1958); on this occasion mortality was found to be higher in the lower social classes for cancer of the rectum and a more definite downward gradient from Class I to Class V was found for intestine, pancreas, prostate, kidney and brain. The occupations with higher mortality from cancer of the lung and bronchus included sandblasters, gas producer men, showmen, cutlers, riveters, glaziers, caulkers, rag and bone and bottle sorters; and those with higher mortality from cancer of the stomach included glaziers, electro-platers, paint sprayers, and various groups of labourers.

16.6 In a valuable summary Kennaway and Kennaway (1937) have shown that 'there is evidence from several sources that association with alcohol increases the incidence of cancer in an area (back of tongue, pharynx and larynx) which is not so affected by tobacco' an agent that has been (especially cigarette smoking) associated with cancer of the lung in numerous studies, notably that of Doll and Hill (1954)—a prospective enquiry into the deaths of medical men with known smoking habits, which has demonstrated a rising death rate from lung cancer proportional to the amount smoked. Table 16.2 is reproduced from this paper.

TABLE 16.2 *Standardized death rate per annum per 1,000 men aged 35 years and above in relation to the most recent amount of tobacco smoked*

Cause of death	No. of deaths recorded	Death rates of non-smokers	Death rates of men smoking a daily average of			Death rate of all men
			1g.—	15g.—	25g.+	
Lung cancer	36*	0·00	0·48	0·67	1·14	0·66
Other cancers	92	2·32	1·41	1·50	1·91	1·65
Respiratory disease (other than cancer)	54	0·86	0·88	1·01	0·77	0·94
Coronary thrombosis	235	3·89	3·91	4·71	5·15	4·27
Other cardiovascular diseases	126*	2·23	2·07	1·58	2·78	2·14
Other diseases	247	4·27	4·67	3·91	4·52	4·36
All diseases	**789**	**13·61**	**13·42**	**13·38**	**16·30**	**14·00**

* One case in which lung cancer was recorded as a contributory but not a direct cause of death has been entered in both groups.

16.7 The Doll and Hill study was a classic demonstration of the prospective or longitudinal method. The manner in which the results were presented, carefully disposing of possible artefacts one by one until the conclusions became abundantly clear, is a model for every statistician. The evidence against cigarette smoking, initially derided as 'statistical', has mounted. A later paper (1964) based on a longer term follow-up has confirmed the preliminary results. The association between cigarette smoking and lung cancer is now rarely questioned even if in individuals it fails to deter.

16.8 Other classic associations with specific agents are: the high incidence of skin epithelioma in cotton mule spinners which led to the appointment of a Departmental Committee (1926) whose investigation corroborated the suspicion that the lubricating oil used was carcinogenic and was followed by protective action, viz. the use of oils of different composition and modification of machinery to prevent oil splash; cancer of the scrotum which was at one time prevalent in chimney sweeps due to concentration of soot on the skin (one clear example of the value of soap and water—as Clemmensen (1951) remarked 'the Danish Chimney Sweepers' Guild which in 1778 ruled that journeymen and their apprentices should have a daily bath, may, whatever their motives, have done more to prevent human cancer than many research workers'); tumours of the urinary bladder in certain sections of the chemical industry (Case, Hosker, McDonald and Pearson, 1954) have been found to be associated with specific aromatic hydrocarbons—in one important instance the isolation of the agent, an antioxident used in the rubber industry, led to its immediate voluntary withdrawal and the cessation of its manufacture (Case, Hosker 1954), but in other instances, too, there has been modification of handling processes or abandonment of production as a result of these clear statistical analyses; high incidence of lung cancer in those working with arsenic, asbestos dust (Perry, 1947) or chromate dust (Brinton, Frasier and Koven, 1952).

16.9 In women the incidence of cancer of the breast and of the uterus seems to be related to marriage and childbearing. Death rates from cancer of the breast in women who have passed the childbearing age are higher in single and in infertile women than in fertile married women. At childbearing ages, married women, whether they have had children or not, have higher death rates from cancer of the breast than do single women. In women over the age of forty-five the reduction in the risk of mammary cancer seems to be proportional to the number of children borne (Smithers *et al.* 1952). Death rates from cancer of the uterine cervix are higher in married than in single women at each age. Marital status alone, apart from childbearing, seems to be a factor causing this higher mortality (Logan, 1953). Death rates from cancer of the body of the uterus tend to be higher in single and infertile married women than in married women who have had children. The causal relationships involved here have not been clearly established; as Logan points out 'is it the marital status that conduces towards death from cancer of the cervix, or does a tendency toward ultimate death from cancer of the cervix, due for instance to some hormonal diathesis, render a woman more likely to marry?'.

The natural duration of the disease

16.10 Greenwood (1926) made a study of the natural growth of untreated tumours which throws much light on the nature of the disease. Greenwood began by appreciating that the 'cure' of malignant disease could only be defined in relative terms of increased survival and that some standard was required against which to make such relative assessments. A study was therefore made of the natural duration of life of untreated patients suffering from cancers of tongue, breast, cervix of uterus, rectum and oesophagus. The results were (in months, with standard errors):

Tongue and mouth	$16 \cdot 5 \pm 0 \cdot 46$
Breast	$38 \cdot 3 \pm 1 \cdot 15$
Uterus	$20 \cdot 9 \pm 0 \cdot 28$
Rectum	$26 \cdot 7 \pm 0 \cdot 58$
Oesophagus	$12 \cdot 0 \pm 0 \cdot 42$

Age at onset was not found to be an important factor in determining the natural duration. The results were also expressed in terms of the proportion of patients surviving 1, 2, 3 . . . years after onset. At the time at which it was made this investigation was extremely valuable in establishing the value of surgery in cancer therapy, then in an earlier state of development than now.

Registration

16.11 Where diseases represent a grave social problem society has usually reacted by making them notifiable. It has been recognized that public anxiety can be allayed and the public health service efficiently organized only on the basis of public information. This procedure of notification has become customary for the various pestilences which have afflicted this country in turn; at one time cholera, typhus and enteric fever, more recently tuberculosis and poliomyelitis—and lately even scabies. Most of these diseases, with the particular exception of tuberculosis, have fulminating symptoms and recovery is usually rapid (though in some instances sequelae may be severe as in cerebrospinal meningitis or poliomyelitis). Where the disease runs a long chronic course, something more than mere notification is required.

Inevitably, treatment is protracted; in some cases radical and in others palliative. There exists, instantaneously, a large population of patients in various stages of disease. In the absence of a specific cure of unquestioned efficacy there is at any one time not only a large volume of treatment in process but also a large programme of research into new forms of therapy, and for a large number of individual patients there is the pressing need to decide upon the continuation of the present regimen or the choice of some other course of action. All these activities involve recourse to information of aetiological significance, of response to treatment and of ultimate survival, for different sites, and stages of disease, for different methods of treatment and for different sections, socially or geographically sub-divided, of the population; and this information must be compiled on a *comparable, i.e. a uniform, basis*. Inevitably there must be not only notification, but registration of cases of disease.

16.12 The need for registration was recognized by the Ministry of Health when it prescribed in 1946 Standard Cancer Registration and Case Abstract cards for use in all areas where there was a cancer scheme approved under the Cancer Act of 1939. In 1947 the General Register Office became responsible for the analysis and interpretation of such treatment and follow-up records in England and Wales. A system of registration already existed before the war for cases treated by radiotherapy. This had been re-organized in 1945 by the Radium Commission in accordance with the Ministry's proposals and was taken over from the Commission as a first step towards the full Registration Scheme. When the National Health Service Act came into effect in 1948, the continuation and extension of the plan for cancer records became the responsibility of the integrated hospital service. Registration of all cases of cancer is not at present compulsory, but the Minister of Health on the advice of his Cancer and Radiotherapy Advisory Committee expressed the intention that all cases of cancer should eventually be covered by the National Registration Scheme. Many hospital boards and individual hospitals have recognized the advantages of such a scheme and an increasing number of hospitals have participated each year since 1945. Participating centres have been urged to make the registration of cases as complete as possible. The objective is the registration of every new case of malignant disease, including those which are too advanced for effective treatment, and the surveillance of all those actually treated.

Method of registration

16.13 For every case of suspected malignant disease a registration card is completed by the treatment centre. The card contains identification details and the provisional diagnosis. It is sent to a Regional Registry. A duplicate copy is retained by the centre. The registration cards form a central alphabetical index, a means of obviating duplicate registration, and a means of checking the movements of the basic records—the abstract cards. The abstract card follows the Registration Card and contains the confirmed diagnosis with histology, treatment history, dates of first symptom and of registration and provides for the recording of follow-up details to be furnished at future registration anniversaries by the treatment centre. This card is sent to the General Register Office.

Objectives

16.14 In a preliminary review of the working of the scheme, Stocks (1950) indicated that the purpose of registration was to provide information on the following—

(1) Incidence of cancer in relation to site, age, and sex.
(2) Interval between earliest symptoms and the patient's coming under observation and treatment.
(3) Extent of the disease when first diagnosed.
(4) Methods of treatment employed.
(5) Reasons for absence of attempt at radical treatment.
(6) Survival rates by different methods of treatment.
(7) Survival rates as affected by the extent of disease when first diagnosed.
(8) Comparisons between survival rates of all radically treated cases and of those in which there was histological diagnosis of malignancy.
(9) Effect of treatment on the primary growth.
(10) Interval between earliest symptoms and death.

Registration in other countries

16.15 In Denmark a system of registration covers all cases diagnosed in hospital and cases who do not attend hospitals are identified by analysis of death certificates. France has a similar system. In the United States of America the problem has been tackled by local surveys and in Canada a local scheme of registration has been instituted in Toronto.

International recommendations

16.16 In 1950 the WHO Expert Committee on Health Statistics appointed a Sub-Committee on the 'Registration of Cases of Cancer as well as their Statistical Presentation'. Their first report recommended that cancer deaths in vital statistics should be based on rubrics 140–205 of the International Statistical Classification of Diseases, Injuries and Causes of Death, but that for comparability with the past the following sub-groups should be shown separately—

(i) Cancer excluding Hodgkin's disease, leukaemia and aleukaemia (140–205 except 201 and 204)
(ii) Hodgkin's disease—(201)
(iii) Leukaemia and aleukaemia—(204).

16.17 They stressed the need for improving the accuracy of diagnoses recorded on death certificates especially where multiple causes including cancer were involved since omission of mention of cancer in such circumstances would lead to the understatement of cancer deaths.

16.18 The Sub-Committee also recommended—

'(1) that efforts be made to determine the total incidence of cancer in the populations of sample areas within several countries during a year or period of years using for that purpose all available sources of information (e.g. doctors, pathologists, hospitals, death certificates);
(2) that cancer registration projects aiming at ascertainment of following histories of patients should be encouraged with a view to eventual

274

inclusion in such registration systems of all persons affected by cancer, thus eliminating selective bias, so as to arrive at true morbidity, survival, and apparent recovery rates.'

Statistical measures used for analysis of cancer statistics

16.19 Apart from the calculation of death rates for cancer of various types and sites as part of the normal analysis of mortality statistics (which do not measure incidence because of differential recovery rates) the most useful rates based on cancer cases identified either by a national registration scheme or by a single treatment centre are—

Crude survival rate, i.e. number of persons known to be alive at the end of a period of observation (as defined below) divided by the total number who were alive at the beginning of this period, i.e. $SR_{\text{cru}} = \dfrac{A}{A + D + L}$

where A = number alive at end of period. [This number may be sub-divided into

A_0—with no evidence of disease

A_c—with cancer present

A_x—with presence of cancer uncertain]

D = number known to be dead (the condition at death may be denoted by the same suffices as are used for the sub-division of A)

L = number untraced at end of period.

16.20 This crude survival rate cannot be judged by its departure from unity since even for patients completely cured of cancer there will be some natural mortality. It is, therefore, usual to calculate the ratio of the crude survival rate to the natural survival rate, p, for a comparable period and for a population having the same age distribution as the cancer patients. [In this context 'natural' means excluding mortality from cancer of the site under review. Normally, this exclusion is unimportant and it is safe to use, as an approximation to p, the probability of not dying from *any* cause.] This ratio is referred to as the *corrected survival rate* $SR_{\text{cor}} = \dfrac{SR_{\text{cru}}}{p}$.

16.21 The *crude apparent recovery rate* is the number of persons alive with no evidence of the disease at the end of the period of observation divided by the total number who were alive at the beginning.

$$RR_{\text{cru}} = \frac{A_0}{A + D + L}$$

16.22 For the first five years the denominator is the original number of patients alive at the beginning of the total period of observation but for annual intervals after five years it is the number alive with no evidence of disease at the beginning of the particular annual interval.

16.23 *Adjustment of the apparent recovery rate.* The crude apparent recovery rate makes no allowance for the fact that some of those who died in the period had some duration of life with freedom from evidence of disease or for the fact that some of the patients whose condition at the end of the period in question was uncertain were in fact free of evidence of disease.

16.24 If we assume that A_x may be split between 'cured' and diseased in the proportion of the known cases, then $A_x\left(\dfrac{A_0}{A_0 + A_c}\right)$ must be added to A_0. If the deaths are evenly distributed over the period then on the average the deaths have half that period of life, or, what amounts to the same thing, we may redistribute the deaths so that half die at the commencement and half at the end of the period (the mean point of death still being at the middle of the period). It remains to decide upon the number of deaths to be used. We require not only D_0 but on analogy with A_x we can assume that a proportion $D_0/D_0 + D_c$ of the unknown cases D_x and L died free of evidence of disease, i.e. we increase D_0 by $(D_x + L) D_0/D_0 + D_c$. The adjusted rate becomes

$$RR_{\text{adj.}} = \frac{A_0\left[1 + \dfrac{A_x}{A_0 + A_c}\right] + \tfrac{1}{2} . D_0\left[1 + \dfrac{D_x + L}{D_0 + D_c}\right]}{A + D + L}$$

16.25 Other methods of adjustment may be made on slightly different assumptions; for example it might be possible in certain conditions of intensive post mortem examination to regard D_x as zero, or it might be decided to assume that L should be omitted from the calculation altogether on the ground that they survived in the same proportion as the traced cases. The general principle of the adjustment however is not affected by these variations.

Observation period

16.26 Comparison of survival rates is not possible unless the period to which they relate is carefully specified not only as to length but as to the starting point. This might be the date of first examination, of final diagnosis, of commencement of treatment of any kind, or of radical treatment. The choice may be made according to the purpose of the analysis so long as it is specified. The WHO Sub-Committee suggested that for comparison of treatment the date of commencement of treatment should be used, while for public health purposes the date of first diagnosis might be more suitable. In the latter cases this will be the date of visit to clinic or admission to hospital during which the diagnosis was established.

Classification of cases of cancer

16.27 Since tumours may be primary or secondary, are diagnosed at different stages of growth, and have different degrees of malignancy, it is equally important to specify, and to establish the greatest possible degree of homogeneity in relation to, these qualities in respect of any group for which survival rates are quoted. It would be misleading for example to compare the survival rates for two different types of treatment, if one of the treatment groups consisted of very advanced cases and the other consisted of early cases.

16.28 The WHO Sub-Committee recommend in their Second Report that classification should be based on the primary neoplasm first diagnosed (a second primary being treated as intercurrent disease) in relation to site (anatomical location) and the following stages of growth.

Stage 1. Tumour strictly confined to the specified organ and of relatively small size.

Stage 2. Tumour limited to the organ of orgin but of relatively large size or with limited extension beyond the original organ.

Stage 3. Tumour with wide infiltration reaching neighbouring organs.

Stage 4. Tumour with considerable involvement of adjacent tissues or having spread to neighbouring organs.

16.29 The Report also provides a decimal breakdown of the neoplasm section of the International Classification of Diseases to provide for greater specificity of site.

Fixed reference

16.30 It is important for assessing the prognosis of a particular class of patients that the classification of a patient (and the period of observation) should be fixed as prior to first treatment and should not be disturbed by later recurrence or further treatment otherwise considerable bias may be introduced into the calculations. If for example all recurrences were treated as new cases then the original group from which they were transferred would show spuriously high survival rates and the group to which they are classed on recurrence would show high mortality at apparently short durations of treatment.

Statistics of incidence

16.31 It is only in areas where registration is almost complete that it is possible to use registration statistics to estimate the prevalence of disease and the incidence of new cases. Rates of registration of new cases per 1,000 population ranged, in 1964, from $2 \cdot 3$ in Wales to $3 \cdot 0$ in the South Western Region. It has been estimated (who 1966) that there should be $3 \cdot 3 - 3 \cdot 5$ new cases per 1,000 in a highly developed population.

Statistics of particular treatment centres

16.32 Several specialist cancer treatment centres maintain their own rigorous follow-up investigations. Of these probably the best known is the Christie Hospital and Holt Radium Institute whose statistical reports are of a very high standard.

REFERENCES

BENJAMIN, B. (1954) *Monthly Bulletin of Min. Health and P.H.L.S.*, December 1954, p. 214.

BRINTON, H. P., FRASIER, E. S., and KOVEN, A. L. (1952) Public Health Reports 67.835 (Washington).

CASE, R. A. M., and HOSKER, M. E. (1954) *Brit. J. of Prev. and Soc. Med.*, 8, 39.

CASE, R. A. M., HOSKER, M. E., MCDONALD, D. B., and PEARSON, J. T. (1954) *Brit. J. Ind. Med.* 11.75.

CLEMMENSEN, J. (1951) *J. of Nat. Cancer Institute*, 12.1. (Washington).

Departmental Committee (Home Office) (1926) Report of Committee appointed to consider evidence as to the occurrence of epitheliomatous ulceration among Mule Spinners. H.M.S.O.

DOLL, R., and HILL, A. B. (1954) *Brit. Med. J.*, i. 1451.

DOLL, R., and HILL, A. B. (1964) *Brit. Med. J.*, i. 1399.

General Register Office (1938) Registrar General's Decennial Supplement for England and Wales 1931, Part IIa 'Occupational Mortality'. H.M.S.O.

General Register Office (1958) Registrar General's Decennial Supplement for England and Wales 1951, Part II H.M.S.O.

GREENWOOD, M. (1926) Min. of Health Report No. 33, H.M.S.O.

KENNAWAY, E. L., and N. M. (1937) Acta of the International Union against Cancer, II. 101.

LIPWORTH, L. (1965) *Lancet*, ii. 1072.

LOGAN, W. P. D. (1953) *Lancet*, ii, 1199.

PATERSON, R., TOD, M., RUSSELL, M. (1950) *The Results of Radium and X-Ray Therapy in Malignant Disease.* E. & S. Livingstone (Edinburgh).

PERRY, K. M. R. (1947) *Thorax*, 2.91.

SMITHERS, D. W., RIGBY JONES, P., GALTON, D. A. C., and PAYNE, P. M. (1952) *Brit. J. Radiology* Suppl. 4. p. 19.

STOCKS, P. (1950) 'Cancer Registration in England and Wales', General Register Office, *Studies in Medical and Population Subjects*, No. 3. H.M.S.O.

WHO Sub-Committee on Cancer Registration (1950) WHO Tech. Rep. Series No. 25. Geneva.

WHO Sub-Committee on Cancer Registration (1952) WHO Tech. Rep. Series No. 53, Annex 3, Geneva.

WHO Expert Committee on Cancer Treatment (1966) Tech. Rep. Series No. 322. Geneva.

CHAPTER 17

MENTAL HEALTH STATISTICS

17.1 In England and Wales at the end of 1963 there were 131,568 mentally ill patients in residence in hospitals and units administered by the Regional Hospital Boards and there were in addition 55,792 subnormal (Ministry of Health 1967). These figures though only of hospital patients, indicate the importance of the mental health service of the community.

General practice

17.2 In the General Register Office survey of general practitioner records referred to in Chapter 18, it was found that the number of patients consulting their doctors, per 1,000 of the practice populations, for psychoses, anxiety reaction, asthenic reaction, other psychoneuroses, alcoholism, mental deficiency and other disorders of character were (annual rates)—

	Males					Females				
Period	*0–*	*15–*	*45–*	*65+*	*All ages*	*0–*	*15–*	*45–*	*65+*	*All ages*
1951–52	15	41	37	34	33	19	77	100	63	68
1952–54	19	40	43	39	34	18	84	98	66	77

17.3 These figures are not necessarily representative of the country as a whole but the rates are impressively large, especially for adult females.

17.4 Of 4,732 patients consulting for psychoneuroses only 473 or 10 per cent were referred to hospital for inpatient or outpatient treatment. Hospital statistics only touch upon the hard core of a very large problem.

Hospital outpatient clinics.

17.5 For all teaching and non-teaching hospitals in the National Health Service the following statistics have been extracted for the year ended December 31, 1966 (Ministry of Health 1967).

Numbers in thousands

Department	*Annual number of clinic sessions held*	*New outpatients during the year*	*Total attendances during the year (new and old patients)*
Psychiatry—children	59	30	192
Subnormality and severe subnormality	2	2	5
Mental illness	142	180	1,261
Chronic sick under psychiatric supervision	—	—	2

17.6 A large proportion of these patients are treated by psychological or physical treatment methods and never become inpatients of hospitals.

Mental health statistics—National scheme

17.7 Arrangements have been made by the Ministry of Health to compile statistics derived from all the National Health Service hospitals in England and Wales.

17.8 Uniform index cards are used in these institutions and the cards relating to admissions, discharges and deaths are sent in monthly batches to the Ministry of Health.

17.9 The cards are divided into two separate parts. The first part is completed when the patient is admitted. It contains personal information about the patient, the diagnosis and some administrative details about the admission. The second part of the card is completed when the patient leaves or dies. It contains the personal information about the patient and the diagnosis recorded on the first part with, in addition, details of the length of stay, type of discharge and diagnosis on leaving. If the patient dies the certified cause of death is also recorded.

17.10 The index cards relating to mentally ill or subnormal patients admitted to an NHS hospital for the first time are filed at the Ministry of Health in an alphabetical index. Information from the cards relating to subsequent discharges or readmissions of these patients is added in code form on the back of the first admission cards, so as to build up a 'history' of periods spent in hospital by each patient. Such an index provides a comprehensive central register of mental patients who have had hospital treatment. In the past patients who have been discharged after treatment and who have later suffered a remission have often been admitted to a different hospital from that to which originally admitted and the absence of a central register has prevented any linking up of medical records and has, therefore, mitigated against the proper evaluation of treatment at the hospital of first admission. Proper provision for the follow-up of a discharged patient has become increasingly necessary as the variety of physical treatments, many of which achieve dramatic reduction in mental disturbance, has increased.

17.11 The base date for this system is December 31, 1963 when a complete census of patients in psychiatric beds in England and Wales was carried out (Brooke 1967). A psychiatric bed was defined as a bed under the care of a psychiatrist. The census asked for particulars of sex, marital status, age, date of admission, type of resident (physically present, on leave etc.), legal status under the Mental Health Act 1959, first or other admission, mental category (mental illness, psychopathic disorder, subnormality, severe subnormality, other), and diagnosis of mental illness or clinical type of subnormality.

17.12 The numbers given in 17.1 are of those physically present in psychiatric beds; in addition there were about 4,300 mentally ill and 4,000 subnormal on leave or still on the books though no bed was reserved.

17.13 The resident mentally ill varied from $2 \cdot 1$ per 1,000 population in Sheffield and Oxford hospital regions to $3 \cdot 2$ in the metropolitan aggregate and $3 \cdot 4$ in the Wessex region. For the country as a whole the figure was $2 \cdot 8$.

17.14 Of male mentally ill patients in hospital 71 per cent had been there for two years or more, and 48 per cent for ten years or more; the corresponding proportions for females were 68 and 44.

17.15 Detailed diagnostic analyses were made in relation to age, length of stay and other factors.

17.16 The census of 1963 could be compared with an earlier census of 1954 to show that although the number of mentally ill patients decreased by 20,000, the number aged 65 and over increased by 6,300 from 45,400 to 51,700. Many of these were long-stay patients, especially those suffering from schizophrenia, admitted to hospital before the development of modern therapeutic methods. The older long stay population was ageing and was not being replaced.

17.17 It is intended that the census will provide a base for an index regularly updated by movement data (the record cards of admissions and discharges and deaths). From this will emerge a series of studies analysing the progress of patients admitted in successive years. In Nottingham an experiment is being made to extend the index to all patients in psychiatric care in the community regardless of whether admitted to hospital or not. Such an extension will be desirable in view of the clear trend towards community rather than institutional care.

The standing mental hospital population

17.18 A census is an essential benchmark but does not of itself indicate the pace and direction of change. It is possible to examine the situation more closely by a simple use of a life table, given rates of admission (per unit of the general population) and rates of exit (discharge, departure and death per unit of the mentally ill population) and assuming that the general population itself is stable and follows the distribution of the L_x column of the current life table. The following table shows an illustrative calculation for males only. The admission and exit rates are those experienced in 1951, i.e. before the current classification of mentally ill was introduced and related to all categories in hospital. The number of males out of 1,000,000 births who are admitted to hospital before attaining age 10 is simply $0 \cdot 000011 \times 9,631,200 = 106$ where $0 \cdot 000011$ is the average admission rate over the ten years of age and 9,631,200 is the number of years of life lived by the 1,000,000 births up to age 10. If m is the central exit rate from x to $x + h$, P_x is the number in hospital at exact age x, and $\bar{P}$ is the number of years life lived in hospital from age x, to $x + h$ then

$$\frac{1}{h}(\bar{P}) = \tfrac{1}{2}[P_x + \overline{(P_x + \text{admissions } x \text{ to } x + h} - m.\bar{P})]$$

where P_x, h m are known and hence $\bar{P}$ can be derived.

In the first interval $P_x = 0$, $h = 10$, $m = 0 \cdot 476$,

i.e. $\qquad \dfrac{1}{10} \cdot \bar{P} = \tfrac{1}{2}[0 + (106) - 0 \cdot 476.\bar{P}]$

or $\qquad \bar{P} = \dfrac{106}{0 \cdot 2 + 0 \cdot 476} = 157$

281

whence the exits in the first 10 years of age are $157 \times 0.476 = 75$. We must now go back and correct the 9,631,200 years of life lived (outside hospital) by subtracting 157, the years of life lived in hospital. This reduces the figure to 9,631,043. At later ages the reduction is large enough to affect the admissions which have to be recalculated affecting in turn P, etc. and a certain degree of trial and error has to be adopted to achieve consistency.

17.19 The final values (Table 17.1) are obtained by first estimating the admissions as the life table population $75+$, i.e. 2,521,700, multiplied by 0.00285. This gives 7,187, and since there were 3,337 in hospital at exact age 75 (the difference of admissions and exits prior to age 75) there must be $3,337 + 7,187$ or 10,524 exits. But the exit rate is 0.353 so that the standing population must be $10,524 \div 0.353 = 29,813$. This number must now be subtracted from 2,521,700 before recalculating the admissions as 7,102. Whence the exits are 10,439, and the standing population 29,572 and no further adjustment is necessary.

TABLE 17.1 *Hypothetical and actual Standing Population—males only*

Age	Annual direct admission rates per unit general population	Exit rates per unit of psychiatric population	No. of years of life lived (outside hospital) in age interval in population generated by 1,000,000 births a year*	Admitted during age interval	Discharged during age interval	Standing psychiatric population No.	Hypothetical per 10,000	Actual 1951 per 10,000
0 –	0·000011	0·476	9,631,043	106	75	157	6⎫	35
01 –	0·00014	0·596	5,739,968	804	555	932	33⎬	
16 –	0·00085	0·591	3,812,114	3,239	2,060	3,486	124	72
20 –	0·00154	0·518	4,731,085	7,286	5,758	11,115	396	260
25 –	0·00169	0·375	9,342,451	15,789	14,193	37,849	1,350	1,268
35 –	0·00133	0·260	9,138,852	12,154	12,050	46,348	1,653	1,922
45 –	0·00137	0·219	8,671,574	11,880	11,109	50,726	1,810	2,289
55 –	0·00171	0·230	7,474,087	12,780	11,848	51,513	1,838	2,028
65 –	0·00205	0·280	5,153,367	10,564	13,617	48,633	1,735⎫	2,126
75 +	0·00285	0·353	2,492,128	7,102	10,439	29,572	1,055⎬	
Total				81,704	81,704	280,331	10,000	10,000

* Using the England and Wales Life Tables 1950–52 (Abridged).

17.20 It will be seen that the actual male psychiatric population was more concentrated at ages 35–65 and contained relatively fewer patients aged 65 and over than a stable population. It thus appeared likely that just as the general population was likely to 'grow up' (see p. 34) so, in 1951, the mental hospital population was also likely to grow older—a fact to which Norris drew attention (1952) and which has been confirmed by the comparison between the censuses of the 1954 and 1963.

Diagnostic classification

17.21 There are difficulties in isolating psychiatric entities especially in conditions where outward expression of derangement may take a variety of forms. For example it is difficult to make a clear separation of psychotic depression from neurotic depression; conditions involving fears are spread over five rubrics of the International Statistical Classification and allocation is affected by the extent to which attention is paid to physical (somatic) symptoms; distinction between immature personality and pathological personality is not clear; the line of demarcation between hysterical reactions and somatization reactions is open to question; neurotic disorders are pluralistic. Precision and comparability in classification and terminology is however improving.

17.22 A special problem arises in connection with the treatment of elderly psychiatric patients where mental illness is often less permanent than the background of physical infirmity of old age and where in order to ensure efficiency in the allocation of heavily loaded services it has been suggested that the diagnostic classification should involve some degree of prognostic categorization, viz. (*a*) dementias of old age, i.e. irreversible disorganizations of the personality due to degenerative brain changes, (*b*) long-standing neurotic, psychotic or character disorders, and (*c*) recent reactions either affective or toxic-confusional (Norris and Post 1954).

Efficacy of therapy

17.23 It might be thought, since mental disease follows a long chronic course in many instances, that follow up investigations, employing statistical techniques analogous to those used for tuberculosis and cancer, would provide a means of judging the effect of treatment. There are, however, difficulties. For tuberculosis and cancer the method is appropriate because the failure of treatment is marked by objective measures of deterioration, viz. radiological evidence of spread of disease, other visible signs of incapacity, the need for further surgical intervention, and—most objective of all—higher mortality. In mental disease mortality is not necessarily affected except for specific disorders such as neurosyphilis, and epilepsy and for forms of disorder where the risk of suicide is raised. [Psychiatric long-stay patients, as members of a closed and sick community, have higher risks of mortality from tuberculosis, bronchitis and heart disease but this is a general factor arising partly from the select character of the population and partly from difficulties of control.] The ultimate test of success of treatment lies in the ability to return to the stresses and strains of full social responsibility, i.e. normal participation in community life, but there are many degrees of marginal improvement reflected by the disappearance of symptoms. In some cases of acute tension the benefit of treatment might be seen only in the facilitation of nursing without any reduction in the need for institutional care. There is also a distinction to be drawn between clinical symptoms and the actual quality of improvement in terms, for example, of ability to resume employment. There seems to be a need for a method of recording 'profiles' or 'complexes' of symptoms with sufficient succinctness to permit practicable grouping of cases but with sufficient specificity to allow sensitivity to small changes as a result of treatment.

17.24 Rees (1949) stressed other difficulties, viz. the difficulty of providing satisfactory control groups and the fact that standards and criteria for diagnosis vary among different workers and hospitals. He tried to overcome some of those difficulties by using a very detailed but standardized description of symptomatology for each patient which permitted point ratings of mental status.

Statistics of Mental Health in the USA

17.25 In addition to excellent reports from the departments of mental hygiene of individual States, the National Institute of Mental Health of the

283

United States Department of Health, Education and Welfare, compiles national statistics of patients in hospital for mental disease, of patients with mental disease in general hospitals with psychiatric facilities, and of patients in institutions for mental defectives and epileptics, based on annual censuses. While there have been inquiries into the incidence of mental disease as part of the population census as early as 1840 the first census in the present form was carried out in 1923. In 1926, annual enumerations of patients in mental institutions were begun, first confined to State hospitals and institutions and in 1933 extended to cover all types of hospitals and institutions specifically for the mentally ill, mental defectives and epileptics. In 1939 the collection of data from general hospitals with psychiatric facilities began on an annual basis. The statistics present a picture of the flow of patients into and out of hospitals and institutions. The data cover:

All hospitals
   (1) Movement of hospital population by sex of patient.
   (2) First admissions by age, sex, and mental disorder.

Public hospitals
   (3) Resident patients at end of year by age, sex and mental disorder.
   (4) Discharges by condition on discharge, sex and mental disorder.
   (5) Personnel by sex and occupation.
   (6) Expenditure by purpose of expenditures.

17.26 The National Centre for Health Statistics have published (1965) the results of a survey of a probability sample of 172 long-stay mental hospitals during April–June 1963. These results comprise a geographical distribution of hospitals and patients, characteristics of age, sex, and colour, length of stay, extent of disability.

REFERENCES

BROOKE, E. M. (1967) Ministry of Health Rep. Pub. H. and Med. Subj. No. 106. H.M.S.O.
Ministry of Health (1965) Annual Report of Chief Medical Officer for 1965. H.M.S.O.
NORRIS, V. (1952) *Lancet*, ii. 1172.
NORRIS, V., and POST, F. (1954) *Brit. Med. J.*, i. 675.
REES, L. (1949) *J. of Mental Science*, 95.625.
US Department of Health, Education and Welfare. Public Health Service (1965). Characteristics of Patients in Mental Hospitals. Nat. Center for Health Stats. Reports Series 12. No. 3.

CHAPTER 18

GENERAL PRACTITIONER STATISTICS

18.1 Most medical care services have their focus in the family doctor and it is natural to look to the records of the family doctor for comprehensive statistics of morbidity. The potentiality of general practitioner records was enhanced in Great Britain by the establishment in 1948 of a comprehensive health service which brought medical care within the reach of all, irrespective of means. Ideally, the general practitioner would be making regular observation of families within his care and would be in a position to record the incipience of the earliest symptoms of even minor degrees of disease. This ideal is, however, some distance from attainment; first, because medical manpower does not permit practices to be small enough for such observation to take place except in a few rural areas—typified by Wensleydale and epitomized in the name of Dr William Pickles (1939), whose classical study of the work of a country doctor has done so much to stimulate interest in the scientific value of such patient recording of sickness in families; second, because, except in rural areas where choice is restricted by distance the general practitioner is not a *family* doctor, i.e. he is not reponsible for every member of the family in all cases—the following figures have been given by Backett, Shaw and Evans (1953) in respect of a practice in North West London:

Type of family	Per cent of families in which the whole family was registered with the doctor
A group containing at least a mother and children	96
Parent, or parents with children; married couples	60
All related persons living at the same address	47
Families with children *and* other relatives living at the same address	27

18.2 It has, therefore, to be accepted that the general practitioner does not see all members of the family except in a proportion of cases, and he does not see them regularly but only under present conditions of pressure, when they are sufficiently unwell to demand his attention.

18.3 A further difficulty is that general practitioner records by their very nature do not lend themselves easily to statistical analysis. When a patient enters the surgery of a general practitioner it is by no means usual for an immediate diagnosis to be made; if it were so it might simplify statistical analysis but it would *not* be good medicine. Very often the record card of a patient will show a series of visits with notes of various symptoms and reaction to prescribed treatment, and the patient may then be referred to hospital without a formal diagnosis necessarily being recorded (though most hospitals now endeavour to keep general practitioners fully informed about the progress of patients referred to consultants) or alleviation of symptoms may cut short attendances and the record may not be completed unless the doctor has the opportunity to review his records for that purpose. Patients sometimes attend for minor degrees of discomfort or for advice for example about fitness for jobs or about marriage and in such cases there may be a great deal observed but little to record.

18.4 It would be possible to supply the general practitioner or even the patient with a check list of a range of symptoms on the lines of the Cornell Medical Index (1949) which facilitate the approach to a diagnosis and would certainly render statistical analysis easier since it would merely be a matter of collecting the ticked list. This would be bad medicine, for patients do not attend for statistical analysis but often urgently need reassurance—a very real component of medical care; to ignore this vital fact is not only bad medicine —it is bound in the end to lead to bad statistics.

Early experiments

18.5 Despite these difficulties, a number of important studies of illness in general practice have been made. Pemberton in 1949 reported an experiment in which eight general practitioners in Sheffield recorded the age, sex, and the diagnosis of all patients, National Health service and private, who consulted them in the course of one winter week and one summer week. They also indicated whether the patient was seen in the surgery or at home, and which cases it was necessary to refer to a hospital or local authority clinic. In the two weeks there were 4,656 consultations involving 4,814 complaints distributed as follows—

Group of illnesses	No.	Per cent
Respiratory diseases	1,601	33·3
Digestive disease	379	7·9
Cardiovascular disease	364	7·6
Mental ill-health	312	6·5
Obstetrics and gynaecology	276	5·7
Chronic rheumatism	264	5·5
Accidents	247	5·1
Acute specific fevers	224	4·7
Skin diseases	165	3·4
Abscesses and cellulitis	140	2·9
Ear, nose, throat	87	1·8
Anaemia	79	1·6
Neurological	75	1·5
Uro-genital	62	1·3
Senility	56	1·2
Eyes	51	1·0
Cancer	46	1·0
Vaccination	35	0·7
Miscellaneous	351	7·3

18.6 Almost one-fifth of the consultations were for patients over the age of sixty.

18.7 In 1950 McGregor published a review of his own practice of 2,486 patients in a small industrial town on the Scottish border. This report gave the age, sex, and occupational distribution of the practice and rates of incidence of complaints in sex and age groups in a year. It also stated the average number of surgery and home visits for each complaint. The complaints were classified in broad disease groups. Information was given about hospital referrals.

18.8 This was followed by a study in morbidity as experienced in general practice by Fry (1952) working in the outskirts of South London, an area 'closely populated by persons of the lower middle classes, whose occupations are chiefly in local industry or in clerical duties in London'. The practice was a large one covering 4,456 individuals of whom 3,373 or 76 per cent required a consultation in 1951, the year of review. The study was important for many reasons but especially for the fact that it gave the view of a general practitioner as to the most convenient method of keeping morbidity records. Cases were coded directly to quinary age groups and to twenty-one broad disease groups.

18.9 Meanwhile persistent studies in methodology were carried out by the Social Medicine Research Unit of the Medical Research Council (Backett et al., loc. cit.) and the General Register Office (Logan, 1953).

18.10 The Medical Research Council study concerned a large general practice in North West London and was designed to determine the nature and extent of patients' needs both medical and social, the pattern of work of the general practitioner, and relationships with other services. The doctor was asked to complete a separate record care after each consultation. On this card which took less than one minute to complete, were summarized the data necessary to identify the patient, to distinguish the diagnosis which had been made and the services rendered by the doctor, and to fix the time and place of consultation. At six-weekly intervals for one week, members of the unit staff attended all consultations and made more intensive records which were used as a source of additional detail. Because general practitioners do not see all members of the family nor all ailments in those patients who are registered with them, it was decided to supplement the information drawn from the practice by direct case study of a group of families carried out by a visiting social worker; in this way comprehensive *family* health records were built up. A broad disease code of some thirty-eight groups was used with a breakdown by chronicity (three months or more except for certain obviously chronic conditions, e.g. tuberculosis) and by seriousness, and a treatment code was added. Detailed results have been published (Backett, et al., 1954) showing that half the work of the practice was concentrated among 16 per cent of the population who consulted the doctor on ten or more occasions during the year. Of all the diagnoses made during the year 16 per cent were of serious disease and the work involved in treating them amounted to 43 per cent of the total work of the practice. Chronic disease caused 30 per cent of the work and acute infections accounted for another 43 per cent.

18.11 The General Register Office study began early in 1951 with the primary objectives of determining to what extent general practitioners' clinical records could be used as a source of general morbidity statistics, and examining the problems associated with the use of those records. Eight general practitioners in different parts of the country volunteered to record by a method of their own choosing the following basic information in respect of every consultation—

(a) date of consultation
(b) place of consultation (surgery, patient's home, or elsewhere)
(c) certificates issued (type)
(d) referral (hospital outpatient or inpatient, clinic, etc.)
(e) diagnosis or other reason for consultation.

18.12 Four different methods of recording were used.

Method I

A medical record envelope (E.C.5 males, E.C.6 females) is issued to practitioners by the Ministry of Health, through NHS Executive Councils, for each NHS patient. The envelopes are filed by the practitioner and constitute a register of his patients. On the front of the envelope is recorded the patient's name, address, date of birth and NHS number. The reverse is ruled in three columns providing for (1) date of consultation, (2) whether a surgery attendance or a home visit or if a certificate was issued and (3) clinical notes. Continuation cards (E.C.7/8) similarly ruled, are provided for continuing records after completion of the space on the envelope. The continuation cards are kept, together with correspondence, inside the record envelope.

One practitioner completed a line of the appropriate envelope or card for each consultation, recording in order, the five basic elements of information. (Surgery attendances were entered at the time: home visits were noted in a visiting book and dates transferred to the envelope.) The same method was used by another practitioner who, however, used Method II for continuation cards.

Method II

Four practitioners used the NHS continuation cards overprinted with columns for the five basic questions, a single line being used for each consultation.

Method III

One practitioner used a specially printed self-coding card on which he ticked the appropriate numbers or letters in code lists for the five items.

Method IV

One practitioner used a specially printed form of paper for each consultation providing for a manuscript note of the essential information in appropriate spaces.

18.13 Method II, using modified continuation cards, was most popular. The serial record of past consultations could readily be reviewed and the record of a particular illness could easily be selected.

18.14 During the twelve months, April 1951 to March 1952, 27,365 patients were registered in the eight practices and two-thirds of them consulted their doctor at least once. Women consulted their doctor more often than men, 74 per cent of the women and 67 per cent of the men seeking medical advice during the twelve months. For each woman patient registered practitioners gave an average of 4·2 consultations as against 3·4 for each man.

The average for both sexes combined was 3·8 but this ratio varied considerably in the different practices.

18.15 Several different rates are shown for separate diseases, the most important being 'consultation rates' and 'patients consulting rates'. The former reflect the number of consultations given and the latter the number of patients affected, without consideration of the number of consultations. Consultation rates, therefore, show the amount of work each disease caused the practitioner (at least in so far as work can be measured in terms of consultations) and patients consulting rates measure the morbidity from each disease.

18.16 The *individual* diseases causing most consultations were bronchitis (68·7 per 1,000 total consultations for all diseases and conditions), the common cold (60·9), influenza (26·5), acute tonsillitis (22·1), otitis media (19·7), benign hypertension (16·3), fibrositis (16·0), boil and carbuncle (15·6) and undefined rheumatism (15·0). Maternal conditions, without complications, were responsible for 26·8 of each 1,000 consultations.

18.17 For *groups* of diseases, those of the respiratory system were by far the most frequent cause of consultation, occasioning 24 per cent of all consultations. Diseases of the digestive system were the next most important cause (9 per cent) followed by diseases of the nervous system and sense organs (8 per cent). The predominance of respiratory diseases was common to all sex-age groups, except elderly women (65 years and over) who sought medical advice most frequently for diseases of the circulatory system.

18.18 The Report gives consultation rates and incidence rates (persons consulting) per thousand of the practice populations for a wide range of diseases and injuries, in sex and age groups. Information is also given of the frequency of consultation (per patient for particular diseases), of certificates issued and referrals to hospital. Multiple diagnoses (more than one diagnosis at a consultation) were dealt with by counting all the diagnoses separately in the tabulation with fractional weight, viz. one of three diagnoses would be given one-third weight. An alternative which would have required more judgement at the coding stage would be to select a primary diagnosis.

18.19 The study did not provide information of the duration of treatment (not to be confused with the duration of illness owing to the lag before consultation). It is difficult to define the point of time at which medical care ceases since a patient may not continue to attend when expected and the record is then incomplete. For the present the main morbidity measure emerging from general practitioner records is the rate of new cases of particular disease groups per 1,000 persons registered in a practice, within a specified interval.

The College of General Practitioners

18.20 Interest in the importance of the work of the general practitioner has led to the establishment of a College of General Practitioners with its own Research Committee and resources for encouraging co-operative effort. The first fruits of this action have been the institution of a larger morbidity enquiry based on nearly half a million patients in more than a hundred practices (in collaboration with the General Register Office) and the conduct of research into problems of special interest to general practitioners. A study of acute chest infection as seen in general practice based on a 'clinical reconnaissance' by fifty-five general practitioners (1956) has provided valuable information of the various syndromes seen and their meaning. A number of valuable studies of individual practices have been produced by College members. The most important development has been the institution of a voluntary system of morbidity reporting. The system is based upon the completion of an 'episode' card carrying details of the patient, the diagnosis made and the service given in terms of surgery attendances or house visits and referred to hospital. These cards are forwarded to a central office for data processing.

Community Health Records

18.21 Mention has been made (15.58) of the potential of the computer for storing and retrieving clinical data in respect of hospital patients. There is no reason why the bounds of the hospital system should not be extended to embrace other agencies which may have care of the patient, especially the general practitioner. The present fragmentation of the National Health Service means that in many instances the record of an episode of illness is equally fragmented. If medical information about an individual could be stored as it arises, in a single magnetic tape record, capable of retrieval at any stage to the full extent of its current accumulation by any contributor of any part of this record, this fragmentation would be overcome. The retrieval is the vital part of the system. Without a feedback of this kind, i.e. the provision of complete medical histories when required, there would be no incentive to collaborate. At the very least the feeding in of information could be by paper e.g. the present morbidity card of the College of General Practitioners could be adapted for the purpose. The technical means exist to achieve something more sophisticated. It would be possible to connect a typewriter head in the general practitioner's surgery to the computer by ordinary telephone line for the direct 'reading' in and out of information. A number of experiments in the establishment of community record systems are already at the feasibility study stage.

Failing a comprehensive record system of this kind there have been attempts at record linkage, viz. bringing together by matching techniques the fragmented parts of the medical history (Acheson 1967).

Administrative statistics

18.22 Statistics of the number and structure of general practices are published in the Annual Reports of the Ministry of Health. In 1966 in Britain there were some 4,740 practitioners practising 'single handed' and 15,050 in partnerships (mostly in partnerships of two). There were some 900 assistants and trainees. Tables are provided showing the size distribution of practices for each type of 'firm' (and age of practitioner). The average number of patients per principal, in 1966, was 2,531 in urban areas and 2,223 in rural areas. The size distributions were very wide. For example in urban areas for partnerships of two principals, the size of the practice ranged from 400 to over 5,500.

Inflation of lists

18.23 A difficulty which has not been entirely solved and which affects the

290

accuracy of populations at risk used as the denominators of rates, is the inflation of doctors' lists arising from the lag in, or omission of, notification of removal. Arrangements exist for the notification of removal on death even where the general practitioner is not in attendance but in cases of change of practitioner the old list will not be corrected until the removing patients register with new doctors and they may not sign the necessary cards until some ailment brings them to the new doctor's surgery. In the meantime the doctor to whom they transfer has patients actually at risk for whom he has no records and this helps to offset the inflation due to unnotified removals but on balance it is found that lists are subject to *net* inflation, to an extent which varies according to whether or not a practice is growing.

18.24 In the study of Backett *et al.* (1953 loc. cit.) the size of the practice was checked by writing to every name on the register and by home visits in some cases. The following figures were recorded—

	Number	Excess
Individuals registered and found to be present	3,037	
Individuals registered according to Local Executive Council	3,483	15 per cent
Individuals registered according to the medical record envelope held by doctor	3,611	19 per cent

18.25 Of the 574 (i.e. 3,611–3,037) 'missing' persons, 59 were found to have died, 178 had transferred to another doctor, 284 had no local record and could not be traced, and 53 were accounted for by duplicate cards.

18.26 It is clear that any extensive use of general practitioner record smust be matched by continued improvement in the efficiency of the machinery used to keep the lists up-to-date. Such improvement depends very largely on public education. [The general practitioner service is administered through local executive councils who regulate the size and disposition of practices and maintain records of doctors' lists. A doctor passes on to the local executive council the record of a patient who registers with him and the council adjusts its own index; it also notifies the doctor from whom the patient has been transferred if this is a doctor within their own area, or, if not, it notifies the appropriate executive council. The General Register Office acts as a clearing house for the notification of deaths to local executive councils.]

REFERENCES

ACHESON, E. D. (1967) Medical Record Linkage. Oxford Univ. Press.
BACKETT, E. M., SHAW, L. A., and EVANS, J. C. G. (1953) *Proc. Roy. Soc. Med.*, 46, 707.
BACKETT, E. M., HEADY, J. A., and EVANS, J. C. G. (1954) *Brit. Med. J.*, i. 107.
BRODMAN, K., ERDMANN, A. J. et al. (1949) *J. Amer. Med. Assoc.*, 140, 530.
College of General Practitioners (1956) *Brit. Med. J.*, i. 1516.
FRY, J. (1952) *Brit. Med. J.*, ii. 249.
HILL, A. BRADFORD (1950) *J. Roy. Stat. Soc.*, 114. 1.
LOGAN, W. P. D. (1953) *General Register Office. Studies on Medical and Population Studies*, *No. 7* 'General Practitioners Records'. H.M.S.O.
MCGREGOR, R. M. (1950) *Edin. Med. J.*, 57. 433.
PEMBERTON, J. (1949) *Brit. Med. J.*, i. 306.
PICKLES, W. H. (1939) *Epidemiology in Country Practice*. John Wright & Sons. Bristol.

CHAPTER 19

FIELD STUDIES

19.1 It will have become clear to the reader that vital registration records and other standard sources of health statistics (infectious disease notifications, hospital discharge records, cancer registration systems, etc.) may from time to time require to be supplemented by specially organized studies involving direct observation of disease incidence or of social and economic characteristics in the section of the population in respect of which information is desired.

19.2 On occasion these studies will be designed to reveal clinical features of individual cases of disease, for teaching or for therapeutic research purposes, but for the most part they are essentially statistical surveys. It is important therefore that the statistician should be competent to take a responsible part in the planning of such a study at the outset. No amount of recondite mathematics can rescue from failure an investigation which has not been properly designed to answer the questions to which answers have been sought.

19.3 Two main problems normally arise: (1) if, as is usual on the grounds of cost, the survey is limited to a sample of the population, the need to ensure that the sample is truly representative of the population and likely to yield reliable estimates of the factors to be measured, (2) the need to train and instruct the observer team to ensure uniform adherence to technique and accurate recording. A subsidiary problem is the recording method itself.

The use of sampling

19.4 The advantage of sampling (as compared with a total survey) lies primarily in the fact that for a sufficient amount of information smaller resources are required or, what is often more important, for the same resources more information can be sought under more time-consuming but more rewarding conditions of contact and general supervision. Families are mobile and are not always where you expect to find them and even if the subjects for a particular survey are at their usual address they may be out a good deal so that several visits would be required to establish contact. It may take more than one interview or at least a very long interview to question the respondent with such a degree of carefulness and penetration as would be required to attain a desired level of accuracy. In health surveys it may be desirable to carry out medical examinations or make diagnostic tests. All these procedures are expensive in time and manpower. High quality response over a restricted (but representative) field is more useful than poor quality response from larger numbers and in fact larger coverage may be impracticable. There may often, too, be a considerable reduction in the time taken to produce results, for the processing of data takes longer than most people expect especially where complex classifications have to be made and applied.

Requirements of a good sample

19.5 Since the ultimate object is to generalize about the total population, the sample must be so chosen as to be likely to reflect correctly the distribution of characteristics in the total population. The sample must cover the whole distribution in proper proportions and must not be biased, i.e tend to contain one part of the distribution more than another. For example, in any survey of physical measurements of men the sample must be likely to contain short and tall men in the same proportions as in the general population and not be biased in such a way as to contain more than a fair share of tall men or short men. The words 'be likely to' are important. No system of sampling can ensure perfect correspondence. There are bound to be chance differences between the constitution of the sample and that of the parent population. The possible extent of these differences, or sampling errors, can be estimated in advance and can be reduced to any desired level by increasing the size of the sample. Bias, if inherent in the system, is not reduced by increasing the size of the sample.

19.6 Bias arises when the system of selection itself does not give equal likelihood to the representation of members of the population, i.e. fails to follow a random process, or where the rules for that process are not strictly adhered to.

19.7 As an example of the first source we may refer to the practice of selecting a particular drawer or drawers in an alphabetic card index of the population. This will tend either to select an undue proportion, or to avoid a proper proportion, of for example Scotsmen whose names so often begin with 'Mac' or Welshmen whose names are so often Davies, Jones, etc. Less obvious associations between name and nationality or other characteristics also occur. Another example would be the selection of a random sample of nursing mothers from those attending a child welfare clinic. While this might yield a good sample of the clinic attenders it would not be representative of all nursing mothers since it is likely that only the more intelligent mothers or the more anxious will bring their infants to the clinics.

19.8 Bias of the second kind arises when for example an interviewer substitutes the neighbouring house if there is no immediate reply from the selected house. This leads to over-representation of houses where there is usually someone at home, e.g. houses with families. Further, if no attempt is made to minimize non-response, there will be over-representation of the more willing responders, i.e. those more especially interested in the object of the survey. If houses are not selected at random but are taken systematically (e.g. every tenth address) then if some other characteristic also occurs cyclic-ally (e.g. large corner houses also occurring at every fiftieth house) these will be over-represented.

19.9 Sometimes an element of bias is unavoidable and has to be accepted as inherent in the conditions in which the survey has to be carried out. For example, in the census of 1951 (General Register Office, 1958) in England and

Wales an attempt was made to check age statements in the census against birth dates shown in the birth register. A sample of persons recorded on the household schedules was selected systematically for convenience, economy of effort being a paramount consideration. Further, because of the sheer improbability of identifying within a reasonable time the correct birth entry for a name which was likely to occur very frequently in the index to the birth register, certain names such as Smith, Jones, Davies, etc., were 'forbidden'. There was no reason to suspect that accuracy in age statement was correlated either with order of enumeration or surname so that the systematic selection and the omitted names were not serious sources of bias, nevertheless, these sources were unavoidable in the circumstances of severely limited staff resources then obtaining.

19.10 It must be emphasized that it may be wasteful to adopt too purist an attitude to bias. A commonsense approach must be maintained. If the amount of bias is known to be small in relation to the sampling error, or if absolute values are not required but only changes over a period of time (so that in subtracting successive values the bias is eliminated) then the bias could be accepted if its avoidance would make inordinate demands upon resources or would call for a much more complicated scheme.

Sampling errors

19.11 In this textbook matters of statistical theory have been eschewed because there is no shortage of the requisite elementary and intermediate statistical textbooks. The reader is recommended from this point on to refer for guidance on theory to any of the books listed at the end of this chapter and in particular to Yates' book on *Sampling Methods for Censuses and Surveys.*

19.12 In general, the sampling error is approximately inversely proportional to the square root of the number of units included in the sample. The size of the sample must be quadrupled in order to halve the sampling error. Moreover, the contribution to variability of groups of units can be reduced by different procedures.

19.13 A restraint on variability can be imposed by stratification, i.e. the population is split into strata or blocks of units in such a way that within each stratum or block there is as little difference as possible between the units. The blocks or strata are then randomly sampled. For example, if it is desired to sample the heights of men, then sampling separately from blocks 1, 2 and 3 known to have strong representation of tall, medium height and short men respectively, would diminish the likelihood that the total sample will contain an undue number of tall or short men. If the same proportion were taken in each block then the blocks will have the same representation in the sample as in the population, as can be seen from the following figures—

	Population	10 *per cent* sample
Block 1.	2,000	200
Block 2.	7,000	700
Block 3.	2,000	200
	11,000	**1,100**

19.14 Within each block, as in the total sample, the variability can be reduced by increasing numbers and it may be desired in the more extreme and less numerous blocks to use larger proportions. Conversely, it might be possible to accept a smaller proportion in the larger blocks. The use of variable sampling fractions in order to vary the intensity of sampling accordance to the variability of the different blocks is a common practice. In order to restore correct proportional representation of the different strata, the results from each sub-sample must be weighted before combination, as indicated below.

	Population	Sampling fraction (per cent)	Sample	Weight	Product	Product per cent of population
Block 1	2,000	20	400	1	400	20
Block 2	7,000	5	350	4	1,400	20
Block 3	2,000	20	400	1	400	20
	11,000				**2,200**	

19.15 Sometimes the population sampled may itself be a sample from some larger population, again with the object of ensuring that at each stage the selection is carried out under conditions of greatest possible homogeneity.

The mechanics of selection

19.16 In any sampling operation the procedure consists of the selection of sampling units from an array of such units, called the frame. In public health and medical social work the unit is usually a person, or a household, or an illness, or an event such as a marriage or a death. The frame might be a list of people or of households on a register (e.g. the electoral roll, or the local list of rateable hereditaments) or, for illnesses,the records of hospital admissions or doctor consultations, or, for vital registrations, the relevant registers.

19.17 The method of selection should be random but may have to be adapted to practical convenience. For random selection use may be made of tables of random numbers, i.e. of numbers arranged in a completely unordered or random way.* The units of the sampling frame are serially numbered and such random numbers, taken successively from the table, as are less than the total units in the frame, indicate the units to be selected.

19.18 For example, in order to take a sample of 20 from a population numbered from 1 to 910 we would use the following unbracketed random numbers, rejecting those in brackets (i.e. greater than 910): 34, [977], 167, 125, 555, 162, 844, 630, 332, 576, 181, 266, 234, 523, 378, 702, 566, [994], 160, 311, 683, 745.

19.19 It will be seen that these are well spread over the population.

19.20 The representation in the nine portions of the range is uneven. One would expect an average to get rather more than 2 in each portion but some deviation from regularity is likely to occur by virtue of the very laws of chance to which we are appealing. As indicated in 19.5, if the sample is truly random the probable extent of the deviation can be estimated in advance.

* A table of random numbers has been published in *Statistical Tables for Biological, Agricultural and Medical Research* by R. A. Fisher and F. Yates. Oliver and Boyd. Edin.

Numbers	Selected units
0—	1
100—	5
200—	2
300—	3
400—	0
500—	4
600—	2
700—	2
800–910	1
	20

In this example the number in a portion will be expected, in the long run of repeated selections, to exceed 4 rather more than once (i.e. one of the nine portions) in every two such selections of twenty numbers. So this occurrence of 5 in one portion is not surprising.

19.21 Where the population is grouped in some way, e.g. numbers of houses in different streets, a different procedure may be adopted. Suppose we have ten streets containing 32, 21, 64, 51, 12, 70, 35, 60, 82, 26 houses, and it is necessary to select 8 houses. We first derive the accumulative sub-totals, 32, $32 + 21 = 53$, $32 + 21 + 64 = 117$, $32 + 21 + 64 + 51 = 168$, etc. up to 453. Eight random numbers are then chosen between 1 and 453 rejecting any which occur more than once. Selection of the number 110 for example would mean that a house in the third group must be taken. This could either be the 110th, if the streets have been strung out and the houses numbered serially or, in the table of random numbers, a fresh random number between 1 and 64 could be used to select a house within the third street.

Non-random sampling

19.22 The use of random numbers is, in practice, much simpler than it may appear in theory, but there are many occasions where either the material is not in serial numbered form or the circumstances are such that a more rough and ready procedure may be acceptable. The important consideration is that the observer should acquire a sound knowledge of the iodiosyncracies of his material so that any procedure chosen on the grounds of convenience should make as close as possible an approach to randomness.

19.23 Possible methods are—

(i) *Systematic sampling*

In this method, a common one, the units of the population are listed or are otherwise arranged in order (the case notes in a file, or a pack of record cards) and every r^{th} unit is selected, a start being made with the sth entry where s is a number chosen at will between 1 and r. The sample will be as random but no more random than the ordered list of units; provided there are no cyclical features in this order the sample will be satisfactory. It is an easy method to explain to medical auxiliary workers who find it difficult to follow more stringent rules of selection. For a good example of the method see Durbin and Stuart (1951).

(ii) *Purposive sampling*

As a time saving device it may be decided to build up a sample which replicates in miniature the characteristics of the parent population. This will involve first setting out the requirements, for example 10 children of each sex under 15, 20 adults of each sex aged 15–44, etc. Then 10 children of each sex are identified on a list or among a standing file by some quasi-random method—systematic or haphazard selection—and so on.

(iii) *Quota sampling*

Even quicker (and therefore commonly used in market research where speed is more valuable than a high standard of precision) is the adaptation of method (ii)—quota sampling—such that the desired groups or quotas are secured by accepting the first suitable units to come to hand subject to fairly crude safeguards to guard against intolerable bias. The safeguard would be to give the phrase 'come to hand' some definition; for example, telling interviewers where or where not to look.

(iv) *Block sampling*

It may be satisfactory to take a consecutive block of new additions to a case register, a section chosen haphazardly from a large numerical card index. For vital registrations one might take all the births or deaths registered in a short interval of time under average conditions. An example of the block method is presented by the survey of the work of child welfare clinics in Birmingham and Coseley in 1951–52. (George, Lowe and McKeown, 1953.)

Administrative planning

19.24 We now turn to the second main problem, the organization of work in the field.

19.25 The first essential is a clear idea of the questions which the survey is to be designed to answer. The questions will be in terms of particular characteristics and will relate to a particular population. For example, if we desire to know the normal blood pressure in old people it is necessary to define 'blood pressure' and 'old people'.

19.26 So far as the first is concerned, i.e. the type of information to be collected, it is sometimes a question of accepting an established technique as in this particular example of blood pressure. More often the very need for a survey arises from a lack of knowledge, and therefore of standardization, of the characteristic to be measured. For example, in the report of a survey of the prevalence of bronchitis in Newcastle in 1955 (Ogilvie and Newell 1957) it is stated that 'chronic bronchitis, confidently diagnosed day by day, and recognized throughout the United Kingdom as a major cause of death, has not so far been found to be susceptible of clinical definition'. It was found necessary to erect certain criteria into a definition, viz. 'For the purpose of this inquiry, chronic bronchitis is recognized as a long-standing condition, the essential features of which are cough with sputum, persistent through the winter or throughout the year, in the absence of other causative respiratory disease. A minimum duration of two years is essential for its recognition.'

297

19.27 Definition of the population will at the outset be made strictly in relation to the problem in hand. If the investigation is concerned with all persons aged sixty-five and over, or all who have retired from normal employment, or all persons resident in homes for the aged, then whichever it is becomes the field for the survey. But it is important to bear in mind that the definition of the population (and the objective of the survey) may have to be adapted to meet practical difficulties in the selection of the sample (if the whole of the desired field is not available) or in response to interviewing (it might be expedient to restrict the survey to a section of the population in respect of whom reliable information could be obtained). Here experience and common-sense are invaluable. If there is no previous experience it is advisable to carry out a small trial before making a final decision. Such a small trial, which need not be strictly random and may cover only a few cases, has other advantages; for example, it provides opportunities for training interviewers, practising any clinical tests to be used, and testing record forms.

The frame

19.28 Before the sample is drawn a decision has to be reached as to the frame from which the units have to be selected. If the object is to produce a representative sample of a population that is already registered but is too large to survey in its entirety then such a register, be it in the form of a list, cards, or a strip index provides the ready made frame. There may be some restriction, e.g. to new patients registered within a given period (if recently diagnosed cases are the focus of interest) or to patients who have been given a particular form of therapy (if the survey is concerned with treatment). If the object is to survey the general population a choice may be made from (i) the electoral register, (ii) street maps on which dwellings have been serially numbered, (iii) addresses in a postal directory (though here there is an element of incompleteness due to absent addresses and these may have to be dealt with as a separate stratum to be identified from [ii]). An excellent account of possibilities has been given on behalf of the Social Survey by Gray and Corlett (1950).

The method of selection

19.29 These have already been discussed. If the units in the frame are serially numbered then random numbers are clearly to be preferred. If the frame is decentralized (e.g. case records of individual field workers) and the field workers themselves (with little knowledge, if any, of sampling theory) have to be depended upon to select the sample, it may be easier to get them to take a systematic sample (every r^{th} case). Even if the records are not numbered it may be possible to ask them to run through the records manually to take every r^{th} case (in this case r should be a small number for reasons that will become obvious to anyone who tries it).

Size of sample

19.30 The size of sample will depend on the margin of tolerance to be permitted in the estimate to be made. For example, if it is required to find the proportion of people, *p*, possessing a certain characteristic, e.g. a previous history of poliomyelitis, then the sampling error of p for a sample of n is $\sqrt{\dfrac{p(1-p)}{n}}$ and as a percentage of p, this is $100\sqrt{\dfrac{1-p}{np}}$. The meaning of this sampling error is that in 95 per cent of occasions the estimate of p will differ from the true figure by less than $200\sqrt{\dfrac{1-p}{np}}$ per cent. If this limit is fixed at 10 per cent we have:

$$200\sqrt{\frac{1-p}{np}} = 10$$

$$\text{or } n = \frac{400\,(1-p)}{p}$$

So that if p is small, say $0 \cdot 05$, n is approximately 8,000.

19.31 Such a calculation of course assumes that there is some prior knowledge of p. If there is no such prior knowledge then it would be advisable to carry out a small trial survey to get at least an appreciation of the order of size of p. Such a trial would also provide an opportunity for testing the proposed administrative arrangements (records, interviewer technique, etc.).

19.32 In the case of a characteristic such as mean weight of a group $(\bar{w})$ with standard deviation σ a similar calculation can be carried out. The sampling error of the mean is $\dfrac{\sigma}{\sqrt{n}}$ and the percentage error $\dfrac{100\sigma}{\bar{w}\sqrt{n}}$. If we wish to impose the same restraint of having a 95 per cent confidence of obtaining values within 10 per cent of the true value then

$$10 = \frac{200\sigma}{\bar{w}\sqrt{n}}$$

$$\text{whence} \quad n = \frac{400\,\sigma^2}{\bar{w}^2}$$

19.33 Here again we must obtain some prior knowledge of the order of size of $\bar{w}$ and of σ, either from other surveys or from a pre-test. It must also be emphazised that the expressions used in 19.30 and 19.32 are simplified for ease of illustration. The formula for the estimate of standard error of the statistic measured requires the introduction of a factor $\sqrt{1-f}$, where f is the sampling fraction. Complications arise in stratified and multistage sampling; for adequate treatment of these it will be advisable to consult specialist text books.

Records

19.34 It is next necessary to decide upon the form of record and method of completion of the record, for obtaining the desired information.

19.35 In some cases the survey is to be made of some existing records, for example, hospital case histories, in which event provision must be made either for a simple transcript form or for the direct preparation of punched cards from the medical histories.

19.36 In most cases an *ad hoc* record will have to be devised. Here the rules laid down on p. 139 will apply with very great force. The essential requirements are a clear idea of the precise object of the survey in terms of the information needed to deal with the underlying problem. The record and the accompanying instructions should indicate without any shred of ambiguity:

(i) who is to be included in the survey;
(ii) the identity of the individual unit if there is any likelihood of reference back or linkage to other records;
(iii) the precise facts to be recorded arranged in an order which represents a logical flow in questions and is also convenient for statistical processing.

19.37 It is important in field investigations to pay particular attention to the compactness and attractiveness of the layout of the form. To a greater extent than is generally realized standards of reporting are adversely affected by poor stationery, and clumsy or complicated form design. The aim should be to produce something simple and straightforward; which has been clearly well thought out and gives the impression of authority. This is true irrespective of whether or not sampling is used.

19.38 In the Family Census of 1946 (Royal Commission on Population, 1950) a good form design combined with a well prepared approach yielded a comparatively high response rate of 87 per cent, even though the census was entirely voluntary.

19.39 Even where the records are to be completed by trained interviewers, good form design will yield dividends in accuracy and expedition.

Training of investigators

19.40 In any field study other than that carried out by postal canvass it is necessary to give careful instruction to those who are to collect the information. In medical surveys it is especially important to standardize any procedures, e.g. tuberculin testing or radiography, that are to form part of the investigation. The aim is to reduce the additional variability which may be injected into the data as a result of lack of uniformity.

19.41 It is desirable to bring field investigators together at a meeting where instruction on methods of interview can be given, rules laid down for dealing with such matters as non-response, and guidance provided for the completion of forms. Questions can be asked, emphasis can be laid on points of particular difficulty or importance and misunderstanding can be corrected. Such meetings would be in supplementation of and not in substitution for written rules and instructions.

19.42 There would be a trial of the records and procedure to ensure that no practical difficulties have been overlooked. A small sample trial in the field would be more reliable but if this is not practicable, then even a test carried out among the investigators themselves or the staff of the authority carrying out the survey would be better than nothing. Whether or not a test has been carried out, the first few records of the survey should be carefully scrutinized to ensure that the prescribed procedure is being adhered to and that the standard of recording is adequate. Any deviation can then be quickly corrected before irreparable harm has been done. Periodical spot checks throughout the progress of the survey would also be advisable; investigators have been known gradually to adapt themselves to difficulties in a way that ultimately detracts from the validity or accuracy of the results.

Analysis of results

19.43 It is worth while drawing up draft tables *before* the forms have been designed. Having a clear idea of the actual statistical tables that are required is a great help, if not essential, in actually designing the questions to be asked, and the way in which they are to be asked.

19.44 Analysis of the records is essentially a matter of allocating each unit record to the appropriate cells of these tables. If only tens of forms are involved these may easily be counted as they stand, but with more than a hundred or so it is advisable to transfer the information to cards for ease in handling. If the detail is considerable or the numbers large, mechanical aids to classification should be considered. The use of edge-punched cards is very effective up to about 1,000 cases. Beyond that number there is difficulty with sorting and counting becomes laborious so that it is preferable to have recourse to punched cards suitable for counting by conventional machines or by electronic data processing methods.

Surveys of sickness

19.45 A useful account of methods adopted in various countries to conduct morbidity surveys has been given by Logan and Brooke (1957). For the British survey of 1943–52 a multi-stage sample was used, i.e. one in which a sample of first-stage units is selected and then within each first-stage unit, a sample of second-stage units is chosen, and so on. The scheme was as follows:

(*a*) The total number of interviews was divided among eleven regions of England and Wales in proportion to the regional population.

(*b*) In each region the allocation of interviews was sub-divided in proportion to the urban and rural population of the region, obtainable from the Registrar General.

(*c*) For rural districts:

    (i) They were arranged in descending order of industrialization index.*

    (ii) The cumulative total of their population was formed and a range of numbers allocated to each district, proportionate to the size of the population.

    (iii) If N was the total population a number was chosen at random between 1 and N, say x. The rural district was then selected in whose range of numbers x lay, and a second rural district by taking $x + \frac{1}{2}N$ as the range-number. Thus two rural districts were selected, with probabilities proportional to their populations.

(*d*) For urban districts:

    (i) All towns of 300,000 and over were included in the sample. In selecting 4,000 out of about 40,000,000 the ratio is about 1 in 10,000. Any town of 300,000 would therefore provide about thirty or more interviews.

    (ii) The remaining urban districts were then divided up into the required number of strata, in descending order of industrializa-

* The ratio of industrial to total net annual rateable values in each district.

301

tion index and with equal populations. Within each stratum the urban districts were regrouped on a basis of geographical zoning, for example, coalfields, woollen manufacturing areas, dairy farming regions.

(iii) Two districts were then selected from each stratum in the same way as for rural districts.

19.46 Somewhat different arrangements were made for Greater London, based on the rateable value per head of population.

19.47 The last stage of sampling, which consisted in determining whom to interview in a chosen district, had to be based upon some list or record of the population. The lists employed were the National Register from October 1, 1944, and later the Electoral Register. Each had its advantages and drawbacks. The National Register was compiled from an enumeration of civilian residents made on September 29, 1939, on the basis of which identity cards and ration books were issued. A card was filed at the local National Registration Office for each resident in the district, the index being adjusted for births, removals or deaths immediately after these events. The cards in the adult register, which contained the names and addresses of people aged sixteen and over, were pushed together and the total length measured. This length was divided up so as to provide the requisite number of names for interview by drawing cards at equal intervals starting from a card selected at random. By this method it was found that the proportion of cases in which no one in the household could be contacted and for which a substitute had to be taken was only fourteen per cent. The advantages of using the National Register were that it was kept continuously up-to-date and administered uniformly throughout the country.

19.48 The National Register was discontinued in 1952; the Electoral Register was used instead for interviews in February, 1951, and onwards. The lower age-limit of the sample was therefore twenty-one instead of sixteen. The electoral register had the further disadvantage that it excluded aliens and that, since it was only revised at yearly intervals, it was not as up-to-date as the National Registration maintenance register.

19.49 For further development of this subject, reference might be made to Moser (1958), or to any other textbook on survey methods.

REFERENCES

BRADFORD HILL, A. (1956) 'Medical Statistics' 6th Edition, Lancet, London.
COCHRAN, W. G. (1963) Sampling Techniques. J. Wiley and Sons, New York.
DURBIN, J., and STUART, A. (1951) J. Roy. Stat. Soc. Series A. 114, 63.
GEORGE, J. T. A., LOWE, C. R., and MCKEOWN, T. (1953) Lancet, i. 88.
GRAY, P. G., and CORLETT, T. (1950) J. Roy. Stat. Soc. Series A., 93, 150.
KISH, L. (1965) Survey Sampling. J. Wiley and Sons, New York.
LOGAN, W. P. D., and BROOKE, E. M. (1957) General Register Office. Studies on Med. and Pop. Subj. No. 12 'The Survey of Sickness 1943 to 1952'. H.M.S.O.
MOSER, C. A. (1958) Survey methods in Social Investigation. Heinemann. London.
OGILVIE, A. G., and NEWELL, D. J. (1957) Chronic Bronchitis in Newcastle-upon-Tyne, E. & S. Livingstone, London.
Royal Commission on Population, Papers (1950) Reports of Statistics Committee. Vol. II, p. 87. H.M.S.O.
YATES, F. (1953) Sampling Methods for Censuses and Surveys. C. Griffin & Co. Ltd., London, 2nd Edition.

INDEX

Printed and bound by CPI Group (UK) Ltd, Croydon, CR0 4YY

24/10/2024

01778493-0003